THE
PERSONAL SESSIONS
Book 4 of
The Deleted Seth Material

Sessions
8/27/77– 8/28/78

THE EARLY SESSIONS

The Early Sessions consist of the first 510 sessions dictated by Seth through Jane Roberts. There are 9 books in *The Early Sessions* series.

THE PERSONAL SESSIONS

The Personal Sessions, often referred to as "the deleted sessions," are Seth sessions that Jane Roberts and Rob Butts considered to be of a highly personal nature and were therefore kept in separate notebooks from the main body of the Seth material. *The Personal Sessions* are expected to be published in 6 to 9 volumes.

"The great value I see now in the many deleted or private sessions is that they have the potential to help others, just as they helped Jane and me over the years. I feel that it's very important to have these sessions added to Jane's fine creative body of work for all to see." –Rob Butts

THE SETH AUDIO COLLECTION

Rare recordings of Seth speaking through Jane Roberts are available on audiocassette and CD. For a complete description of The Seth Audio Collection, request our free catalogue.. (Further information is supplied at the back of this book.)

For information on expected publication dates and how to order, write to New Awareness Network at the following address and request the latest catalogue. Also, please visit us on the internet at www.sethcenter.com

New Awareness Network Inc.
P.O. BOX 192
Manhasset, N.Y. 11030

www.sethcenter.com

THE PERSONAL SESSIONS
Book 4 of
The Deleted Seth Material

Sessions
8/27/77– 8/28/78

© 2004 by Robert Butts

Published by New Awareness Network Inc.

New Awareness Network Inc.
P.O. Box 192
Manhasset, New York 11030

Opinions and statements on health and medical matters expressed in this book are those of the author and are not necessarily those of or endorsed by the publisher. Those opinions and statements should not be taken as a substitute for consultation with a duly licensed physician.

Cover Design: Michael Goode
Photography: Cover photos by Rich Conz and Robert F. Butts, Sr.
Editorial: Rick Stack
Typography: Raymond Todd, Michael Goode

All rights reserved. This book may not be reproduced in whole or in part, without written permission from the publisher, except by a reviewer who may quote brief passages in a review; nor may any part of this book be reproduced, stored in a retrieval system, or transmitted in any form or by any means electronic, mechanical, photocopying, recording, or other, without written permission from the publisher.

ISBN 0-9711198-7-2
Printed in U.S.A. on acid-free paper

I dedicate The Personal Sessions
to my wife, Jane Roberts,
who lived her 55 years
with the greatest creativity
and the most valiant courage.
-Rob

A NOTE ON THE COVER DESIGN PHOTOGRAPHS

June 2003. A note about the photographs Michael Goode used in his striking cover design for The Personal Sessions *series.*

The central colored photograph of Jane and the lower right-and-left-hand shots of her and myself were taken by my father, Robert F. Butts, Sr., in Sayre, PA a year or so after our marriage in December 1954. The upper right one of Jane in trance for Seth was taken (among many others) by Rich Conz, a photographer for the Elmira, NY Star-Gazette, *while he witnessed Session 508 on November 20, 1969. (See Volume 9 of* The Early Sessions.*)*

I don't know who photographed the young Jane shown on the upper left, but she saved that picture all of those years for me to inherit upon her death in September 1984, when she was 55.

My inventive and versatile father had always taken photographs, and in his later years turned professional, photographing many weddings and other events in the Sayre area (and also Jane's and my wedding at the home of my younger brother Loren and his wife Betts in Tunkhannock, PA). To help my father, my mother Estelle trained herself to hand-color his black and white photographs, for color film was not available then—and so she colored Jane's portrait. Now I wonder: do my long-deceased parents, and Rich and the unknown photographer of the young Jane, all know that their creativity will grace the covers of a series of books that I so lovingly dedicate to them, as well as to Jane and each reader? I believe that they do, each in his or her own way.

—Rob

DELETED SESSION
AUGUST 27, 1977 9:52 PM SATURDAY

(Jane lost an eye tooth early this morning, before we got up. It became abundantly clear that she was going to lose the tooth a couple of days ago, as it began to visibly descend from its socket; I could see it wobble in its socket as we ate breakfast Friday morning, and she expected to lose it at any minute. I found this very discouraging, and once again began to question the whole bit about symptoms, recovery, Seth, etc.

(Yesterday we also had two unexpected visitors, as well as a brief call from a young man who had called on us unannounced with a friend, last week. The two women were from Arizona and Massachusetts; the former had flown here to see Jane unannounced. I turned her away at the door with a promise that Jane would call her at the Holiday Inn. Shortly after she left, the second caller, a "parapsychologist" from a college in Massachusetts, was camping in Pine Valley with her family. I arranged that both women would meet here at 4:00 PM to talk with Jane for an hour before supper time; Sue Watkins was also due that afternoon with some typed material for Psyche—*which is why I made the arrangement to begin with.*

(Jane and I almost had an argument over the setup, though, for I had mistakenly assumed that she'd be glad to see everyone at once and get it over with, so we'd be free the rest of the day. Instead, Jane was counting on being free for the day and didn't want to see anybody except Sue. I decided that henceforth I would turn visitors away, since I didn't see how I could know in advance whether she felt like seeing anyone or not. I mention these details to show something of our situation re Seth's last deleted session on "intruders" when we want privacy. We haven't resolved such dilemmas then, obviously.

(It follows that Jane did keep her tooth during the women's visit, losing it while still in bed early Saturday morning. Strangely, she could eat and chew better with the tooth gone than while she still had it. I'm very sensitive to tooth troubles, of course, and probably project some of this upon others; but Jane's losing the tooth reminded me of Seth's very recent declaration that she might lose more teeth because of the relaxation taking place in her jaws. We'll see whether she can retain her two front teeth, which shifted their position at once after the eye tooth dropped out.

(Tonight I didn't know whether it was worthwhile having a session or not. Yet Jane reported more walking changes today; we thought they were good changes, so eventually we sat for the session. I might add that although Seth said losing the teeth was a minor thing, comparatively, it doesn't seem so to us. Also: when Sue arrived, she reported that on her visit to the dentist this afternoon a large cavity was discovered that she didn't know existed. She remarked upon her own beliefs about teeth—

something she'd had no trouble with for many years.)

Good evening.

("Good evening, Seth.")

A session was a good decision.

It would be silly for a violet to wonder why it was not a grape. You have certain natures, then, that are your own. It is somewhat beside the point to wonder why your natures are as they are. You have always been loners, in reincarnational terms and otherwise.

Suggestion, so-called, is little understood. The word perhaps is a poor one. Yet to an important extent your world runs by suggestion. Suggestion is simply an impetus to act in given directions. Your social, political, religious, economic and medical areas of life are all built upon certain assumed suggestions that people agree to accept as standards of behavior. The word "standards" is important, for in certain terms through such "obedience, " through such compliance, they are given recognizable patterns into which their most personal experience can flow.

They are given recognizable patterns through which their experience with others, and with the community, can flow. They are given certain more or less predictable frameworks in which to experience their lives.

Those experiences may at times be quite jarring, tragic, frightening, but they will happen within a framework provided by the accepted suggestions of the society. People may question the precepts, but generally speaking they live and work within organizational frameworks, each one ruled by various assumptions or suggestions.

Students go to schools, patients go to doctors, criminals go to jail. Experience, then, is largely programmed in that respect, so that you know where you belong. Your experience, no matter how joyful, bizarre or frightening, can find a category. Few people <u>stray</u> from those frameworks, and few creative people, even of high quality, operate outside of the accepted disciplines, schools, and organizations.

Because of your natures, to a far greater extent than most, you and Ruburt have strayed in such a fashion. Because of your natures, you are seeking answers to the most difficult problems of <u>life and death alike</u>, on your own, so to speak. This is because your natures require it. You <u>want</u> to do it. At the same time you provide a new group of suggestions, an alternate way for others. In the meantime, however, you have no cozy categories in which to place your experience.

In a way everything is new. This of course requires on your parts energy, self-reliance, faith in what you are doing, and a certain stubbornness. At the same time you are everywhere surrounded by the suggestions of your culture.

Those who come here often <u>are</u> questioners of it. They certainly are not ready to go all of the way, as you are. They may appear quite bizarre. They may form odd theories, but they are between worlds.

There is no doubt that improvements have occurred in Ruburt's condition. You would have to be blind not to realize that his ankles and feet, his hands and wrists, his neck and jaw, have all improved. Frank is correct: many ligaments have stretched to allow him to sit down—*(leaning forward, and loudly:)* <u>I would say 50% better within two weeks</u>.

You are, however, blazing your own path, and confidence at times will unfortunately lag. You should not let those periods collect, however. I am helping out here, to give you some extra support, and I will tell you that my word in this area is far more dependable than any other information you could receive.

Today <u>could have been</u> a day of relaxation and some mild enough triumph. It was not, of course. It was not because Ruburt's confidence failed, and so did yours. Then Ruburt did not communicate because he did not want to worry you, since he knew your confidence was no better than his.

What happened is this: the large neck ligaments considerably loosened further, releasing important areas of the jaw—unfortunately enough dislodging a tooth. While unpleasant, that is not a tragedy. That release allowed further relaxation so that vitally important areas in the arm and in the backs of the legs were further released. These permitted some new rotation of both knees, and also loosened some ligaments to the feet.

(10:20.) Those areas tried to work together today. The trembling *(in the legs)* is indeed a sign of new life, new sensation, as large areas of the body try the new positions. Had you both trusted the body, had you believed that it did indeed improve to improve, then Ruburt would have been more aware of the new balancing sensations and positions, and would not have added anxiety on top.

It is highly important that you do keep up your communications with each other, and that you begin each day in one way or another by stating your faith in the body's processes. This would take but a few moments. It is also important, now, that you concentrate upon your own creative works, both of you—Ruburt particularly, so that he takes his mind off of his body, and focuses elsewhere. Since you are doing this alone, more or less, it is natural to be upset at times, but when your confidence is greater than your doubts, Ruburt always improves.

(Intently:) There is no reason to fear a prolonged period of improvements that "go nowhere." Only those fears slow down your success.

His body is responding extremely well, despite the mental anxiety that both of you place upon the process. Ruburt's condition is in no way reprehensible *(repeated twice)*—there is no reason why you should consider it in such a fashion. There are more people than you know, relying upon the best medical knowledge of the society, who are in far worse shape, whether or not the condition is observable—millions, incidentally, with false teeth.

It does no good to exaggerate Ruburt's condition, and if you do <u>not</u> exaggerate it, then you must admit the improvements that have lately occurred.

Forget worrying about visitors, one way or another. Dedicate yourselves to your joint and private creative pursuits, to providing a mental climate in which you can produce while Ruburt's improvements continue. Anything else now is beside the point.

If you were different people, you might of course have done other things. You are yourselves. If you accept those selves you will not waste energy comparing yourselves with others, particularly in negative fashions.

(10:35. Seth held up a bottle of beer.) Open this for our friend.

I will not keep you long—but you need this session.

Each morning, briefly together in whatever way you choose, dedicate yourselves to your creative pursuits. Imagine a calm and peaceful aura surrounding the house. Tell yourselves that your work will be productive, and that Ruburt's body will improve as the day goes on. Such suggestions are immensely important. Suggestions are always impetuses toward action, psychological sets that can indeed program your day and set up reminders.

Because you do not rely upon mass suggestions and mass frameworks, it is then highly vital that you learn to set up your own alternate patterns. You do this from scratch, where of course most people have not set themselves such challenges or opportunities for creativity.

Because you were born in this culture, it is not surprising that you still fall prey to lack of trust in yourselves, or in the body's abilities to cure itself. Teachings to the contrary have been deeply imbedded. You do have something extremely valuable when you realize it, though this is often lost to you in practical terms because of your fears and negative projections. The large majority of people are confused, besieged, and struggling without any clear idea of why they are in such a state, and with barely a hundredth fraction of your insight or understanding, unable to form their own framework, yet aware that the conventional one is sadly lacking. Your sense of direction may be far more obvious to <u>them</u> than to you, because they sense it so vitally in contrast to their own condition.

The suggestions I gave about the morning should be followed. Everything in the session is important—keeping up your communication and so forth.

The trembling will not last—at the most two or three days. It is no copout to keep a chair handy, or whatever, nothing to be afraid of when that is understood. The legs will want then to exercise. He can stand up and hold on to something, and exercise them, even if he has had to have chairs about while walking from place to place. The balance of the body is changing. The eyes will continue to improve. Fear, his and yours, makes him concentrate upon the body's sensations too much, and that prevents him from the frame of mind necessary for his writing.

His eyes <u>are</u> changing. They are not protruding as much, and they will far less. Nor generally will they be as red. They are still not fully synchronized, however. There are long periods where he can read properly. He can copy *James* then —an hour at a time—however. In other periods he can work on his preface and his own to notes for the book, and leave himself open to new inspiration.

Dedicate yourselves as I have said. Be honest. If someone comes to the door and you do not want to see them, make a polite excuse. If you feel so inclined, see the person. Make a decision, however, whatever it is, and stick to it in any case—that is, in any given case: you follow me? You will learn that way, and your decisions will be in league with your inclinations at the time.

(10:56.) These will <u>naturally</u> even out. You can trust those inclinations. They will be built upon your own inner knowledge and your feelings about your state at the time, and your inner knowledge about people at the door.

When you go against those feelings you cannot be satisfied with any decision. There are issues involved that you are unconsciously aware of—concerning, say, the people. The knowledge will merge with your own conscious feelings at the time. You are tinged by conventional ideas and judgments—natural enough, but they often contradict your intuitive feelings, and make you act counter to them.

You, Joseph, were initially annoyed by Lady Caroline *(from Arizona)*, who came in the taxi. You felt she intruded. Quickly, however, you felt sorry for her. Conventional attitudes began to speak: you should be kind to guests. The woman had come from so far away. Your original feelings of intrusion represented your own attitude, and your instant recognition of her character. Your original feelings were the correct ones, so to speak.

Ruburt's were the same. Each of you felt that you <u>should</u> see the woman regardless of your feelings. The woman would have accepted a no. She halfway expected it, as you both unconsciously realized. A yes to her would mean far more than yes to a brief interview.

To her, if you saw her at all, it meant that you would accept her as a student, or rather as a clinger. Ruburt was not hiding *(as I suggested)* in that particular instance. The other woman was an entirely different matter, yet you saw her also because you thought you must, or should. She benefited by the interview. If you follow your inclinations you cannot go wrong, for they are acutely tuned to each instance and each person, and take into consideration your own circumstances at the time.

When you do not trust your inclinations then you must indeed make rules to follow instead. It takes but a moment to check with each other, though so far you usually answer the door, but state your feelings to Ruburt clearly, then ask for his, and make your decision jointly. One of you may want to talk to the person involved, or both of you, or neither. There is no strain that should be involved. The affair is taken care of in a few moments.

When you do not trust your own feelings, however, and do not have specific rules governing such issues either, then few decisions are clearly made, or are even halfway agreeable. The visitors that you honestly feel like seeing you will also help the most, and there will be something about them that will benefit you, so that the encounter is creative overall.

Do you have questions?

("No, I guess not.")

Now I hope before too long to get on with our book, but I am also highly interested that you put our ideas to work to better your own daily lives.

Part of the book will deal with mass suggestions and their effects, <u>and</u> benefits. If Ruburt had gone to a doctor, he would have been a different person after a certain point in his life—so in a way it is meaningless to ask what would have happened. Had you insisted that he go to a doctor, you would have been a different person also.

Please remember that many people get in physical difficulty. They are indeed the norm rather than the exception. People who are not questioning necessarily the nature of life or of reality, creative people, unimaginative people, dumb people, athletes—all get in physical difficulties. What I am saying is that questioning the nature of reality does not cause physical difficulties <u>per se</u>. You cannot justifiably say, then "Had we not taken this route, everything would have been hunky-dory *(loudly)*." You should know better than that.

(I didn't know I <u>had</u> said that.

(Loudly again:) Now: had you not taken this route, you both would have been in far greater difficulties. Of course, you would not be the same people—but your understanding and knowledge has drastically changed the future that could have been expected, say, from your backgrounds in this life, now.

To some extent the York beach images held what might have been expected of you. In the terms of which we're speaking, now, having attained a certain but quite limited artistic career that you felt was more of a prison that no technique could help you escape.

The career would have fallen into conventional pattern for money's sake. Your understanding, stretched somewhat by earlier ideas, would have fallen backward, so that you ever strained against it. You would have had physical difficulties of quite important natures.

Ruburt would have been stifled, unable to find a writing niche, having written out early personal, autobiographical material, but not able to make the new important creative leaps that were actually taken.

He might have died of heart trouble by the age of 40, for literally his heart would have been broken, and communication between the two of you would have quite fallen away. His heart is as strong as an ox (definitely). Do not think then that your creative endeavors have caused you difficulties, or that without them life would have been a bed of roses.

The solution to your problems is within your knowledge, and <u>consciously</u> so—something few people can say.

(And I'd say that Seth's material on Jane and me represents a probable reality for us—that those things DID happen elsewhere....

(11:33.) You are trying out highly creative, innovative, imaginative, and truthful concepts—not just theoretically and artistically, but applying them to your lives. You have again fallen into the habit, negatively, of considering your achievements in other areas as insignificant—*(louder:)* <u>in light of Ruburt's condition</u> as if they caused his condition. They did not. His condition was caused by a set of beliefs, and so was everything else in your lives.

<u>Luckily</u>, those beliefs allowed the possibility of achievement even if they did also permit experience most dismaying. But watch the center of your focus. We are setting up an alternate framework. Your focus must be upon your abilities, your achievements; the realities—all of them—of the moment. You both have <u>great</u> powers of concentration and energy. I want those directed toward the issues just mentioned. <u>Reinstate the library</u>, together. Only your poor habits and lack of confidence stand in the way. When you worry all day then the library goes out the window, and so does your feeling of creative adventure, in your own creative hours, both of you.

When you feel the sessions do not help, it is of course because you doubt yourselves, and you doubt yourselves because of the very cultural reality you are in the process of changing for yourselves and others.

Do you have questions?

("Well, your last line reminded me of my question about the acceptance of

"Unknown" Reality *by others."*)

When you say others do you mean—

("Generally.")

The general acceptance.... First of all, our books would frighten many people. They run directly counter to the many beliefs by which the masses live their lives. Our ideas will filter through the masses. Directly, however, in a manner of speaking, our books are subversive. They will sell continually through the years, and the readership will grow.

College people in particular will promote our ideas. Many people who seem quite strange or cultish, bizarre, and possibly offend you, read the books because they are often acutely aware of society's lacks. They try to show their dissatisfaction through highly individualistic or strange behavior. Since on their own they are not creatively gifted enough to find other expression.

The books also find their way, however, to the serious questioners within the establishment itself. Often they are not in high positions—because they <u>are</u> questioners. Yet they deal with the young quite directly, and with the arts and sciences in unconventional ways, but within the system.

There are also a core of individual thinkers who straddle all social or academic categories, who follow our books. There is no overall general reaction, therefore, in the terms of your question. But the effects will be, and are being felt. *Cézanne*, for example, will reach some people who have not read the other books, and some historians will read James, and hence be led where otherwise they would not go. *Psyche* will mention my ideas about sex, for example, and will be bought by some people because of that subject alone, who will be again led to the other books.

Hopefully Ruburt will finish his other *Seven*, for beside regular readers he will pick up readers of fiction, who again will be led where otherwise they would not travel.

Please reread this session, and a hearty good evening.

("Thank you very much, Seth.")

Put this session to work, and see the difference in your lives.

(11:54 PM. "Good night."

(A note: The woman from Arizona sent Jane a telegram late Saturday afternoon, asking that Jane see her again, saying that she would wait several days at the Holiday Inn. etc. Jane called her at the Holiday Inn. only to be told.< that the woman had left. She must have done so soon after sending the wire. A change of heart? We had been out earlier Saturday, but evidently the woman had not been here. In any event, Jane was prepared to tell her that she would not see her again.)

DELETED SESSION
AUGUST 29, 1977 9:45 PM MONDAY

(Jane received her first copy of Cézanne *Saturday morning. Tonight she began reading the appendix material I've done on Volume 2 of* "Unknown" Reality. *The evening was very hot and humid.*

(Generalized body changes since the last session Saturday night: More loosening in neck, ligaments, chin and face area; walking is easier but still requires support – legs tremble and have trouble supporting weight, but knees move better. "Shitty," Jane said with a rueful laugh. Right foot looser and looser, but no help walking. Head and back more flexible; eyes not quite so red—"in and out" of focus in a period of minutes, yet Jane could see to work part of the time today, as Seth suggested.)

Now—good evening.

("Good evening. Seth.")

The practical experience of reality is formed through the suggestive psychological idea-shapes that appear in the guise of theories, dogmas, and assumptions.

The theory of evolution represents a magnetic organizing suggestive hypothesis. It can, even in scientific terms, never be proven. Under its banner of suggestion, however, the great parade of men and other living creatures are observed so that the hypothesis brings about its own hypnotic focus—so that creatures, man, and indeed the universe itself, seem to behave in certain highly ritualized fashions.

(Appendix 12 for Volume 2 is on evolution; I was surprised to realize that Jane's reading it today had apparently triggered Seth's material here.)

In a manner of speaking, the motives familiar to men are applied to the smallest microbe. More than this, however, the theory's vast suggestive nature forms a framework through which people then view the experiences of their lives, and through whose focus the behavior of their own species seems determined.

The theory, then, is a way of organizing experience, a suggestive hypothesis. It is indeed no more than a point of view. It has colored man's societies and cultures since its inception. It has dominated economical systems. In that regard, for example, James was quite correct: certain religious societies interpreted the theme so that it read "evolution of the soul"; but there is no soul in Darwinian theory and hereditary, and certainly none in the environment.

I do not think you understand yet the importance of suggestion, for once you said to me "Suggestion cannot be all that important."

("I said that?" I didn't remember doing so and I certainly wouldn't say so

today.)

You did indeed—not in that context. There is little difference, however, between private suggestion in your personal lives, and the power of mass suggestion in your society.

Suggestion not only impels toward action, but causes you to interpret action in a given manner. In strict Darwinian terms, man and animal alike had to be turned aggressively outward in the most competitive of physical ways. A new achievement on the part of a species, or any mutation occurred, occurred as the direct result of personal experience—and of course no information was available otherwise.

In deepest terms the world had an outside only. It was empty inside. The soul or any remnant of it vanished, so that all of the action had to occur in an arena where competition ruled. Life was not trusted. You could be betrayed by your genes. There was no purpose in nature except its own mechanical reproduction. The individual had no importance, once it served its part in reproduction.

(10:05.) These ideas went a long way to justify later scientific experiments that involved giving pain to animals, for example: nature itself had no feeling. It was seen in human terms as inhumane: life without reason, life with no purpose except its own repetition, life in which the individual was dispensable. Many people cannot operate under that kind of system. The individual shouts that his life does indeed have meaning, while the scientists until now have vehemently stated otherwise.

Why then did such a theory originate? Darwin was initially a religious man. Like many others, his religious background held out nonsensical propositions. It saw a good God, a just savior, who nevertheless never thought twice about sending down death and destruction as punishment for sin.

Darwin was faced with the proposition of a kind god who was more cruel than any human being, and with supernatural power behind him to boot—so Darwin tried to justify God's ways to man.

Nature took the place of the devil in an insidious sleight-of-hand that initially Darwin himself never expected. He wanted to show that God was not responsible for the world's cruelties. Darwin loved nature in all of its aspects, yet he could not reconcile its beauties and splendors with the course of its events. He could not bear to see a cat play with a mouse, without blaming God who would permit such cruelty. He tried to wipe God's hands clean, as he understood the nature of God through his early beliefs—but in so doing he wiped the soul from the face of nature.

To a large degree, however, and for many people, he did remove the idea of God's injustice, even if he removed the image of God in the process. The idea of one God as a superman would not carry again the same weight as it had before. For your species, the questions behind the conventional God the father were at least brought out into the open.

Those theories of Darwin, however, formed part of the suggestive background in which you and Ruburt and millions of others matured. Each person interpreted those beliefs in an individual fashion. Sexual, economic, social and even religious behavior became tinged by these concepts.

The value of the artist was deprecated. Contemplation had little part to play. As per James, it was no coincidence that the beliefs of Freud and Darwin merged so well to form western society's idea of the self, physically and psychologically. The ideas of financial competition, advocated, came into direct conflict, Joseph, with your own inclinations to be an artist. The ideas of manliness in your society, particularly in past years, were directly tied in with Darwinian concepts and Freudian theory. They operated as suggestion that directed the actions of millions of people, and provided a framework through which they experienced their reality.

Now when either of you, or both of you, feel that there might be something wrong in spending your time thinking, writing, painting, or worse, daydreaming, you feel that way because your way of life meets some conflict from old Darwinian and Freudian beliefs: you should be out there in the world—active, competing, or even just riding bicycles.

In other kinds of systems, great premiums would be put upon your work. I want you to understand, personally, the importance of such suggestions—particularly when they have authoritative backgrounds.

For example, Ruburt's latest status, and your somewhat natural concern with the temporary walking difficulty—you know what I am referring to—I say to you that the concern is natural; for it certainly seems so to both of you. You have little idea, however, how sometimes the most natural-seeming reactions are not natural at all, but programmed. An animal, say, in Ruburt's position, feeling as much new activity in the body, new motion in the knees, new elasticity in the ligaments, would quite naturally accept the improvements with physical elation, even if it had more difficulty one day, or two, than it had in days previous. It would sense the body's interstate condition. It would not worry, but would exercise whatever new motions were possible. It would take it for granted that its body knew what it was doing. It would not be hampered by remnants of Darwinian or Freudian concepts.

(10:36.) I want to show you where culture and cultural beliefs meet with your private experience. Ruburt's body needed more challenge. Before this lat-

est episode that upset him showed, Important releases in the hip sockets occurred, with hardly any notice on his part. Little inconvenience. The amount of new motion there was minute but vitally important if his stance upward were to improve.

That small alteration, however, immediately altered the legs' position, however minutely, placing new challenge upon the entire leg and foot region. That challenge further activates additional motion: it is <u>almost</u> impossible to explain how intimately your psychological beliefs program your experience of events, or to tell you how to interpret them.

Any animal would rather be running and physically vigorous than not. But when an animal's improving, he goes along with the improvement. If Ruburt suddenly walked more poorly than usual, as for the last few days, showing no other signs of obvious beneficial change, then that would be something else. There are natural bodily reactions, however, and psychological reactions that may seem natural, but that often are contrary to the body's knowledge, and that can block that knowledge with the sense of reassurance that it can bring.

Ruburt's eyes change constantly while improving overall. It may seem to you that this is indeed a very strange condition. Ruburt certainly finds it disconcerting at best, and at worst worrisome. The eyes, however, quite naturally in their motion are connected with all of the body's other motions. They are <u>healthily</u> (underlined twice) responding.

Ruburt's new attitudes and intentions to be responsive <u>are</u> renewing the body. The fears and anxieties of course do not help. They add tension. You are going ahead in spite of the worry. The entire jaw is being realigned to its natural and most ideal position. This is allowing all of the other bodily beneficial changes.

Animals have their own culture. They understand it differently, however, but it is taken into consideration in physical terms. You are doing very well, and your own beliefs are changing, Joseph, perhaps in greater fashion than you realize. The idea of Ruburt's teeth should be dropped, however. The concern over the matter becomes far more an impediment than any actual loss of his teeth. Yes, beliefs <u>could</u> save the rest of them—but both of your interpretations about teeth at this point hold you back.

The work of the jaws necessitates the actions occurring, and if the new jaws end up with new teeth *(humorously)*, that must not be considered a failure or a tragedy. That fear is precisely what keeps Ruburt from saving the teeth so far. The teeth business has to do also with Darwinian concepts of age, with thought of the animal not surviving, and in your world that is ridiculous. The fears behind the fears are groundless. He must not be so afraid, then, of losing the teeth—and then perhaps he can save them. But in any case you both lay highly negative and unwarranted suggestions in that area.

(10:58.) Darwinian concepts allowed the passage of no knowledge from one generation to another that was not genetically transmitted. It did not understand the inner communication of the animals, and certainly it did not admit any altruistic animal intent.

To some extent the Freudian self, as per *James*, more or less followed the same pattern. A man could scarcely trust his neighbor if he agreed with Darwin or Freudian concepts. Behind any altruistic impulse there had to be a selfish gain. Before all of this, however, nature was seen as primarily passive—put here by God for man's purpose, but without possessing the uniqueness or even approaching the status of man.

Darwin managed to bring out nature's complexity, though this had been mentioned by other men—I believe by a man called Mendel in particular. But Mendel did not catch man's imagination. Darwin then brought nature to man's focus in a new way, for before neither science or religion had dealt with it in a meaningful manner. The full sweep and extent of the natural world , with all of its seeming ambiguities, cruelties and splendors, had to be accepted as more than a passive package delivered into man's hand.

Darwin's theories, and Freud's for that matter, will in the future be seen as any other antiquated, outmoded system—yet from their ashes will rise new ways of interpreting and experiencing reality.

You may take a break or end the session as you prefer.

("We'll take the break, then."

(11:10–11:43.) Now: even before you met each other many of your private abilities, and the thrust of your intellects and intuitions, made no sense in Darwinian or Freudian terms. This applies to you both.

In those terms, what value is there in any love of contemplation for its own sake? You hastened, Joseph, to put your talent to the proper Darwinian and Freudian goals: to make money, and to compete. Understand, I am not saying there is anything wrong with making money or in competition, say—only when these become primary so that other stronger individual drives must necessarily be put in secondary or third place.

Ruburt went from a strict religion, embracing both Darwin finally, and Freud also, as liberators from old doctrines—not realizing of course that he was substituting one dogma for two, period.

In Darwinian and Freudian terms, certainly later your joint and private pursuits literally made no sense, nor did they conform to any organized religious framework. Many of your difficulties came as your own natural impulses and natural inclinations conflicted with both Darwinian and Freudian concepts.

Your own behavior with your parents, with Ruburt, your attitudes toward your painting and outside jobs, Ruburt's attitudes toward children, his work and you—all of these were so influenced. You set up defenses, privately and jointly, providing justifications, so that you could do your own thing, and "hold your head up" in the world of those beliefs. When you wanted to quit your job you became ill so that no one could blame you. That was years ago, when you were working full time. This would give you parental acceptance.

Illness is a face-saving device, socially, often occurring where private beliefs and feelings find irritation with mass beliefs. Our sessions began, and you managed to make other changes or compromises: you worked part time, and so did Ruburt. This had some advantages, but also many points of conflict. When either of you were offered jobs with advancement, you avoided them like the plague—idiotic behavior in Darwinian and Freudian terms.

Yet those terms influenced you both. You were involved in work that required growing trust of the self. Your painting required it, but Ruburt's position required it still more. The self could be trusted least of all, however, so that Ruburt felt a necessity to criticize his procedure and performance, lest he was leading you and he both down a Freudian garden path.

That young psychologist brought all those doubts to the surface. He was young, and following Darwinian and Freudian concepts both, he was therefore vigorous and to be trusted, where Dr. Instream was in his dotage.

As a woman Ruburt was in a worse position than you from both theories. He took greater precautions, therefore. Now that is the climate in which you began our work.

(*12:01.*) You have learned much, but until lately you always interpreted your position in the light of Darwinian and Freudian concepts. You want the books to sell well. That <u>is</u> natural. Your natures however are not particularly competitive. There is no reason to feel that you <u>should</u> (underlined three times) "be out there selling books." You naturally both concentrate on ideas. Left alone, that concentration will naturally seek expression, amplification, and might result in, say, if you wanted it, some tours. But many of your ideas there are your attempts to bring your work into Darwinian terms.

In the more important ways you have left those frameworks, and your hearts were never in them. Now it is necessary that you, consciously, and with greater understanding, set up your own alternate framework. Rededicate yourselves, as per my last session, together each morning. Reinstate the library at least twice a week.

Ruburt's return to his writing will again trigger psychic response and creativity. With that work the comparatively few visitors will fall by the wayside in importance, and Ruburt's condition will improve more smoothly, with his main concentration elsewhere. Your preoccupation with such matters has certainly hampered your creativity.

Your preoccupation with Ruburt's condition, however, was beneficial for a while, because it upset the status quo, shook him up, and started him more firmly in the proper physical direction. It should not continue, however. It was necessary to unite you both.

Period. End of session. My heartiest regards and a fond good evening.
("Thank you, Seth.")
Unless you have questions—
("No.")
Some of this can be used, if you want to, in an appendix to the new book.
("All right." 12:12 AM.)

DELETED SESSION
SEPTEMBER 3, 1977 9:35 PM SATURDAY

(I had several questions for Seth: they'd grown out of our activities in recent days, and I read them to Jane now.

(1. More on her eyes, and other physical conditions.

(2. Last Thursday night, kidding around with Frank Longwell, Jane said I could have all the reincarnational material on my own lives that I wanted, but that she wasn't interested in her own. So I asked that we get some info on my Roman captain life, since we'd been talking about that one.

(3. During a conversation Jane and I had wondered why the members of the human species were so woefully ignorant of the internal structure of their own bodies. Not that we wanted or needed conscious <u>control</u>—but why didn't we have the conscious visual knowledge of the workings of our various bodily parts, be they heart, liver, or whatnot?

(4. Why does Jane sometimes feel so blue when she wakes up from a nap?

(Another question I'd meant to ask but forgot to list, had to do with our failure to do certain things, regardless of how often Seth mentioned them: viz.—using the hot towels, trying for the library, etc. Seth does go into those questions tonight.)

Good evening.
("Good evening, Seth.")
Now: in answer to, in partial answer to, your question concerning conscious knowledge of the body's workings, I have several things to say.

Perhaps primarily the answer lies in the necessity that man recognize the spontaneous source of his being. I will come back to that. More than that, however, your question of course reflects your cultural beliefs and assumptions, and so you do not realize that in some ways such conscious knowledge of the body's workings might limit rather than expand concepts and experience of the body and the self.

I assume that by your question you mean, why does not man understand how his heart works? I confess that I do not quite know how to explain what I mean. In all the terms of common sense, of course our body is composed of organs—heart, liver, and so forth, and I mention them at times. You must understand, however, that the very terms are arbitrary <u>to a certain extent</u>.

In your terms, early man felt his body to be a living, independent extension of the earth itself, and of the land. His head, to him, was like space or the sky. His feet were like moving roots. He believed that his feelings were like the world's winds that swept through his body. To him, his spirit was inside his skin. Blood flowed through him with refreshing life, as water flowed through the rivers, refreshing the land. In your terms of course he had a heart and liver, but those terms are still arbitrary.

Early man related to his insides, then, symbolically in a way that is now quite outside of your comprehension. He knew he needed rain and sun and food as the land did. He felt so at one with the land, he and his body, that "a conscious knowledge of it," it in your terms not only would have inhibited his identification with nature, but his agility within it.

Such a knowledge as you suggest in <u>actuality</u> would not have added to his comprehension of his body, for he comprehended it very well. It would not have added to his health for example either, for he listened to his body so acutely that natural healings followed as he sought from nature what his body needed. Perhaps a more recent example would help. There have been articles *(in the newspapers)* about people dying of broken hearts after long periods of time, when hearts were simply regarded as mechanical pumps. No man's knowledge will alone save him from heart failure, or heart difficulties, if such knowledge is not backed up by comprehensions of an entirely different order.

If you understand that people can die of broken hearts, however, in symbolic terms, then practically you may be able to use that knowledge. There have been many concepts of the body. You can deal as effectively with the body by regarding it in entirely different terms than you do.

Native cultures, believing that the courage or fleetness of an eaten animal became part of the hunter's mental and physical acquisition, handled the body in entirely different terms, and did very well. You can say that you have a brain and heart and liver and appendix, and so forth, and muscles and bones, and insist that all of these work in a certain fashion, as of course they do. Cutting the body open will show those organs. You can say with equal validity that the body holds a man's ghost, that it is filled also with the organs of all the animals a man has consumed—that one man has the heart of a lion, and in that framework that is true.

I cannot explain this at all adequately. All I hope to do is to show you the assumptions behind your questions. And <u>that</u> is important.

(10:00.) Physicians, perhaps, can be used as an example of men who do have a conscious knowledge of the body's workings. They should indeed then be the healthiest of men. Obviously this is not the case. Man must be free to experience the body as he wishes, and to be aware of its spontaneous order.

Medically much can be done in your framework to alter bodily parts. The body is not just a physical entity, however, nor is its working completely the result of the condition of all of its parts. People in seemingly good health, for example, all parts functioning normally as far as you know, medically, can suddenly die, or become ill, while no reason can be found. Such cases can occur, among other reasons, because of relationships between or among bodily parts that in your terms do not have a physical status.

Give us a moment.... There are for example pressures that do not show, strained relationships between, say, organs that are not apparent medically. These can best be symbolically stated, and would always represent states of mind or feeling. They affect bodily behavior, however, and bodily experience, and are far more important to health in basic terms.

Give us a moment.... For example, in your culture some people <u>feel</u> that there is a struggle between their hearts and their heads, a conflict between emotion and reason, in other words. In many cases, now, meaning not in all, such feelings set up quite invisible but definite alienations, or lacks of balance, between the heart and the brain, so that <u>delicate relationships</u> between them are upset. Those relationships affect physical organs, but the medical profession is not used to thinking in terms of relationships that cannot appear under a microscope.

Early man, "stupidly" knowing nothing of the body's organs, did not feel that particular kind of disorientation. Man has an inherent knowledge of his body. On some occasions specific knowledge of the various parts leads him to forget other issues, and leads to a mechanistic approach.

(10:18.) Give us a moment.... You have categorized by part, certainly it seems, the great part of emerging knowledge, when in your terms taboos were broken and medical men were allowed to dissect corpses, to see what was before

hidden. Yet again, men who felt they had the fleetness of the gazelle, the heart of the lion, or whatever, did not need literal knowledge in your terms. It is quite correct to say that your body is composed of everything you have consumed, also—each bird, animal, and plant—that those qualities form your flesh, ever change their form.

A conscious knowledge of the eye's working will not necessarily give you better vision. To a certain extent that system, while it has its advantages, is also limited and differently slanted in certain directions that <u>can</u> at least at times mitigate against the body's health and well-being.

The body is given mechanistic qualities. The heart is a pump, for example, but everywhere there are examples where people act in an entirely different fashion. Medical men are taught that certain muscles or organs do thus and so. People who should have died ten years ago by such prognoses, still live, while others who it seems should have lived, died.

Man has a knowledge of his body. This need have nothing to do with detailed information about its parts. Each man feels his relationship with his body. Your belief structures have clouded the practical use of that knowledge, however.

Give us a moment.... As to Ruburt: the relationships between his bodily parts are being corrected. I am not speaking of stance here, but of those invisible relationships mentioned earlier, for he felt earlier as if he were literally a self divided, so that one part shouted discipline, and one shouted spontaneity. One shouted go ahead, one shouted slow down, be cautious, and these feelings of separateness were reflected in the body.

There have been considerable changes even since our last session, and I hope you have noted them. Feelings and emotion caused tensions under certain conditions that are not necessarily physically apparent, but that change the body. In your terms the body grows in time. So do beliefs. Ruburt is completely changing emotional and intellectual beliefs of long standing. His poor mobility did not exist alone, but reached back to an archaeology, say, of beliefs that affected his sinuses, jaw pressure, and so forth.

That archaeology is winding backward. The body is making excellent progress in an overall way. He goes through new stances quickly now. Even the smallest alteration of stance and muscular attitude affects the eyes. A child's eye level is a tabletop. Ruburt got along well looking straight in front of him. The visual area is enlarging. The jaw pressures are constantly being minimized. This also requires changes in the eyes.

The entire posture required a tightening, however, of all muscles, including eye muscles. The body is letting down. You <u>can</u>, and you have, helped him by reminding him that this is safe, that the body's protection and his own lies precisely in the body's agility and quick response.

You have changed your own beliefs. This is reflected in your household, but you did not have Ruburt's backlog, so to speak. Your table *(pointing)* is an excellent idea. The further changes in his position will take place far easier. Reinforce that idea of safety, and comfort him, as you have.

(10:47.) Now: making love encourages feelings both of safety and spontaneity. It decreases the feeling of isolation, it promotes spiritual and physical ease, it encourages communication. It is a boon whether or not you know what hormones are stimulated, or have a conscious detailed knowledge of its effects.

It should play far more a part then than it does in your lives, whether it amounts to a quiet half hour, simply lying together; but touch is vital. You see how your cat needed it *(who stood in Jane's lap as she spoke for Seth).*

Now take your break, or end the session as you prefer.

("We'll take the break.")

(10:50—11:05.)

Now, as to the blueness after naps.

There is no one reason. There are several issues involved, however, and if all of them are activated at one time, then the blues results.

If he feels that he has not done enough that day before his nap, he then compares himself to those who come home from work around five, after "putting in a good day." If he has worked enough in his terms the comparison is not so bothersome. Beside this, there is sometimes a feeling of isolation, since you nap separately, and at times he has felt that to be a rejection—not in deep terms, but important enough so that that feeling is combined with the first one mentioned.

Also, he uses his energy differently than you, and needs to eat oftener. Coffee cake is no answer. Either he may be hungry and take his nap, or he may eat coffee cake for example that initially supplies energy that quickly depletes itself—just about the time his nap is finished.

Give us a moment.... On occasion then he feels isolated, guilty, and is in a period of depleted energy. This state, added to his physical condition, is responsible for his feelings. They often fade after eating—in fact, they usually do, or after a friendly comment from you, or whatever.

Noises outside the bedroom, of neighborhood activity, sometimes add to this, making him think he should be out in the world in a more gregarious, competitive manner, so he feels more isolated from other people and the community also at such times, as a result of the Darwinian concepts mentioned in our last session. If all of these issues click in one day, then his mood is more severe, but usually one or two operate.

He should not go from lunch until 6 o'clock, however, without some other nourishment.

Give us a moment.... I will go into the other material at our next session, because I want to emphasize a few points here. When you reinstate the library, that reinstatement will represent other certain stages in your private and joint states of consciousness and intent.

You have not done so yet, and that means something also. The same applies to the hot towels, and to the extent to which you are willing, even in small ways, to alter your way of life, to achieve desired ends. It means something that you do not make love more often, also, and I am not necessarily referring to hours of rollicking passion, either, but to an allotted time to the simple pleasure of body and mind together, and to a kind of communication that is important for its own sake.

(11:21.) You watch television. Perhaps this is an odd suggestion from me, perhaps not even practical, but a television set in the bedroom also invites intimacy. Be more creative in your living patterns.

I mention some things again and again, so you do not have to go back to old sessions, though you should occasionally. Then let Ruburt encourage his spontaneity. He will find himself writing well—inspired, with time for new work and typing manuscripts, with periods of relaxation and ambition.

I will begin your other questions at the start of our next session, and I bid you a fond good evening.

("Thank you, Seth, very much." 11:25 PM.)

SESSION 810 (DELETED PORTION)
SEPTEMBER 10, 1977 9:30 PM SATURDAY

(The following material is from the 810th session.)

(10:24.) You have abilities as a leader, as Ruburt has. To some extent or another each of you has played this role for the other at various times, in this life and in others. This has to do with a brief conversation the two of you held recently. You can indeed now, <u>to some extent,</u> serve as a leader to Ruburt in certain areas, where before you feared that might inhibit his independence, and you felt he needed the freedom to grow.

You each have literally incredible power at your command—as each individual does. You should both be able to sense that power, however, more than others, and to direct it where you want it, both together and individually.

When you see Ruburt going too far in one direction, and see him trying to alter that direction, you can indeed exert your energy, leadership and direction there, for the two of you also operate jointly as well as individually. So his overt action also represents latent action of your own that you are not expressing because you have too much sense. Each of you should now and then try to sense your individual power, for it goes out creatively in the books. It comes back to you as evidence when through the mail you see the books help people change the directions of their lives.

Ruburt must realize that his power and energy can, and indeed is, changing his body for the better. That confidence is important, and it is only where he, first of all, and you secondarily, doubt it that difficulty occurs.

You are still both in the habit of minimizing improvements, and negatively projecting into the future, although at times you have spurts of confidence that are responsible for Ruburt's quite definite physical improvement.

The lack of confidence is what you must both work at, and the old habits of thought. Ruburt is back at writing again, which is excellent. When I make recommendations, such as the library, I make them with the knowledge of their implications, and their importance in the entire picture. This is not an original statement, but the past only has the power that you give it.

Ruburt's entire body is more pliable. His balance is continually working toward normality. Confidence can vastly accelerate the process, and definitely smooth the way. I suggested that you both use your creativity in that regard—again, a suggestion not lightly made. I want you to understand your power, individually and jointly, in that regard.

(10:40.) You are doing fairly well, but you can do better by far.

Give us a moment.... I want to stress that nothing is wrong with Ruburt's physical body except for applied tension. The feelings of relaxation and mobility can frighten him—though they do so far less than previously, and less often. The entire body is releasing tension. It is important that both of you stress the safeness of the procedure. The massager is very beneficial now, for his body is pliable enough now to respond—but more, as he used it recently the intent to relax is there. The mechanical aid is good: he is safely seated, and he has also used the occasion to relax his mind.

The relaxed tendons. And muscles can cause a sinking sensation that is quite natural, and a beneficial sign that should be psychologically interpreted as such.

Released tension in the head area can also change both Ruburt's depth perception and head pressure, as it lessens. The eyes will at times have a further range—that is, an increased range—while not focusing as clearly as they should, necessarily. The entire picture is as I have given it. Concentrate upon your creativity, both of you, and your power, with the morning suggestions I gave you, and the library. He should not concentrate upon his body.

The eyes have improved enough so that he can work near normally enough at his writing, and they will continue to improve. The morning eye condition results from the sinuses. The draining is beneficial. If you understand your power and <u>exert</u> it, and you <u>can</u>, then you can accelerate the process. You must not focus your attention upon past failures. You do not think of any paintings that you did not succeed at. Ruburt does not think of books that he did not finish. All of those things are lost in the light of new achievement. You can coax Ruburt more and encourage him, and exert your power more in that direction. You have not believed you could do that.

You have not thought it would have an effect. I am not telling you to take responsibility for Ruburt's progress at all, but saying that it is certainly to your advantage, and his, that you exert more energy there in terms of active encouragement. There will be times when you are discouraged, each of you, but when one has confidence at any time, the other can use it. It is that one area where each of you believed you had no power to change events, and that belief could impede your progress, at least, even when both of you want a change.

Ruburt has obviously progressed. He is quite ready for more observable improvements, however, and that is why I am making these suggestions.

(10:55.) Give us a moment.... Have Ruburt give himself suggestions that he will dream of his Turkish life, for there is information there that can help him now. Overall, you are <u>both</u> doing well. In your painting, remind yourself of reincarnational selves, for there are more portraits ready, and in your nap time, beside rest, both of you give such suggestions:

I want you united, so to speak, with your powers focused psychically, creatively, and toward bettering Ruburt's physical state. Do you have questions?

("No.")

I bid you then a fond good evening—

("Okay, Seth.")

—and there is more meat here than may appear.

(10:58 PM.)

DELETED SESSION
SEPTEMBER 12, 1977   9:48 PM MONDAY

(We had three questions for Seth:

(1. We were concerned about Jane's continuing eye-sinus condition—the protruding and drainage. We didn't want it to become a lasting thing. What, we wondered, was necessary to bring about a reasonable remission?

(2. Something about Jane's Turkish life. Seth mentioned this in the last deleted session. I wondered if there could be clues there related to Jane's symptoms.

(3. Something about my Roman life in the first century AD. Although Seth discussed reincarnation in the last regular session, he gave nothing on that life per se. I was curious.

(We were visited after supper this evening by Leonard Yaudes and Ann Kraky. As we waited for tonight's session, Jane said she thought that Seth was organizing material about the four of us, our years together at 458 West Water St., and the flood of 1972—but that when we decided upon the questions listed above, Seth changed his tactics: he began to organize that *material instead—"reorganizing what he'd already planned, in order to put it all together," as Jane put it. She could feel the process. I suggested to Jane that she make some notes about the phenomenon.)*

Now—good evening.

("Good evening, Seth.")

I was going to give you some material that you could use, with some name changes, in an appendix for my latest book.

("Okay.")

Instead, as Ruburt supposed, I will reorganize that material somewhat, so that some of your questions are also answered. Give us a moment.

There are biological families. There are also all kinds of other groups which are not necessarily family substitutes, but different kinds of families. Social organizations, clubs, and other frameworks of course to some extent apply here, and supply for many people frameworks in which certain relationships can be encountered that are specific—limited in some ways, perhaps, to certain specific interests, and yet they give a sense of belonging.

All societies are different. The tenants at 458 at one time formed a kind of family, and to some extent that relationship continues, as far as the two of you are concerned, with Ann and Leonard. You remember past tenants together as people recall distant or dead family members. And in particular you chose the conditions of the flood and took part in a joint history.

<u>To some extent</u> you all have characteristics that are similar, while of course there are differences. In one way or another, however, you have not accepted the traditional social roles. Neither Ann or Leonard married. You married, but not at the usual age—later. You did not have children. Leonard and Ann also have a certain stubborn independence. When they look at your relationship with Ruburt they still assure themselves that it is after all not the traditional marriage.

I will at some time go into the reasons why all of you chose that house and the flood situation, for it fit into your joint and private purposes. The Walls were also involved. They served as house parents to some degree.

In Turkey you dealt with an order rather than a family—a tribal order, so to speak, with males predominating. It was of a religious and warlike nature, in which the sword predominated. Women had no part to play. Ruburt was the leader of such a group, and you were what could be considered his lieutenant, or closest at hand. The group was given to mystical practices, in which the dictums of Allah were followed—but also those dictums were enmeshed with some old Jewish practices and beliefs.

(On file: see "A Life in the Talmud," New York Times Magazine for September 11, 1977, on oral history of Jews as well as the Talmud itself.)

Moses was considered a saint, for example. The sect was a strange mixture of Mohammedanism, Christianity and Judaism, but it went under the banner of Mohammedanism, and considered Christians in conventional terms as enemies. The Jews were sometimes considered allies, and sometimes not. It was a rich pageantry of beliefs—almost an Oriental Christianity despite the fact that the Christians were considered the true infidels.

(From page 914 of the dictionary: Mohammed I. 570—632 AD; Arabian prophet, founder of the Moslem religion. 2. Mohammed II, 1430—81; Sultan of Turkey (1451—81); captured Constantinople (1453).

Ruburt was used to the unbridled use of power, and at least among the sect his word was law. Reincarnation was also part of the belief structure. It was considered a blight of the gods, for example, to ever return as a woman.

You were Ruburt's younger brother at that time, and both of you engaged in many bloody religious battles. You were blunt men, yet highly emotional, living for some time near Constantinople, but ranging far, even to Afghanistan, and on several occasions meeting bands from Rome.

You were great riders, horses being wealth, and collectors of fine gold ornaments. Ruburt was just, as he understood justice. To some extent he felt it a comedown to be born as a woman *(as Jane)*. He also played down physical abilities, for toward the end of that life he became hungry for knowledge, and wondered at his own unbridled use of power.

You were the man again, so for some years he was confused because he felt himself to be, as a woman, in an inferior position to you.

He accepted you as a mate and teacher, however, and put such weight upon your words because in that old context you were a male. You both decided to use power indirectly, however, to affect your civilization through thought rather than through combat. In early years Ruburt found it difficult even to contradict you, even while he insisted upon his own independence of mind, and upon his use of his abilities. At times, however, you refused to lead in this life when circumstances might have warranted a more active role at particular times, because in that previous life you would not buck Ruburt, and because you also were more cautious this time about the use of personal power.

(10:16.) You had excelled, as he had, in all areas of that experience—as warriors, religious leaders, chieftains. In this life, therefore, you always felt sorry for those you felt could not achieve, and often held back your own abilities or criticisms for that reason.

You have been hard on yourselves, for you were used to the instant recognition of your peers, and accepted none as your superiors. In this life you concentrated upon the search for knowledge—and even in that particular past life, power was important only because it was considered the gift to believers from God, and therefore the natural result of knowledge.

In many ways then you have refused to show others your true presences, except through the books. Yet through the books you obtain followers, though you say you do not want followers. Of course you do, to a certain extent. You do not want blind followers, as once you had them, but you do want to create your own kind of inner civilization, and you are.

This time those followers are provided with information you did not have then, and they are taught to be true to themselves. They are told not to be cruel or fanatical, not to die for the sword, or by the sword. Yet they look to you. Ruburt became overly cautious, however, and your own attitudes helped. To some extent you felt, both of you, that a woman, gifted, needed greater protection. She was not as dependable, nor should she really show her face in public— <u>so to some extent, now</u>, the symptoms took the place of the veil.

All of that occurred in the background in which you chose an artistic ability that did not fit into the accepted male role, and Ruburt possessed a drive that did not fit the feminine picture, either. You quite concurred with the attitudes involved. Each of you dislike fanatics because you were once so fanatical. Ruburt went to battle with all of his men, and only as he grew older did he begin to wonder at his own motives, or the beliefs that were the structure of his life.

You also questioned. You set up a system of balances so that you would think before using your power. This was overdone, however. On the other hand it was reassuring now because in that other life you were afraid of your own impetuosity, together, and had to know you could control it while using your abilities. You have each controlled it. There is no need then to further show yourselves that you can indeed be understanding and compassionate leaders. In that <u>joint</u> venture it made little difference which of you accepted the role that would in one way or another prevent the both of you from misusing power, for the one role would be passive while the other was active.

You simply decided to know what you were doing this time, and an over-conscientiousness on both of your parts led you to rein in your joint spontaneity.

Ruburt's condition in late years would fluctuate. You would use it, the two of you, as a measuring yardstick: if he began to improve considerably enough, particularly a few years ago, you would instantly, Joseph, become negative and guarded. Instead of being thankful when he began to go out again, you became frightened, and felt that everyone noticed his condition. After all, the two of you rode horses at the head of the pack.

On those occasions when he improved, and you did not become negative, then he instantly became frightened and negative himself. On other occasions, when he improved, you began with a variety of assorted symptoms of your own, as if to say "One of us must do it," and he would think "Well, I had better keep things as they are. Better that one of us at least should be happy."

This time you have maintained your health equilibrium, and you have not become negative. Ruburt's improvement has been steady, but guarded, as he watches for your attitude, and to make sure that it is indeed safe now.

To some extent, I do not want to overstate. You initiated the procedures years ago, and decided you would not be the one. Now Ruburt could have refused that role also. Nothing said that either of you had to accept it.

(10:40.) Give us a moment.... Partially it was the belief that women were more vulnerable, and the social conditions—Darwinian and Freudian concepts—that led him to accept that position, and all the material I have given fits in here. There was also the feeling that contemplation and action were self-contradictory.

You also both felt that you needed isolation from society, and a position from which you could examine it with some solitude, while still maintaining contacts—and while still affecting it through your works. You did not want to sell your paintings because you did not want that much direct contact with that society or marketplace *(intently)*.

Prentice served your purposes for the same reason, and because of reincarnational contacts with Tam.

Ruburt's condition has also served as a framework in which he is the opposite of the conquering hero. It is an attempt to play down his presence, to be the absent leader—and in this, again, you heartily concurred. You also played down your own leadership role, while of course maintaining it, and the two of you operate as a team now as you did then.

In that life women were expected to be decorative, and most of all compliant, so in his relationship to you, when Ruburt felt decorative or compliant, he felt you would have no use for him. You each decided to have no children—you, of course, as well as Ruburt. Your children are the people you influence, help, and guide.

In any case, in the context of this discussion, had you not married Ruburt, you would have remained single, or possibly married to a woman who also would not want children. You were both used to the idea of attaining knowledge and influencing minds. In the Turkish life that meant following Allah and the dictates of holy battle. Now you know that no wars are holy, only regrettable.

In that life you did not understand, however, the true independence of men's minds. You went overboard, trying to influence their minds, and not influencing their minds at the same time in this life, lest they follow you blindly.

Very briefly: as a Roman, you pretended to be a follower while you were a man of rank in the military. You had no belief in the conventional gods, yet you were supposed to be conquering lands in their name. You traveled even to Africa. You had a disdain for leaders as liars, and of the masses as followers, and so you were always in one kind of dispute or another, with your fellows, and even with the authorities. You were of a querulous nature, yet highly curious, and again physically involved.

Your curiosity did not involve philosophies, but had to do with the physical world, and particularly with its water passageways—an interest that did indeed find you and the Caribbean, later, in either the 14th or 15th century, directly involved with piracy—and I believe with some controversy involving the French government at the time.

Take your break.

(10:59—11:06.)

In connection with the Turkish life, you decided upon certain handicaps this time. You were the adored sons of a Turkish chieftain, following the social patterns of your times, gifted at birth with power and position.

In this life Ruburt chose poverty as a background, a mother who was not physically fit, a broken family. You chose parents who in their way were culturally deprived, ignorant of fine music or literature, and temperamentally poles apart. Then you chose a prime ability, not overly valued by society. When the two of you took up together for the reasons given, you decided upon a further handicap, though you had not specifically chosen one.

You were the elder this time, where before you were the younger. Ruburt looked up to you in those days as once you looked up to him. There is no need for a handicap of any kind. You both also had from other existences strong drives toward privacy and secrecy. The television program you saw about monasteries and privacy to some extent applies here, for in the hurly-burly of medieval life there was no privacy for thought.

Only monks could afford it, and there were thousands of different groups scattered throughout Europe. There were equally as many long-forgotten communities, in which hermits of every sect imaginable squatted in caves in given areas. People of solitary nature born in medieval times had to make their own structures, and if they were not hermits or monks, they were outlaws of one kind or another, frequenting the woods, which were often full of semi-permanent but isolated communities—men and women who preyed upon travelers, for example.

In some ways the monks and the outlaws had much in common: a desire for privacy, a bent for independence, an unconventional curiosity, and yet a need for some kind of communal existence, for there was no technology to support such people.

Often there was little difference between the outlaws and the monks, and fanatic roving bands of monks often went through isolated communities or farmlands with a vengeance.

You both had existences in which you combined the traits of each in medieval Europe. Sacred manuscripts were often stolen from one monastery and taken to another, where they were exchanged for the goods of this world, and for sanctuary. Some of those experiences led you both to desire a certain privacy while remaining in the midst of a community, and here again Ruburt's condition came into service, giving you a built-in reason for not going out into the world.

He is obviously more restricted in that regard, but neither have you had a woman you had to escort, so your times were spent thinking, writing, exploring the nature of reality, and affecting society while not being infected by it, according to your concepts and beliefs. More than this, people come to _you_, as befits your Turkish condition. You do not go to them. Nor do you set up a school for fools—again, according to your beliefs and concepts.

To some extent, then, the situation has served you both well for years. Ruburt finally became so depressed, however, about the symptoms that his work was involved—an intolerable situation, presenting an instant dilemma. Neither of you really <u>miss</u> not traveling, not going on tours, or not mixing with the world. You became embarrassed at Ruburt's condition when others saw it, and you finally became alarmed when you wondered how much the body could put up with.

Above all, neither of you wanted the condition to worsen. That is where you drew the line. No condition is stable, but ever-changing. The entire system of beliefs was based upon, again, fear of the spontaneous self on both of your parts—fear that it would lead you where you did not want to go, as if you and it were separate things, or as if its intents were by nature so divorced from your own that you must set up barriers against its expression except in certain acceptable areas.

(11:30.) Ruburt became the spontaneous one to both of you, therefore the one who must use controls. You became the disciplined one to both of you, which meant of course that you also impeded your spontaneity. The mind cannot be fully used when it is used at the body's expense. You have gone along with Ruburt's improvements. You are <u>beginning</u> to actively encourage it. Your suggestion to Ruburt involving touch is highly important, and represents growing understanding on your part.

To some extent or another you each feel that the world is insane. With his literal mind Ruburt took protection against it, and found in your apartment and home what he hoped would be a safe sanctuary in monastic terms, where each of you could learn and grow. On purposes you both agreed. Carried to extremes, however, the condition became alarming. This is why improvements are occurring, and because you each are beginning to realize that there is a natural world out there for the world of nature to which both the soul and the body relate. Your protections have been against the social world, but in the extremes you end up losing an important part of the natural world as well.

If you really do understand that you live in a safe universe, you need no such protection. If you emphasize your natural selves, and your relationship with the dusk and the dawn, and with the earth itself, you will feel free in that natural world.

(11:38.) Give us a moment.... The eyes and sinus will clear up as you understand what I am saying. The sinuses were not as noticeable before, for the backlog of congestion had caused crystallizations that lodged in tissues. These now become soft and drain away.

The entire session, if you understand it, will help. In healing, hot water, that is steam, can accelerate the process. Though the eyes may initially feel fuller, the material will loosen more quickly, but it will then have to drain. Otherwise, entire bodily relationships are changing, but he needs confidence that I hope this session will give him.

The library, again, is important, and because of your joint participation and purpose.

Encourage him toward physical activity of a kind that in his physical condition challenges him enough, but is not beyond his physical means. This is important. Do not think, again, in terms of absolutes, but of improvement from where he is, and use your creativity there. This is important.

(Emphatically, and with humor:) I bid you a fond Turkish good evening.

("Thank you very much, Seth.")

Take this letter to heart.

("Yes."

(11:47 PM. Jane's voice was now quite hoarse.)

DELETED SESSION
SEPTEMBER 17, 1977 9:25 PM SATURDAY

(Before the session Jane read her summary of the week's events, including her continuing improvements. Her knees especially have shown many signs of loosening. Tam called her Friday; he'd received the James *presentation, and was most enthusiastic, which cheered Jane a great deal. Then Saturday we learned by mail that Bantam is about to contract for the paperback edition of* Politics. *We are also waiting for the September royalty payment from Prentice-Hall, due probably next week. Tonight Jane remarked: "If only I could get my physical condition to work as well as the money one." But she's making progress. And last night we had a congenial group of friends in.*

(Neither of us had any questions for Seth.)

Now: good evening—

("Good evening, Seth.")

—and since I can choose my own topic, let us begin with suggestion.

Ruburt has made some effort to avoid negative projections, and has therefore met with some success. Last evening, however, he became involved in a round of such projections, which operate, of course, as negative suggestions. When he voiced some of these you immediately told him that he was doing so. Previously this round of projections had been almost automatic—that is, he did not catch himself at it, but accepted the worries as worries, without seeing that the situations might or might not occur.

The two of you have been working much closer together, however. Your remark therefore instantly alerted him, and in spite of company coming almost immediately, and in spite of his worries generated by the projections, he did immediately use your remark in such a way that he was challenged creatively to change his approach at once.

He resolved that he would refrain from such projections <u>for the evening</u>, and he did. This required initially some considerable effort, but once he decided upon this a mechanism took over so that for a while he behaved almost automatically in the new manner, as before he had behaved almost automatically in the old way. Your remark therefore operated as an excellent suggestion, that he desist from such activity.

It served to remind him what he was doing—but more, it allowed him to recognize the situation, which you saw clearly while for a time it was invisible to him.

The affair was important because it showed him that such techniques do work, and it is an excellent example of one of the most important ways you have of helping him. You did not lecture him, for example—simply stated your recognition of behavior that you knew he would not want to continue, and was trying to break.

His method of dealing with the affair was also good in this way. He gave himself a time period that he knew he could reasonably handle. There is no use in telling yourself in absolute terms that you will never project negatively. To expect any kind of commitment to an invisible future is too much in that regard. Ruburt can, however, each day tell himself that for that day he will try to avoid such negative projection. That kind of method gives you something to work with, and a time period you can handle.

Since his intents have now changed some, he is able to use any remarks by you that lead him to recognize such behavior.

Your simple remark then was strong enough to completely alter the pattern of his thoughts and behavior last evening, and most of today, so I want you to recognize the importance of your comments. In the past Ruburt might have reacted differently, perhaps with self-pity, but now he is much more amiable to beneficial suggestions, so that one <u>can</u> completely turn him about, back to his course.

(9:41.) Your intimate periods are of prime importance from all angles. Each of you needs to realize the importance of pleasure for its own sake. You always recognize pleasure in work, but the body also enjoys its own creature-reality, as any animal enjoys stroking—and in the past you have stroked your kitten more than you have each other.

This is a way of encouraging Ruburt's physical spontaneity, for his emotions and body each together want to move at such times. It is a way of assuring your own physical selves that you have a right to physical pleasure, as any animal does, whether or not you succeed in the world, or reach work goals, or meet any of the other issues that may concern you. Such periods also provide definite regeneration of the spirit, body, and mind. Carried to the extreme in the past, Ruburt would not even want to take time for a decent shower, unless his other goals for the week were met.

(*It should be noted that this Saturday morning, for the first time in many years, Jane took a shower when she got up—even before breakfast, in other words.*)

Now: his body is continuing to regenerate. The *(typing)* table is still a necessary help. He should not feel worried about using it, or being dependent upon it. It is allowing him to navigate while his body undergoes certain vital readjustments. He knows he can write. He would not think of beginning a book by saying "I cannot write a book." He has been convinced, however, that he could not walk properly, and so we had to work in that context. You have, after all, "the physical evidence" to support that hypothesis. We have concentrated upon the fact that he could walk better, then, and that the body could improve itself —as indeed of course in that context it can, and does.

The belief that he could not walk properly is the result of all the issues we've mentioned. It is indeed a <u>side effect</u>. You saw how well your remark last evening worked. It was hardly a momentous affair, yet it meant that Ruburt could forget his physical problems to a considerable extent, stop worrying about whether he would have to go to the bathroom, or how to get there, or when people would leave so he could get there, and so the evening was effectively altered for the better.

I want, therefore, to reinforce certain points. I must always couch my material for you personally—the two of you, that is—according to your situation and understanding. And there are indeed multitudinous levels, each quite valid, that are involved.

At your present "working level," Ruburt goes through a series of beneficial physical changes, of posture, body alignment, release of muscles. These are all occurring. They are for that matter accelerating. The practical value, for example, of good suggestion finally does accelerate into improved behavior, though some periods of time may be involved. Finally, however, the suggestions accumulate, so to speak, in the realm or level we are speaking of.

For example, you can see this operate in terms of creativity: money comes to you now without new work involved, in terms, say, of paperback sales. Those paperback sales were latent, so to speak, when the hardcover books were sold. In the same way highly significant improvements not yet visible, are in the offing in Ruburt's condition, that will, say, seemingly require no effort when in your terms they do appear. All of this applies in the terms in which you are now working—that is, in your present framework.

(10:02.) <u>I want you to keep this framework as a working one</u>. I also want,

however, to gently introduce another framework, that I want you to use simply as a point of higher reference for now.

In that framework the rules are different. In that framework the truth is that Ruburt can indeed walk normally <u>now</u>, and that nothing prevents it except for the belief that it is not so. Now I would like the truth of this higher framework at least to affect the framework in which you are now operating in this other framework, and I will have to use your points of reference *(with almost a laugh.)*

We will call your working framework, Framework 1 for purposes of discussion, and this higher framework, Framework 2. In Framework 1, time must be allowed for the body to respond, physical time. In Framework 2, and in the terms of Framework 1's understanding, such body work is not really necessary, since the body itself has nothing wrong with it except the application of beliefs.

Even if you think the body <u>does</u> have something wrong with it, then the necessary adjustments would be made in another kind of time that in Framework 1 would take no time at all—or, the amount of time you thought required.

The whole idea of the release of muscles, joints, the physical procedure, involves necessary methods and procedures while you are operating in Framework 1, and there you always are looking for the necessary quite vital evidence of improvement. You are checking to see how you are doing—again, quite necessary when you believe that there is indeed something wrong with the body. In Framework 2, there is nothing wrong with the body, again. It is responding, however, to suggestions almost automatically applied. In <u>that</u> framework you deal with mental patterns, beliefs, and emotions. <u>There</u>, you are confident enough to forget the body entirely, as you work with the nature of suggestion, and with the changing of mental patterns. There, you are so confident of the truth that your beliefs form reality that you need not check the body at every point to see how it is reacting, for you know it will respond as completely to the new suggestions as it did to the old, even though you recognize that practically speaking <u>some</u> time might be involved in Framework 2's time.

You feel, however, the new reality take hold in Framework 1, so that you are not worried: the paperbacks will come out *(intently)*.

The process of recovery that you have chosen, therefore, exists in Framework 2, though you are between both frameworks now, operationally speaking. You are reaching for Framework 2, while doing all you can in Framework 1.

So keep Framework 1 for working purposes, but become more and more aware of Framework 2. In your terms this will cut down the time necessary drastically.

Saying all this, I want to make certain things plain, however. You are still largely in Framework 1, so I do not want you to think in terms of absolutes. I do not want you to suddenly expect in Framework 1 sudden, normal activity on Ruburt's part, or to compare his present behavior against that standard. That operates detrimentally.

(10:21.) Give us a moment.... In terms of creativity, however, Ruburt has long been operating in Framework 2, and this session should help him make certain correlations so that he can automatically begin to use such methods in regard to his physical condition.

The suggestion that he have heating dreams will work now, for work can indeed be done in the dream state that would otherwise take physical time.

I simply want to remind you of that other level, so that you can begin—gently, now, gently—to alter your emphasis, to begin to emphasize the use of suggestion in a new creative way. I have used the word creative before, asking you both to utilize creative methods to the physical situation. What I was actually doing was trying to point you toward Framework 2, where you do each have faith in the nature of ideas, suggestions, and achievement. You know the power of an idea, but you have not applied that to the physical problem. I hope that the session will arouse you both in that regard.

Your introduction of intimate moments, Joseph, is a small example. You have been afraid of dreaming of physical success, for fear you would not succeed, but the dreams are what makes Ruburt's improvements possible.

Plan for a vacation. Dream about where you would go. Open your minds to such dreams, for when you do you do not close your imaginations. You need not set a time schedule, but at least in your minds gives yourselves freedom. You do not even have to decide that Ruburt is completely recovered—but the very plans for motion will definitely have beneficial effects on his condition and on the shape of your daily life.

I will have more to say about suggestion, how it operates personally, and how it affects political beliefs and even economic conditions, for it causes your daily reality. In your lives you see the results of the suggestions you have given yourselves—some extraordinarily excellent, bringing about superior understanding, growth of character, achievements on both of your parts, and a comfortable living in financial terms. Others have resulted in Ruburt's physical condition. Your small suggestion about last night—because he was ready and open—altered the evening. Because you are less affected obviously by the negative suggestion, you can catch him, and he will now respond beneficially.

In Framework 1, it does take some time for new habits to form, but even there constructive suggestions accelerate as beliefs change, so I would like you both to pay particular attention to the suggestions that operate in your lives.

That is what I wanted to say for the evening, so unless you have questions I will end the session.

("Well, let's take a break.")

You may indeed.

(10:37. I thought since the hour wasn't very late yet, we could get some information on other subjects. Jane had no questions. I speculated about my painting of the Italian woman, as I call her, and about a passage I read recently in Seth Speaks; in it, Seth had mentioned that he'd been a black in Ethiopia. Perhaps, I suggested to Jane, we could get some material on his life then.

(Jane wasn't particularly interested, however. There followed a rather complicated discussion between us about the idea of questions for Seth—why I seemed to have them, but Jane seldom did. Much of Seth's material to follow these notes deals with the topics of our discussion. Resume at 10:58.)

Now: you each operate differently.

You think in a more detailed fashion, or you begin from a more specific viewpoint, and then move outward toward concepts and large philosophical issues.

Ruburt begins with the large philosophical issues, and somewhat purposefully adopted a thinking pattern at least, or a method of operation, that <u>to some extent</u> ignored details, lest he become too involved in them—in, say, slaying a multitudinous number of detailed paper dragons. He does not deal with generalities, however, but he does not think in terms of specific questions, allowing specifics to emerge in a fresh way from the larger subjects of his interest.

The two of you often misunderstand your patterns of behavior in that regard, for they operate at many levels of your lives. Ruburt is pragmatic, however, in that he insists upon relating philosophy to daily life—but, again, by providing overall models for behavior, rather than, say, specific detailed method.

(A connection here with the codicils?)

Often your detailed questions, however, will initiate new concepts that will themselves provide, by the way, the required answer. Your specific questions, however, also serve to give necessary ribs to the delivery of the material, so that many aspects are covered, and details not <u>ignored</u>. The two of you together then add to the entire psychological structure, and keep the delivery of the material in an excellent overall balance.

This balance is to a large extent responsible for the fact that the material reaches so many people, and your own joint characteristics in that regard are more obvious to your readers than to yourselves. The entire scope of the material of course reflects your joint questions—but Ruburt's are often unformed, dealing with intuitive issues that he does not trust to verbalization.

He trusts the direction of the sessions to cover whatever detailed information is necessary, and he does rely upon your questions in that regard.

The material follows its own flow: there are certain things I want to say, but how I say those things is colored and tinted by your own characteristics jointly, and your experience daily. Your different ways of working are obvious in your other creative endeavors, and your own questions and appliance to detail are highly important in your notes to our books, serving as important ribs, again.

("Thank you, Seth."
(End at 11:32 PM.)

DELETED SESSION
SEPTEMBER 19, 1977 9:22 PM MONDAY

(We had no questions for Seth in particular, hoping that he would just continue where he'd left off last session. Jane felt there was much more to come on Frameworks 1 and 2, etc.)

Good evening.

("Good evening, Seth.")

Now: Ruburt has been looking through some old papers, and it became obvious that over a period of time his journals show two main concerns—or, rather, main interests and goals: his writing and his attempts "to get better."

Before, earlier, there was a third concern—a financial one, but he did not come across those journals this evening. The two main concerns then instantly caught his attention. He did not see, however, the difference in his approach to those concerns—and in that difference lies the difference in results.

Oftentimes he was not sure what his next book would be, but overall he never doubted there would be a next book. He did not imagine impediments that might rise to prevent a next book being written—nor did he doubt his ability to write one, or any number of books. At times he might think of writing in one area or another, but his imagination did not set up barriers: it was always receptive to new ideas, casting about for new experiences, consciously involved in the process of creativity.

To Ruburt <u>that</u> is taken for granted—for there he operates extraordinarily well, mixing and merging the realities of Frameworks 1 and 2. The practical results of course appear in Framework 1, while the real creativity takes place in

Framework 2. Understand that I make these divisions for simplicity's sake, for the realities are merged. In "trying to get better," Ruburt has taken impediments for granted, not only generally but specifically. In his books he lives in and with the present. Manuscripts that did not jell are simply forgotten, so he is supported in those terms by a background of success.

In his other main concern, "getting better," he looks back upon past failures, and projects impediments into the future. In other words, his approach to these two main concerns is quite different—one opposite the other.

He creates impediments then as in the other area he creates success. To a lesser extent this applies to your own approach also. Creativity <u>is</u> involved. Let us look then at the third area, for at one time you both also to some extent imagined impediments, changed your approach, and found new results. That area is the financial one, that indeed does now seem to come with an almost magical ease.

You changed your approaches indirectly, and Ruburt was always stronger in the financial regard than you, as far as his beliefs that artistic creations could bring financial rewards. <u>You</u> believed that commercial art could give financial results, but not necessarily good writing, or good art.

There were other issues that have been mentioned, concerning you and the marketplace, but Ruburt's creativity straddled poor beliefs finally. He stopped looking for financial impediments. He did not worry about money. Just not worrying about it immediately began to give you some financial gain, for in Framework 2 conditions were reversed, and the imagined impediments were not projected into the future. Finally, in Framework 1 those gains began to show: the evidence, in other words. *(Amused:)* Then, in Framework 1, you had some success to bank upon.

It did not seem particularly practical to stop worrying about money. It could even have appeared quite impractical. Yet Ruburt began to feel more and more that you and he would have whatever money was needed for any of your wants or desires.

He felt that your needs and desires would be fairly reasonable; that is, he approved of them. He did not think you would suddenly become ostentatious, for example. Again: Frameworks 1 and 2 merged, and the beneficial results began with a change of ideas and intents in Framework 2.

(9:45.) Now let us look at Framework 2. Your ideas come and go effortlessly, without impediments, with a sense of ease that is taken for granted. Your freedom to think is so transparent and natural that you are scarcely aware of it. That freedom comes from Framework 2, as does the great creativity it makes possible. So in certain terms everyone exists in Framework 2. Many people,

however, live out their lives, practically speaking, in Framework 1. Ruburt's physical condition has been most troublesome to you both, for in that area you have stressed impediments and felt a lack of control. Many people, however, experience such difficulty in all areas of their lives, with nothing in their own experience that they can trust to give them evidence for a greater reality or control over their own destinies.

Once you asked a question *(recently; on file)*, wondering how those who only believed in the evidence of their senses could try to force that limited reality upon others?—and of course they cannot: they can only blind themselves to the greater dimensions of existence.

Generally speaking, however, in handling Ruburt's condition over the years, until lately you have concentrated your working efforts in Framework 1, while in all other areas you at least had a good foothold in Framework 2.

Framework 1 deals with predictable behavior, predictable results, and dislikes surprises. In all other areas of your lives you have prided yourselves on the unpredictability, the creative ground-breaking concepts. You forgot ideas of being practical in terms of Framework 1, and as a result of course your creativity became highly practical, and in the most profound terms.

You are both doing very well. This information is meant to accelerate that progress through clear understanding, and help you grasp hold of your creativity in this area as well. You can continue, and Ruburt's improvement will continue in Framework 1, but you can also accelerate even further, and grab hold of the threshold in Framework 2, which in your terms will let Ruburt improve as easily as now your money comes.

Saying this, I do not want to make you impatient with Ruburt's progress, for he is naturally improving. He can do more than naturally improve, however, if you understand what I am saying, and does not confuse the rules of the two frameworks. That is highly important.

In Framework 2, extranatural help, energy, impetus, and knowledge are "naturally" available. This should be apparent from the very fact of our sessions and from the nature of Ruburt's writing. In Framework 2, then, the same kind of extraordinary help is available in terms of physical condition. That help is blocked, if in Framework 1 you constantly imagine impediments or concentrate upon past poor performance, or project such performance into the future.

In a manner of speaking, then, supernatural help is available, but only when your own beliefs are clear enough so that the help is not blocked. By supernatural I mean the source from which nature springs, and Framework 2 represents the medium in which the natural and the source of the natural merge in a creative gestalt. That gestalt forms your physical being. Nature, without nature's source, would not last a moment.

In Ruburt's dream last night, he was dancing. His physical body carries that memory. The actual muscles involved were rehearsing. The dream in Framework 2 is as much a definite plan for a normally walking body as any *Oversoul Seven* that did result in the book. The original *Seven* did come from a dream, from a drama occurring in Framework 2—but there were no negative beliefs to block it, no habits of erecting impediments. Other dreams of Ruburt's health did not materialize because their creativity was blocked by an insistence upon following, in that regard, the most limiting of Framework 1's premises.

(10:10.) There is no difference between the idea of a book and the idea of a normally walking body. It is simply that in one area Ruburt, and you secondarily, have insisted upon relying upon the conventional levels of existence. Therefore, your confidence was undermined.

There is, incidentally, a Framework 3 and a Framework 4, in the terms of our discussion—but all such labels are, again, only for the sake of explanation. The realities are merged. A brief point *(with some humor)*: When you moved here you wanted to make "a fashion statement" as per your television commercials, where the gentlemen only cut hair. You are more knowledgeable now, but at the time Ruburt did restrict his abilities, pull in his horns, and to some extent with your implied consent. Those in the neighborhood would know you were not to be bothered. You did not go out to parties. You were, generally speaking, to be left alone.

The move, however, served to highlight some of those beliefs, so that Ruburt could see that he could not afford to carry the process any further.

Frank represents your belief that you must hold on to someone at least medically oriented, if unconventionally so, in Framework 1—a needed crutch, and he has been of some help. He has also however reinforced your conventional beliefs that muscles and joints must behave thus-and-so, that so much time must pass for such processes to take place; he helped you set up a situation that served handily, for you could not leave Framework 1, nor yet really accept wholeheartedly Framework 2.

In between, Frank's help was quite necessary. His assurances were important, and quite valid. They helped Ruburt considerably. To some extent, however, they limited improvement in that area. Ruburt must now take the lead. Frank's knowledge can still be helpful, but it should not be allowed, now, to curtail improvements, or limit them, by conventional knowledge of what muscles and joints can or cannot do, or by projecting any particular procedure—as, for example, Ruburt will do this or that, before this or that.

At this stage I do not want Ruburt to compare his physical performance with yours at all. That would be detrimental. In the physical flexibility area, however, you are operating in Framework 2 yourself, and so you can be of great help by catching Ruburt when he projects negatively on the one hand, and on the other by leading him toward the more creative habits of thought that are your own about your body.

You can also help by trying to utilize your natural feelings about flexibility on Ruburt's behalf. This must be done however in Framework 2—in other words, in quiet moments when you recognize when you are dealing at another level, so that you feel no contradiction with Ruburt's Framework 1 behavior. Such thoughts <u>will be</u> received by Ruburt in Framework 2, and <u>will then</u>, with his present intent, begin to alter Framework 1 through direct action.

Such methods will work now because of the changes in beliefs he has made—that is, he is more open. In your intimate periods, <u>to some extent at least</u>, impediments become minimized through love and desire. This session should help him, so that he can begin to mentally minimize impediments, and then they <u>will be</u> minimized.

Take your break.

(10:31—10:56.)

When Ruburt writes a book the paragraphs take care of themselves. It is his way not to concentrate upon details. He does not wonder how he constructs a paragraph. In the area of his physical condition, however, he does concentrate upon details: how to get up, how to go to the bathroom, how to do thus-and-so—an uncharacteristic mode of behavior.

So in our change of method, have him try as best he can to forget such details. The morning shower, in its way, was a breakthrough, for several years of conditioning simply disappeared—an issue I notice you did note.

He has been trying too hard to some extent in Framework 1, where the spontaneity of motion in Framework 2 will allow for the more or less spontaneous accomplishment of detailed motion in Framework 1. I want to emphasize the importance of the improvements that are taking place in Framework 1. These sessions, however, will result in an acceleration and ease, if the sessions are put to use.

By way of comment, and in reference to this discussion only, without taking other issues into consideration, your own parents for example operated largely in Framework 1 for their entire lives. In portions of our work and your own, you have sometimes operated in Framework 3. Ruburt's initial Idea Construction experience momentarily propelled him into Framework 4, where indeed enough energy, creativity, and power was generated to change his life beneficially, and open his mind to higher levels of understanding and knowledge.

The actual time involved in that experience was minute. <u>In a way</u>—underlined twice—that kind of time use represents the kind of threshold I use in my communications in sessions. If you followed Framework 1's beliefs, the sessions would never have begun.

(Pause.) I am trying to think of an analogy.... That experience of Ruburt's in time terms would be like a concentrated time pill: there are pills you take that are released in timed sequences. So everything I am saying, in a manner of speaking, was made possible in that experience. In the time framework of Framework 1, the time period could not contain such accelerated mental or psychic motion, so it appears in your terms of time during our continuous session. My personality could not be "defined" or contained within that initial experience either—so you see, strung out through the years, what in other terms I "said," or "was," at the time of Ruburt's idea construction experience.

Yet I responded to your experience of the continuing days, so often the sessions reflect "current happening." In the terms of the discussion, and with the terminology I am using, my level of existence is simply such that I can move through time by taking advantage of levels of activity that are too fast or slow for you to follow. They appear to me as patterns that I can put together as I wish.

This does not mean that I have a free hand, or that I can impose patterns upon others. Time has a <u>thickness</u>, however, that you do not perceive. Probabilities are a part of time in those terms.

Probabilities are valid time terminals. Ruburt's accelerated state at that "time" led him to a threshold of experience that could be <u>translated</u> into Framework 1, but could not be sustained here in terms of ordinary behavior. The bridge personality was a psychological result, appearing in time, yet apart from it. Framework 2, however, is quite familiar to you, as stated, in your creative work, and most other areas of your lives, including your own physical experience of your body.

The only place where this has not been applied is Ruburt's physical condition. I hope that these sessions will allow you to move rather easily now into Framework 2 in that regard. I have given you important hints in that direction, and I will also see that Ruburt has help in the dream state.

It takes physical time to write a book, so <u>some</u> physical time must be allowed for the normal behavior of Ruburt's body. The book is being created, however, before it appears, and in an easy manner. This is what can happen as far as Ruburt's body is concerned: forget what you think the body can or cannot do. Forget the details that you think must happen before Ruburt can walk properly. Follow my suggestions, and know that the necessary work is being done completely outside of physical time, so that improvements can occur of a significant nature without any particular conventional expected processes that must first occur.

Our sessions came from outside of time in that fashion. So do Ruburt's books. So did your home. So did your existence—and so can Ruburt's flexibility. Again, I will see that you do have help in Framework 2, and in the dream state.

End of session—

("Okay. Thank you.")

—and I gave you some hints as to your question.

("Very good."

(11:26 PM. I hadn't actually asked any questions of Seth; his material after break came through following my joking remark that I was half afraid to ask any, my reaction stemming from his discussion in the last deleted session, regarding Jane's dislike of details, etc.

(At break tonight I'd explained to Jane that I still thought the 14th session contained some excellent material on Seth's awareness of "something resembling time" to him—and that it was "still a reality of some kind" to him. I'm in the process of quoting passages from the 14th session, held in January, 1964, in Appendix 18, as I write it for Volume 2 of "Unknown" Reality.

(Seth's material offers some new insights, I think, as I type this session, concerning his reality. He may be saying that our entire experience with him was encapsulated in Jane's experience with Idea Construction.*)*

DELETED SESSION
SEPTEMBER 24, 1977 9:33 PM SATURDAY

(Notes for the records On Tuesday, Sept. 20, I received psychically rather strong impressions about Nebene, one of "my" personalities in the first century AD. These were triggered, I believe, as I looked over Seth's material on counterparts in Volume 2 of "Unknown" Reality, *and by his material on my Roman captain life in the same period, as he gave it in the deleted session for Sept. 12.*

(The sketch of Nebene is rather successful and would make a good painting. Most interesting is the pendant I showed him wearing; I did a couple of enlarged sketches of this feature, noting that I didn't understand its meaning or origin. I was quite surprised to find two days later, in the New York Times *for September 12, a photograph that contained strong resemblances to my drawing of Nebene's pendant: an Egyptian pendant possibly dating from around the time of King Tutankhamen,*

circa 1355 BC. It seems that currently Egyptian-motif jewelry is the rage in New York City, at least. My own notes contain a detailed chronology of events between my drawing, when we were given the newspaper containing the photo in question, etc. I asked that Seth possibly comment tonight. It seemed that the similarity between the Egyptian piece shown and my own drawing was a bit too coincidental. Nor do we know that much about the circumstances of the Nebene life to begin with. I thought it interesting that Nebene's land, Jerusalem, say, was geographically next door to Egypt, and not great in physical distance, as far as miles go.

(*Jane had no specific questions, except that "I hope he goes into stuff for me. I still need all the help I can get."*)

Good evening.

(*"Good evening, Seth."*)

Now: the small morning statement I gave you each to read *(in the deleted session for August 17, 1977)* has worked. Why? Because for one thing it was general enough so that it did not bring any immediate details into your minds, and left plenty of room for action in an overall manner. It directed your thoughts and expectations again in an overall manner.

Your house has been calm, Ruburt's body has improved each day, and his work and yours have been productive. Because that statement was couched as it was, it did not bring any arguments to your minds. You read it easily. You did not question how your house was to be more calm, and indeed the suggestion itself was rather innocuous in its way, yet highly effective. The suggestions took hold, uniting Frameworks 1 and 2.

Several times this week, Ruburt imagined the two of you on a trip to Florida, with a trailer by the ocean; both of you working, of course, but quite happily. He began by thinking in practical terms in Framework 1: you could—could—do it now, though it would be difficult; but you could go to Florida. If you had to you could even fix it so Ruburt could eat mostly in the car, or in a van. So his thoughts went.

Framework 1 thoughts, but despite the restrictions they entailed, they still represented an important turn for the better. On several occasions he simply imagined the two of you in Florida, in the trailer as before, with no thought for how you got there.

The first thoughts, with their emphasis on detail, were still important, convincing him that such a trip <u>was</u> possible, even under present conditions. He was then free in his second imagining. Physically his ideas of motion, however, moved from the house—highly important. There was a creative use of suggestion—the second, of course, far better than the first group of thoughts.

A good deal of the time he has been writing well, operating in Framework

2. Whenever you operate in Framework 2 in any area, to some extent you enrich other areas of your life. He was excited last evening about *Seven*, and in that period of physical time he forgot his problems, and he dealt with the challenge of the book in the same way that he can learn to handle the physical situation.

In Framework 2 in your terms, time is foreshortened, and work is done there in a flash, so to speak. Some time may be involved physically for the materialization, but in usual terms the foreshortening effect can be quite startling, for time is affected and used in an entirely different fashion. The ideas for *Aspects*, *Politics*, and the entire library experience germinated one evening in a flash of inspiration just before the flood *(in June 1972).*

The physical time was nothing—a few hours—and physical time had to pass for the writing of the books. Yet those books will also influence future time in an important fashion. They represent concentrated experience in which Ruburt threw aside "for a time" the known beliefs of Framework 1, its laws and regulations.

Even *Chestnut Beads*, written so long ago, published in an obscure-enough—forgive me *(humorously)*—pulp magazine, reaches out into time, and affects a woman's movement that then did not exist in your terms: Ruburt's imaginative act in writing *Chestnut Beads* was that concentrated.

(This afternoon Jane had received a call from Larry Davidson in San Francisco. He wanted her agreement to an interview next Saturday at 3 PM, for a radio show about science fiction, for half an hour. Jane agreed. Larry mentioned Chestnut Beads, *and told Jane that her novel is still well-known, at least in the Bay area. It's also become something of a symbol for aspects of the feminist, or women's liberation, movement, he said—something Jane was quite surprised to hear.)*

On a few occasions this week, that he has already forgotten, he intuitively felt that his physical condition could indeed change so smoothly that he was hardly aware of it. <u>That</u> is creative thinking in the physical area.

He should use large, general suggestions of a positive nature that do not concentrate upon details that do not automatically give rise to contradictions with present behavior. I would like such suggestions inserted when he is already in a Framework 2 situation, for they will have double benefit there.

You had some good points when you told him, for example, to simply think of fixing rice, rather than <u>worrying</u> about how to do it. There, however, he was in his situation, saying "Well, I can do it, though it may be difficult," then leading up to "Well, perhaps, since I know I can do it, I will then be able to do it easier"—needless thought steps to your position.

(10:02.) The thoughts of the Florida trip offered no present contradictions because he knew he was not leaving for any trip tomorrow. The fantasy,

however, involved him in motion, aroused e̲motion, and instantly broadened his mental outlook. The days he had those fantasies he operated better physically here. *(With emphasis:)* Someone who is thinking of going to Florida can get to the bathroom far more quickly. The comparison is ludicrous.

"I can think more creatively and positively in all areas of my life. I can move faster and more surely in all areas of my life. My body can feel better and perform better. I can enjoy each day more."

Those suggestions give room for action. He should use them daily. There is no such thing as hypnosis—or, all thoughts involve hypnosis. In a way each statement is true. Your political campaigns involve hypnosis, which simply means concentrated suggestion.

Suggestions always imply an impetus directing action. Your entire household is a suggestive structure. Your writing room, Joseph, is a physical reminder of your intents, filled with not only books and papers, but the implied suggestion that gives them reality. It is of course no coincidence that you have a writing room and a studio—not simply one or the other, so that the two rooms show the two important interests of your life.

They show how you use your time, and imply what has come from the past, and what is projected into the future. They represent the state of your mind.

Your kitchen is a room you walk through in your house. Ruburt tried to explain this in terms of lighting, though that did not particularly apply. But you are everywhere surrounded of course by your own suggestions, physically materialized.

What you do in those situations is in a way concentrated. It does things to time because of your intents and because of the peculiar nature of Framework 2. Such physical areas are charged in that regard because the mental areas connected with them are. In a manner of speaking they are hypnotic containers, emphasizing what you want emphasized, and cutting off data that do not apply, or that is contradictory. You direct yourselves to concentrate in a particular fashion.

All of this happens quite automatically, yet it is the result of your conscious decisions along the way. Hypnosis then involves concentrated stimulus toward action of a certain kind. Everyone uses it, regardless of the terms. It works well because at the time impediments are intentionally cut to a minimum, and the details involved that are necessary are part of an overall plan.

Ruburt earlier said, before the session, that he suddenly had an idea for a book, called <u>The Beginning</u>. He was creatively aroused. He did not wonder how he would get the paper to write it on. He did not question the mechanics. In the physical area he has questioned the mechanics. He has doubted his ability for reasons given in the past, and in the past, to some extent you helped him, and you did not reinforce his sense of physical ability. Now you are.

I do not want a concentration upon detail, however. He is indeed overall taller. His eyes are improving. His interest and improvement in the writing area will also help his general condition, for many reasons. It is perfectly natural, however, for him not to be happy at certain times, temporarily. When he feels that way he should tell you. That is different from projecting negatively into the future. I would like, however, some hypnosis—of the kind we have been speaking of—in the near future. This involves concentrated work, again, that foreshortens time.

Give us a moment.... I am making the recommendations, for I know what is most effective, but I am not certain of your equipment. At one time, however, he made his own tape recording, with his voice giving himself suggestions in the background of a record, and he played that while he was <u>writing</u>.

Now when he is writing he is often in Framework 2. He did not concentrate upon the record, and that method worked most effectively. Some version of that method would be most effective, for it directs him most effectively toward physical ends. Most of all I want him to realize that his body is improving, and that the improvement can easily accelerate—<u>easily</u>.

Now take your break.

(10:37—10:59.)

Now: the idea of a journey is always highly important, symbolically speaking, so that particular mental fantasy is a good one. It does not conflict with the details of any given day, and yet it acts to generate overall impetus, and emotionally places Ruburt out of the house.

It comes naturally to him, and even done in Framework 1's limited manner, it is beneficial. It would even help if the two of you discussed such a trip as a definite possibility, but without any definite time period involved. Work done in Framework 2, however, is out of all proportion to the effort expended. That is why the taped suggestions are important. An alternative could involve two definite periods of self-suggestion a week, prepared for ahead of time, with a specific physical area chosen in the same way that you choose certain areas for your writing or painting.

Ruburt would either read himself suggestions that he had thoughtfully written out earlier, or listen to a cassette that he had made. Another alternative is for you to give the suggestions in the role of hypnotist. Any of these methods, however, involve little effort, with important concentrated results, for you are taking time aside in the same way that I explained earlier you both do in the areas of your work. This involves accelerated suggestion.

Now: Nebene traveled extensively in early years. He did visit Egypt, and made tours to various esoteric communities. *(Long pause.)* He became disenchanted at a young age with the many conflicting schools of truth, so when he found what he finally settled upon, he would brook no interference. When you operate, practically speaking, in terms of Framework 2, you have a stronger impact upon time and reality. You are more effective in that regard. Nebene and you influence each other because you operate in Framework 2 in the work areas of your lives. You become closer, say, for in physical terms of time there is a foreshortening. Time, then, can be lengthened or shortened, or made to disappear entirely.

The events of time in such a case from the outside might seem to change drastically, while those inside our time structures would not notice any change, in a Framework 1 level. Your historical actuality and Nebene's would never collide. On that level no change occurs, but the foreshortening of time can allow you and Nebene to interact if you want to, or if he does, so that images, ideas, and other interchanges can occur in a way that does not dislodge or disarray a moment of your physical time, or his.

That is what happened with your sketch.

When Ruburt sends out energy he feels no impediment in space, and has felt a straight line go out in whatever direction required. That is definitely a Framework 2 experience.

Now with you and Nebene the same occurs in time—a channel opens up as surely, through which images, ideas, and interchanges can occur. It is interesting that you picked up an older Nebene than earlier, for the elder Nebene, if disillusioned, was also more open than earlier, and more gentle of disposition.

(11:21.) He was looking toward the kind of answers that you are beginning to find.

In Framework 2 the mind affects the physical brain in a more complete and effective manner than usual, and can spark images, thoughts, or correlations that exist in a context outside of the time that is happening in Framework 1. Time happens at a certain regulated rate, then, obviously, in Framework 1. A certain amount of time is needed there to do a certain amount of work, and according to scientific dictates a specific amount of effort is required to perform different kinds of work.

Framework 1, to some extent or another, however, is always influenced by Framework 2. There, the same correlations do not apply between the effort expended and the work performed, or the time required for such procedures. Very little effort, there, comparatively speaking, has an effect here in Framework

1—that is, a small amount of effort in Framework 2 can result in extraordinary work done in Framework 2, and with a foreshortened time effect.

Suggestion, then, purposefully applied while in a relaxed state, which is a connective to Framework 2, can be most effective.

Your impressions of Nebene came while you were relaxed, thinking momentarily of something else, but with an overall desire to know more about Nebene. The creative principles are the same—that is why I am making these connections, so that Ruburt can insert what he wants in Framework 2 with little exertion of effort, and great benefit.

The same applies to you for more material about Nebene on your own. Nebene prayed and meditated often, so his framework, you see, is often the same as yours, and those meditative periods provide the necessary conditions on both of your parts.

His pursuit of truth led his mind outward through time. You use space. I use time. Time, again, can be lengthened, shortened. You can move sideways in it, for example, as you do in space. These frameworks, one way or another, always involve alterations in time, even as Ruburt's *James* and *Cézanne* books from the library involve information not usually available in Framework 1's time sequence.

I will tell you what I can of what you want to know about Nebene's times, for example, but you can also obtain from him, if you understand tonight's material, information of that nature, and "firsthand" data about the various sects he visited. I suggest that for your enjoyment and education. He also obtained some information about you, you realize, for the channel is open. You would not get such information unless both of you consented.

I gave you both plenty to work on this evening—

("Yes.)

—and the suggestions in the session are not for my benefit. Ruburt's eyes are improving, obviously, since he is working at his copy, and so forth. They do not protrude as much, and are improving in their appearance. They are also still adjusting, however, as the whole body posture undergoes changes. This is a quite natural procedure. If you trust the body then you trust that procedure.

Your drawing of the jewelry does represent a piece of jewelry that Nebene wore all of the time. The symbols were then ancient in origin, representing the search for truth and the godhead, but it was an unorthodox piece for him to wear.

It did have an Egyptian origin, but also Hebrew connections. There were no pure sects even then, and the particular one Nebene followed was a curious mixture of ancient Egyptian beliefs and Hebrew beliefs. See what you can find out about it.

And now I bid you a fond good evening.

("Thank you very much, Seth.")

Tell Ruburt I will see, again, that he gets help and inspiration in Framework 2 that directly affects his physical condition. A shove up there is a shove indeed.

(11:46 PM. "I'm out," Jane said....

(A note: When Seth remarked about the pendant Nebene wore being an unorthodox procedure for those times, it reminded me that I'd had the same thought while doing the drawing. However, I forgot to write it down in my notes, and didn't mention it to Jane.

(Additionally, when Seth suggested that I see what I could find out about the particular sect Nebene followed, it flashed through my mind that I could almost start writing out a list of the beliefs, the credo, etc, connected with it. I may try this.)

SESSION 811 (DELETED PORTION)
SEPTEMBER 26, 1977 9:46 PM MONDAY

(The following material is from the 811th session.

(11:47.) Give us a moment.... Very briefly, for your edification: Ruburt's eyes are achieving normal motion, the muscles and so forth being released to normal capacity in the last few days. The synchronization is not accomplished yet. The right side is highly active. New body relationships are taking place, and that activity gives him a sense of disorientation as muscles, released, practice their flexibility, and learn to synchronize it.

He should relax when he feels that body loosening—go with it without worrying, for it leads to better body performance. The sinuses are vastly better, the jaws in the process of returning to normal.

End of session. A fond good evening.

("Thank you very much, Seth. Good night.")

(11:56 PM. A note: The next day—as I type this—all of the changes and improvements that Seth noted above are still continuing for Jane. If anything, they have accelerated. She feels the entire right side of the body especially in new motion.)

SESSION 812 (DELETED PORTION)
OCTOBER 1, 1977 9:33 PM SATURDAY

(The following material is from the 812th session.)

(10:54.) Now Ruburt, because of his beliefs, "artificially" disciplined his muscles so that he would be forced to concentrate upon what it seemed you and he both thought was most important in life—your work.

He felt that for artistic, financial, and personal reasons this was necessary. It was necessary because he believed that the spontaneous self, left alone, would not so concentrate—or that <u>his</u> spontaneous self would not, but would also be tempted by whatever other private pursuits. That belief built up a body of habits so that even when he made <u>headway</u> in changing the basic belief at least, he was left with beliefs about the body that were secondary but habitual; beliefs shared by each of you about his body, so that the evidence was always present.

Those beliefs formed a body stance. That stance is being broken up. It resulted however in an operable but limited fashion with all of the muscles tightened and restricted to some degree, the original tension being applied to the head and neck area.

His eyes did not freely roam, but followed the limited head motions. The neck and throat muscles were held in a particular fashion. Everything fit together. He allowed himself no leeway, or very little, and in that framework the body was limited but predictable.

Now that old framework is shunted aside. The body is not as predictable. The eyes are trying out new freedoms. Those important neck ligaments and head areas are definitely releasing. They are highly active. They relax and tense in great bursts of activity and relaxation, and this affects the eye muscles as well, of course.

It also affects the release of the knees, which is occurring. At this time, the right side is particularly active from the head down, and one eye is therefore sometimes more active than the other, causing the image difficulties. His eyes rarely feel strained, however, or tired. They are enjoying the mobility. His overall balance, or feeling of balance, does constantly change, however, as the muscular pressure pressures, or tensions, do. There is no doubt that this can be disconcerting, as can the eyes' motions under the conditions noted.

The entire balance and posture is in the process of the greatest beneficial alteration. He is allowing himself leeway now. He does need to hold on, walking, with all of these changes. It is highly important, however, that he does not project negatively, as the paranoid does *(as described in the regular 812th session)*. You can be of great help there, particularly now. I suggested the use of suggestion through the framework of hypnosis simply because such techniques can be like mental vitamin pills. They provide for the insertion of the required and desired beliefs for use when needed.

(11:16.) They provide a backlog of psychic well-being to fall back upon. It is up to Ruburt personally, and to the two of you jointly, as to whether or not you want to make that effort.

Ruburt's balance has completely changed in a week, so that his weight can now fall on his heels. He gets up easier, as well as sitting down easier—something he neglected to mention; nor did you observe this.

If you keep Framework 2 in mind, much of these stages can be vastly minimized, and the work with hypnosis that I suggested gives you such a method of inserting data, here, that accelerates motion in Framework 2, and greatly cuts down the time and effort involved in Framework 1. Of course, *(with wry amusement)* if you each are convinced that the venture was important-enough in your lives, and would get the results, you would have clamored to begin such experiments.

Your information was quite correct, regarding Nebene. The plant *(acanthus)* was used for spices and other purposes for some centuries in that part of the world.

Unless you have questions, I will end the session, and hope you found it provocative.

("Well, my tooth has been bothering me. I was wondering if it has anything to do with George Rhodes' tooth trouble.")

Give us a moment... There are correlations in your overall experience with George. Otherwise, regarding the tooth episode in particular, there is only the fact that you have used the idea of the tooth and George's difficulty to organize certain elements of your own experience so that by having the cavity filled a need will be satisfied.

The need is a sexual one—your sweet tooth—for your sexual feelings have been rearoused by your intimate encounters with Ruburt, even while neither of you thus far have even been willing to devote time to sexual gratification in the deepest terms.

You have decided to acknowledge such needs, and to give them token satisfaction, so you have recognized that cavity, which in the past you both tried your best to ignore. Now it needs to be filled.

Does that sufficiently answer your question?

(Yes, and very well.")

My heartiest good wishes.

("Thank you, Seth.")

A fond good evening.

("*Good night.*" *11:30 PM. I thought Seth's data on the tooth mechanisms very acute indeed. Jane and I haven't done anything about the hypnosis suggestions, obviously; we need our recorder repaired. I sometimes think it impossible to do all we want to do, or think we should, in the course of an ordinary day. Even if we could manage this, I fear we'd end up so regimented that half of the tasks would be self-defeating. I do think that on my part at least this feeling underlies some of my own shortcomings. Seth was quite chiding in a gently amused way tonight when mentioning the hypnosis affair, his voice quiet, and, I thought, rather tired. This weekend—it's Sunday afternoon as I type this—we've been literally so occupied that we didn't take the time to go food shopping for the week's supply. This means extra time later in the week to make up. Nor did Jane get her mail answered yesterday, as she had planned to do, nor did she find the time to putter about in the house, either in her writing room, or the studio annex.*)

SESSION 813 (DELETED PORTION)
OCTOBER 3, 1977 9:57 PM MONDAY

(*The following material is from the 813th session.*

(*10:47. During break I wrote three-quarters of a page "from" Nebene. I read it to Jane, who encouraged me to do more. I'd felt the urge to do the same thing yesterday, without going along with it, and had reacted the same way earlier today. My copy of this part of the 813th session is attached to my Nebene material on file.*

(*Resume at 11:15.*) Though I am using numbers and classifications, please realize that I am doing this for the convenience of explanation, and that these realities exist one within the other. We are looking into reality from your viewpoint, therefore, from your threshold.

With that understood, my material comes from beyond Framework 2. Creative material in general, however, has its origin in Framework 2, and when it is perceived in Framework 1, to some extent or another it connects the perceiver to that other source. When you read the reincarnational information, (*about the Roman captain on September 12, 1977*), it triggered the Nebene material because of your own personal situation at the time—your mood, and so forth (*on September 20, 1977*). You felt a path open, and followed it. Earlier this evening I spoke of association as often operating outside of time sequences. At other levels of activity you realized that this could apply between lives also, and the path again opened—at both ends.

Give us a moment.... Ruburt's feather is an aid because of its associative value. Unconsciously it reminds him of a physically vigorous, flexible self. In Framework 1 his recovery is coming along, and yet the ease and quickness of that recovery, again—and <u>again</u>—could be increased, and should be, by greater activity in Framework 2. Once that is begun it accelerates.

Any and all of his doubts <u>can</u> be alleviated by the complete realization that he can indeed trust the physician within, and the ancient wisdom of the body. That trust can be inserted through suggestion. This does not require long periods of time at all—but the intent is all-important. The suggestions concerning hypnosis, therefore, would be of great help in accelerating Ruburt's progress, and thereby relieving both of your minds.

When you write the Nebene material you see how quickly it comes, once a path is opened. The same can apply in Ruburt's physical condition. I keep comparing that to creative activity because the same principles are involved—and impediments do disappear.

He needs you at times to remind him that he can trust the body's ancient wisdom—otherwise he would be in as good physical condition as you are. The body is an artistic creation, and in certain terms you create many bodies, each one perfectly mirroring your beliefs. I gave suggestions that you creatively plan a vacation trip together. That need not take time, yet you have not followed through. That mental planning, however, is important.

Despite that, Ruburt's body is improving, but the rate of improvement mirrors your individual and joint beliefs. You are afraid to use all of your efforts in that regard, for fear they may not work. In your creative endeavors, however, each of you go ahead, and you, Joseph, particularly with Nebene now.

If you think of Ruburt's normal flexibility as a creative endeavor, then automatically and easily, Ruburt first of all, and you, will find your creative abilities coming to the fore in that direction, bringing about results that are far quicker, easier, and executed in such a manner that Framework 2 adds immeasurably to that area of your lives.

You form your own reality privately, yet one cannot <u>enforce</u> a joint reality upon the other. I suggest therefore that each of you, privately or together, open your pathways to Framework 2, requesting simply that further insights will be given you—and so they will be.

<u>Now</u> I bid you a fond good evening.

("Thank you, Seth. Good night.")

(11:39 PM. Without getting up from the couch, I wrote another half page of Nebene material. I finished it at just midnight, then read it to Jane. It contained material on lunar eclipses.)

SESSION 814 (DELETED PORTION)
OCTOBER 8, 1977 9:43 PM SATURDAY

(The following material is from the 814th session.)

(12:13.) Give us a moment.... Your Nebene material is excellent, and shows the development of your own abilities psychically and creatively.

If Ruburt will read the last two or three sessions given for him, then I will not need to repeat them this evening. He did make gains this week in the use of suggestion, so that he understood better <u>how</u> he has been using it to his disadvantage, and how to change that course.

Some of that understanding <u>should</u> flower this week, so that he grabs more fully a hold of that creative stimulus that can greatly accelerate his improvements. The paper that he wrote and you read is important there—he must understand more fully that his mind can indeed direct his body toward flexibility. He made the necessary distinctions in that paper, and he should use it as a basis for whatever work he decides to do with suggestion, whether it is alone or with you.

You see from *(tonight's)* the session the climate of suggestion that is about you, and that had to be conquered. I do not want to repeat myself—Ruburt must read those sessions again. You bury them at your own expense in time and energy.

It is one thing to understand the imperfections of medicine, but quite another if you are not willing to take one to two hours a week to work with techniques that are highly important to improve your own health. I have said enough in my gentle fashion—but there are accelerations, and I want you to take advantage of them.

My heartiest regards to you both—

("The same to you, Seth.")

—and a fond good evening.

("Thank you very much. Good night."

(12:22 AM)

DELETED SESSION
OCTOBER 10, 1977 9:58 PM MONDAY

(These notes will recapitulate two rather surprising events. While we were having last Saturday's session, someone knocked on our door; I didn't answer it and they left. Sunday they returned: Rusty and Dr. Hal from Lancaster, Pennsylvania, on

their yearly visit to us with a cheesecake. As the four of us talked for an hour or so two things emerged. Dr. Hal had a teacher many years ago, a woman, who used to walk with William James; indeed, he read part of his Varieties of Religious Experience to her. James also discussed his own psychic experiences with this woman. Hal told us her name but we forgot to note it down. Interesting, that this information would come to us just as Jane is preparing her James manuscript for Prentice.

(The second bit of news is that Rusty met the president of Prentice-Hall recently. This individual—again, name not recalled—listened to a talk Rusty gave in an auditorium, explaining some of Seth's ideas along with her own interest in the tarot. After the program Prentice-Hall's president told Rusty that listening to her had helped him better understand Jane's own work. But this meeting took place last summer, and we've had no feedback from anyone at Prentice-Hall.

(The second event took place starting at 8:15 PM this evening. We were visited by a youngish couple from London, Canada. They too had knocked at our door earlier —while we were napping this afternoon. The knocking woke me up, but I saw them pulling out of the driveway so let them go. Jane and I ate supper with the lights off and the blinds drawn, but by the time she went to work Jane decided to turn on the lights in her writing room, and see them should they return. A most fortunate decision on her part.

(The couple, Carol and Fred—not married—related to us a most "far-out" series of events leading to their finding out where we lived. The odds against such a series of happenings must be very high. The heart of the chain of events resulted in their meeting Miss Dineen on the sidewalk in front of Rubin's bookstore as they were putting money into a parking meter. Miss Dineen told them they needn't do so on a holiday, and the conversation among the three of them took off from there—culminating in Miss Dineen remembering that she knew us when Miss Callahan was alive, etc.—all of this after Carol and Fred had <u>asked Miss Dineen if she knew us</u>.

(These notes hardly do justice to the string of events that led to Carol and Fred meeting Miss Dineen—from the couple's leaving Watkins Glen, motoring to Elmira, deciding upon how to find us, asking a policeman finally for directions to a bookstore, going to the <u>wrong</u> bookstore—Rubin's—just as Miss Dineen came out of the religious bookstore almost next door, Miss Dineen first directing them to 458 West Water, then remembering that we'd moved, etc. This list is not complete, but could be fleshed out should we ever want to; we have the addresses of Carol and Fred on file.

(It wasn't until after the Canadian couple had left us, actually, that the implications of what had happened began to sink in. I thought the odds alone staggering that it had happened at all. During their visit the woman, Carol, several times expressed the thought that she returned the second time, to see if we were home, *because "it was meant to be," or words to that effect. She also said that if we hadn't been home, that was meant to be also. Carol had met an individual named Ron who had visited us here at 1730 two years or so ago—not long after we'd moved in, incidentally. Jane and I haven't seen Miss Dineen except once soon after Miss Callahan's death at least 10 years ago. Personally, I do not think I would know her if we met.*

(Note that in both cases, involving Rusty and Hal, and Carol and Fred, the couples returned to 1730 after their first visit had failed to make contact with us. Since we have all names on file now, more information can be obtained if we need it. Note: Rusty Carnarius has relatives living on Coleman Avenue. Either Jacobs or Jenkins. [Check boxes.]

(Seth covered both visits in his material tonight. One aspect not covered, and which I forgot to ask about, involved Rusty's meeting with the president of Prentice-Hall; will try to remember to ask about this next session.

(I told Jane after the session that the affair involving Carol and Fred, plus the session material itself, had seemed to give me a firm grasp on the Framework 2 reality; I've already begun putting the new appreciation into use. Half of it simply involves feeling in new ways, I think, an extra confidence... for the coincidence, so-called, of the meeting on the street between Miss Dineen and the couple is just too much as far as I'm concerned.

(The encounter with the Canadian couple was so recent that as we sat for the session it hadn't occurred to Jane and me to hope that Seth would discuss the affair, or to even ask that he do so. I was impressed by the meeting on the street, but equally taken with the fact that Hal had known someone who'd known James. Strangely, in all of this the meeting of Rusty and the president of Prentice-Hall hadn't registered as strongly with us, though we recognized that it could be an event originating in Framework 2. Oh yes—the president is involved with Spiritual Frontiers Fellowship, which may have been his motivation for attending Rusty's talk to begin with.)

Now: good evening.

("Good evening, Seth.")

This is not dictation. Let us look at the simple event involving your two visitors.

I want to use this as a case in point, showing how desire brings about its own fulfillment when possible. Anything possible is probable. The young lady wanted to see the both of you vividly enough so that that desire, with no effort on her part, was a reality in Framework 2. Miss Dineen likes people, and would be quite lonely were it not for the desire to meet with and enjoy other people. She particularly enjoys unusual people, or foreigners, and chance encounters. Otherwise she is a rather solitary person—but her desire for such encounters exists with no effort on her part in Framework 2.

You have then two separate people living in different countries, completely unknown to each other, of different ages and backgrounds. In Framework 2 however, again, time and space are not barriers, and there are no impediments <u>in usual terms</u>. Laws of attraction operate in far too complicated ways to explain with any real preciseness. Emotional computations and associations occur <u>there</u> with incalculable rapidity. Data is sorted out, arranged and rearranged, as if associations were tabulated and retabulated under a million different headings.

Using such "a psychic computer," information was sorted and resorted, probabilities examined, some discarded because the conditions were not apropos. Miss Dineen this evening was looking for a small adventure. She met two delightful strangers—near-foreigners. She will tell the story to friends. The meeting then originally was "planned" in Framework 2. In case your young visitor—the woman *(Carol)* now—did not meet you, she had insisted in her mind that she would meet someone who knew you or had some personal connection somehow.

Remember—<u>you two</u> were involved, with your probabilities and free will. Until Ruburt was at his desk this evening, he did not finally decide whether or not he would greet the strangers you knew had earlier tried to reach you. He played with the idea of checking some notes, and then taking his chapter *(on James)* to the living room table, and darkening his room. In that case, the young woman would still have met someone who had a connection with him.

At the last moment, however, before you left, Ruburt made up his mind and told you to unlock the porch door. *(When Carol opened the screen door, she let Willy Two out, but picked him up easily.)* Miss Dineen remembers you kindly also because of Miss Callahan, of course.

The organization in Framework 2 is entirely different than your ordinary experience. Events are put together in a different fashion. Neither Miss Dineen or the young woman planned the physical events directly as they occurred. They did not think of detail, and details were arranged more beautifully and precisely than would be possible in conscious physical terms. The details just seemed to fall into place.

(10:19.) This sort of thing happens frequently with Miss Dineen, and consciously she is drawn toward areas of town, for example, in which certain individuals are shopping or strolling, so that while she visits few fashionable establishments, she enjoys a series of seemingly unrelated, pleasant encounters with strangers.

She was drawn to shop when she did for that reason, and also because of the personal connection—how strange that she should have anything in common with these visitors from Canada. The whole affair happened like any truly creative event. The methods that the girl used—the young woman—in the various adventures she related to you, occurred in the same way.

(*In a long conversation that Jane and I found hard to follow at times, Carol described how she'd put together elements from various philosophies and belief systems in order to get what she wanted. In some fashion, Jane and I thought as we listened to her, she was able to make it work for her. I kidded her, also, about "saying the heck with the details," I remember.*)

Ruburt's books, your paintings, follow the same overall format. In all cases faith is involved, and the feeling that all in all the means will come or be given. The means are then arranged in Framework 2.

Later, for the book, I will use this sort of explanation to show for example how various groups of people, planning say a vacation to one spot, will all choose two or three airplanes for the journey—knowing unconsciously quite well that one very well <u>might</u> crash, even though the final decision is not made until the last moment.

I am trying to give you different kinds of examples, showing how work is practically done in Framework 2, that then appears in Framework 1 as physical events.

(*10:28.*) In terms of Ruburt's flexibility, I always take your present level of <u>practical</u> comprehension into mind, for I know quite well that your reactions to what I say will vary according to your own situations at any given time.

So far, you have been hesitant—Ruburt particularly, but both of you—to release or express that desire for normal physical flexibility on Ruburt's part. And, also, you would have compared his present condition unfavorably with the desired end, simply involving yourselves in contradictions.

I said that I did not want you to compare his condition to the ideal one, and that certainly still stands. If however you understand what I am saying about Frameworks 1 and 2, <u>then</u> you can express and release that desire fully and without fear, knowing that the meanings or the details—the way—<u>will be found in Framework 2</u> to bring about the desired results.

To do this properly, however, you must not check at every moment in Framework 1. If our young woman of this evening had done that, she would have hopelessly complicated matters. She might have looked at a map and said "Someone in one of those houses must have had a personal contact with the Buttses, in case we do not meet them. I will try every third house, or I will go to the police department—or to the newspaper." All quite practical ideas.

She did in fact go to a bookstore, but in so doing she killed two birds with one stone, so to speak, for she found your address in the phone book, but also just happened to run into Miss Dineen—and that was something that only a thorough canvassing of the town might produce.

The freely-expressed desire will bring its own results—and in retrospect everything will fall into place.

Ruburt's body is expressing as much of that desire as he, and secondly you, have felt free enough to express. Release the desire into Framework 2, remember the examples I have given you. Ruburt is making inroads, learning not to project negatively. <u>That is highly important, and must be stressed</u>.

(10:40.) Give us a moment.... You must remind yourselves that these methods work. Your creative work and all of the other elements of your lives show this, including your financial security. The fear that the methods will not work in any one regard inhibits the process—as if our young woman said "I am sure I will not meet the Buttses, although I want to." Then the connection would not have been nearly as strong in Framework 2.

I am trying to make conscious to you methods that you use beautifully unconsciously and well in other areas of your living. Our young woman selectively interpreted her experience with the interpretation of names, for example, as given this evening—but that selectivity led her exactly where she wanted to go, and in certain terms she actually did ignore any data that did not lead her in a desired direction. So, while it may <u>seem</u> impractical, you do the same thing when you selectively pay attention to Ruburt's improvements and selectively ignore areas of difficulty. You build a new orientation, which then becomes the actual one.

In areas of conflict, you have to learn to do this consciously while in areas of success you have done it unconsciously all along. Many of Ruburt's joints, particularly in the neck, feet, and knees, are loosening considerably. Their motion is all connected, of course. This causes the muscles to change, and in particular their tension is altered. When his weight is on his feet, when they are ready the joints and feet try new positions—that at the time they might not be able to maintain.

It is impossible to be consciously aware of all such motions. There has been new activity in the knees, in those joints that would allow him to kick out in such a fashion *(gesturing with leg)*. This can cause some feelings of instability when he is walking—but the body must also try out its positions when he is on his feet. If you concentrate upon the improvements you will see that some sensations that at first appear uncomfortable are not detrimental at all, but a part of the body's recovery. He favored certain portions of the neck and shoulders. The tension on the neck tendons is loosening, and this definitely affects the eyes. Placing your desire in Framework 2 will automatically, however, minimize stages of change, and automatically take care of many details in a much more pleasant fashion. Again, obviously, suggestion plays an important part.

Give us a moment.... Ruburt should tell you, as you told him, when he finds himself in a particularly blue mood, or projecting negatively, but he does catch such situations better than he did. That release of desire is all important, however. What I have given you this evening can be of the utmost help. And trust your own Nebene material.

Now I will end the session, or take a break as you prefer.

(*"We'll take the break."*)

(*10:59—11:27.*)

Now. Give us a moment....

You must remember that there are no impediments in Framework 2, and therefore that all seeming impediments in Framework 1 will be dissolved.

You must not wonder how, or dwell upon details. It is the overall pattern of behavior we are after here. I am not telling you to be blind in daily experience, but I <u>am</u> telling you how daily experience is formed.

In its own way, the James connection happened in the same fashion, for your desires and beliefs go out in all directions in time. Your context outlive your deaths. The particular connections here are too complicated to try to explain, but they do involve James's intense interest during his life in the future of his own work, and in the state of the psychic field of the future.

I am sometimes at a loss for words, believe it or not, for often explanations make things sound more difficult than they are. All of this happens quite naturally. To some extent or another after death you retain psychic connections with anyone you have ever met during a lifetime. The connections can be strong or weak, some important some trivial, but they form a psychic network, so to speak.

That network can be put together in different ways, and used now, in an analogy, as a communications system. All in all, it will mean that generally speaking you will keep in contact with areas of thought or development in which you were once interested, and will be able if you wish to follow their development in time.

The living people, so involved in this network, will have their own other encounters, of course, but again through a psychological selectivity. You can be aware after death of those encounters also. There are implications I am not expressing adequately, and it may be impossible to do so.

In a manner of speaking, the gentleman's *(Hal)* visit, while Ruburt is doing the James book, completes an intent on James's part that he had in life. The event, again, in a way is even separate from Ruburt's present connection with James, but followed as a result of James's living curiosity regarding highly gifted mediums that might exist after his death.

Had he been living, he would have sought Ruburt out, you see, and they would have gotten along famously. You and James would also have been excellent friends. The three of you missed each other in <u>time</u>. In other frameworks, however, you are friends, hence Ruburt's book, and your first attraction to James's writings.

That James however is, of course, as he says the William James that he was —and yet is no more the same William James, as the child and the adult are one person and yet are not. Consciousness can be put together in many ways, <u>and you use your own consciousness</u> in ways that presently at least escape you, even though the results may be quite objective. The encounter and Miss Dineen and your friends, again, is a case in point. The meeting was real in your terms, yet the manipulations of consciousness behind it were largely unknown.

In those terms James is aware of the Hal connection. It is only because so many of the manipulations of your own consciousness are unknown to you in life that such issues appear odd.

You are indeed colleagues of James, and <u>in a way</u> the unconventional Doctor Hal carries out, in his own fashion, some of James's living intents or questions.

Hal works more directly with the body. It is rather that he accepted some of James's questions as he understood them through his teaching, and allowed these to merge with questions of his own. It is as if you hand on challenges or questions to others, which they accept for their own reasons, and hence follow through for you in areas in which you might be highly interested, even though in some cases they might have been sidelines in your own work.

<u>Now</u> I bid you a fond good evening—

("Okay.")

I do want to mention that relaxation will definitely quicken all areas of Ruburt's improvement, releasing the neck tendons and so forth, so that the eyes will stabilize in good vision. The hot towels will also benefit.

A fond good evening to you both.

("Thank you very much, Seth. Good night."

(*11:56 PM. As I typed the session the next day, I told Jane I was quite enthused by it. Somehow the two incidents described, involving Rusty and Hal, and Carol and Fred, had served to impress upon me the validity of Seth's ideas about Frameworks 1 and 2 in ways that the intellectual understanding of those concepts alone hadn't done. I found myself trying out the concepts as I worked—and they worked. I may regard the session as a key or breakthrough session, then. I told Jane I* wanted to discuss it thoroughly with her when I had it finished. It seems that we can put the concepts of the frameworks to use in all areas of daily life, reinforce longtime goals, etc.

(It may be that I'm quite intrigued by the understanding that in Framework 2 one doesn't have to be concerned with the details—that desired goals are being arrived at in ways we may not easily grasp—but that the work *is* being accomplished. This understanding, faith, if you will, in such a process can then be seen as quite a leap in understanding for me, with my love of detail.

(<u>Not to worry</u> that challenges are being accomplished within Framework 2 can then be an absurdly simple, liberating way of life in Framework 1.)

DELETED SESSION
OCTOBER 17, 1977 9:25 PM MONDAY

(Within the last few days Jane has lost several teeth, necessitating help from our dentist, Paul O'Neill. I called him at the office this afternoon, but there was no answer. When I checked his home phone, Paul told me he'd taken the day off; he offered to look at Jane here at the house. When he'd done so later in the afternoon, he further offered to do the necessary work here at the house, saving Jane going to his office. We were most surprised. After he'd left, we could see that in actuality Paul's visit had offered all that Jane could have desired, under the circumstances; we hadn't asked for any of it, even his preliminary visit to the house to examine Jane this time—although he'd done that on a couple of previous occasions, again without being asked by us.

(Thus, Jane found his offers of help at the house to be just what she'd have asked for, given an "ideal" situation. In many ways, we found the situation to be quite similar to that involving the recent visits of Carol and Fred, from Canada, and of Hal and Rusty, from Lancaster, Pennsylvania—in that it seemed the necessary inner workings to bring about the ideal situation had been carried out in Framework 2. More on this can be added in later sessions. Jane said she thought Paul O'Neill has strong healing abilities.

(No session was held as scheduled last Saturday evening. Jane was extremely upset by her continuing eye condition and the disorienting changes taking place throughout her body; I ended up equally upset after we talked. I'd say we both lost much confidence in the idea of Frameworks 1 and 2 that evening; I still feel that way to some degree; at the same time Jane has felt better. However, she's also learned some things about the eye condition through using the pendulum, and Seth comments.

(This morning I mailed the first three Cézanne books, of the 25 we have on *hand to send out to artists, reviewers, etc.*

(We were visited yesterday by Jane's second cousin, Carol Dudley, of California. Carol is to send us data on Jane's family background.

(For some reason we've had a number of visitors lately, after a long lull late in the summer. I turned one away this afternoon.

(Jane wanted to try a session tonight, while not being sure the tooth condition would permit it very easily.)

Dare I say, good evening.

("Good evening, Seth.")

Your psychic work has given both of your lives an impetus, direction, challenge, and opportunities for accomplishment that in certain terms at least would otherwise be lacking.

Had your goals previous to your psychic experiences been adequate to your natures, and sufficient to you, nothing else would have developed—nor would you have been seeking so avidly answers to the kinds of questions that then and now concern you.

You did not seek goals that could be reached easily by anyone, or even goals that you yourselves could be certain of attaining. You sought instead questions that would stretch your abilities, and develop them, that would bring out all nuances before unknown to you. It is easy enough to at times look at others, perhaps now—for I am not saying that you do this—but perhaps romanticizing them, thinking that you would after all prefer a much simpler, more overtly physical existence, freed of any deep concerns about the nature of reality or the plight of the race.

It is easy perhaps at times to have regrets, to wish that curiosity, the love of learning, the desire for knowledge, and yearning to help your fellow men *(was Seth a bit amused here?)* had not gone quite so far, and to imagine that had it not Ruburt would be in excellent physical condition, and no one would miss the work that then would not exist.

Nothing is worth what Ruburt has put himself through, you both say *(as I did Saturday night)*, yet Ruburt has put himself through nothing, in those terms—that is, his condition is not from the result of, again, your psychic activities. <u>Those</u> he has been eminently able to perform, and has done beautifully.

The beliefs behind the entire affair were far more mundane, and his knowledge and yours has kept away many problems that might otherwise have occurred.

There are many things I want to say, whether or not they can be said this evening. I did, however, have a few comments about the dentist affair.

Briefly, Paul is a good man, quite concerned in his own way about the welfare of his fellows, and trying to help them in a very practical way. *(Humorously:)* Mending mouths will be his pearly gates to heaven. He thinks he cannot change the world—but he can help the individual patient. He does have strong healing abilities. He is independently minded.

Now: Ruburt knew he had to have dental work. He wanted it done. His beliefs were not of the best at all, as far as physically getting to the office. He did not, however, imagine himself, for example, falling, except I believe in one or two very brief thoughts. Had you told him "Never mind, when the time comes you will make it," that would have been adequate enough. You did say, several times, "You'll be able to make it all right"—and that was also adequate and a good response.

To remind him, however, that others went up those stairs without a thought, was no help at all *(intently)*, whether or not it is true, for that aroused instant contradictions. "I will take your hand if necessary," for example, would have been an adequate response.

(I plead being misunderstood here to some extent, however. It should be added that I'd said that I thought it strange Jane was seemingly more concerned about making it to the dentist's office than she was about why she had to be there to begin with.)

What you have then was Ruburt's desire to have his teeth fixed, when it was obvious that he must, and his fear that he could not perform adequately <u>at this time</u>. That data existed in Framework 2. <u>There</u>, computations involving yourselves, Ruburt's conditions, the circumstances, and your dentist, all went on with great rapidity. You know the solution.

Paul's activities over the weekend, yours, the time of your call, the fact that he did have the time today, when ordinarily he would not—all of these issues were juggled in Framework 2, to give you, now, the best possible solution, given the conditions in Framework 1, with the desires and beliefs involved.

(After I received no answer at Paul's office, I thought of waiting to call him at home after supper tonight, with Jane's agreement. Five minutes later, however, I decided to try him at home after all. Jane said she thought he took Mondays off, whereas I'd thought he took a midweek day off.)

It was originally Ruburt's loyalty to you that led him to see Paul in the beginning, because Paul had been friendly to you and you liked him. <u>That feeling</u> dissolved Ruburt's fear of Paul as a dentist. The state of Ruburt's condition is as I gave it. I will clarify. However, the eye material.

(9:50.) The pendulum was correct, in that it was answering the questions Ruburt asked. The eye condition did result from fears, and <u>in a way</u> "compensated" for other improvements, but not in any specific manner. Ruburt's gener-

al uncertainty and fears with the progress of his improvements led him to overcompensate, in muscular terms, causing lacks of balances otherwise unnecessary as the large areas of the neck and jaws began to relax and release.

The fear that the eye difficulty might be a serious disease caused further tension, of course. The knees are definitely continuing to release. The hands, fingers, arms and neck areas also. You both believed for years—and many years—that if you were gifted you had to do all you could to protect yourselves from others. Ruburt believed that people hated you if you were different. Those beliefs existed, and Ruburt felt that he was different, from the time he was a young child.

Those ideas from Freud, Darwin, and even the churches, have been inherent in your civilization. To the extent that you understand this and combat those beliefs, you are free. Whenever you have serious doubts of any kind, they usually arise from remnants of that framework.

There are indeed many questions that we have not answered. In a strange way, the depth of your understanding, to some extent now, determines how much I can tell you, and I am not speaking of personal matters here.

Your remark about the dishes was most creative, despite the way the remark was put: "Soon you will be able to stand and do the dishes, and just enjoy the task." That would have been excellent. To expect Ruburt to do that the next moment, however, brought up instant contradictions. You did remind him of the joy he used to take in that activity, however, and in an important way a conflict was resolved: he enjoys the dishes now, and he can say "Before I know it, I can enjoy it standing up also."

Paul reacted to Ruburt's and your affection for him. That already existed in both frameworks. He rather surprised himself, however, with his suggestion.

Do you have specific questions?

("Are you going to end the session early?")

It will not be as long as usual.

("I was just wondering how the Cézanne *books we've started sending out will be received.")*

Granting that probabilities operate, two people in particular will be quite interested. Rather importantly, however, your own view of the art world is changing for the better as you hear from individual artists in connection with our work, and those more positive feelings will definitely help now, where sometime earlier your feelings would have been somewhat detrimental.

In some circles I believe there will be a small furor, and the book will spread.

It is very important that both of you realize, paraphrasing James, that the universe is <u>with</u> you, that it supports you. That belief will always bring the best possible developments from Framework 2. Ruburt should concentrate on his creative work. You should both help reinforce each other's beliefs, in the actuality of Framework 2, and in the safety in which your existence is couched. There are several good developments coming your way that I will let you discover, and there should be some definite improvements in Ruburt's eyes—I would say, very quickly.

That is the end of this evening's session, and a hearty good evening.
("Thank you, Seth. Good night." 10:20 PM.)

DELETED SESSION
OCTOBER 22, 1977 9:20 PM SATURDAY

(In recent days we've had several conversations about Frameworks 1 and 2, and these have apparently begun to show results. I think the suggestions about the two frameworks that we've worked out are very close to the suggestions that Seth implied we should use in the hypnosis experiments.

(Jane is recovering extremely well from her tooth extractions. Rather to my surprise she suggested having a session tonight, so we thought we'd see how things went.)
Good evening.
("Good evening, Seth.")
Now: as I told you, Framework 2 is the creative medium that is responsible for physical life.

It is not true, however, that positive and negative feelings and beliefs "take" there with equal vitality. It is true that your beliefs form your reality; however you do have a certain leeway, in that those desires that lead to fulfillment and positive creativity are more in keeping with the natural leanings of Framework 2 itself.

Relatively speaking, then, these "take" more quickly, and accelerate in a more direct fashion. Limiting beliefs have to meet certain resistances, for they are not in keeping with the overall creative framework. It is easier for a body to be healthy than ill, and in the terms of this discussion, for example, old age does not basically bring with it any particular diseases or susceptibility.

Practically speaking, now, negative beliefs often finally catch up with an individual, leading to various diseases. I want to emphasize however that Framework 2 is not a neutral medium.

Negative beliefs have to be inserted there with great repetitiveness before you meet their physical results. To that extent also, energy is not neutral, as is often said, to be used for good or evil, for example. Energy is a positive force, ever-inclining toward creativity and fulfillment.

You are learning. The simple change of dish routine shows you how a change of attitude can break a negative pattern overnight. The pattern was actually broken by the simple remark that you made earlier, that led Ruburt to think of the stool for dishes.

Your suggestion about the bathroom *(sitting down)* is another instance of creative action which takes. Ruburt's previous position about the dishes was black or white. He would make no concessions. The more you enjoy life, and your daily moments, the less difficulty you will be in in <u>any</u> area, for your thoughts become naturally pleasant, and naturally attract good to you from Framework 2.

The stool at the sink reminded Ruburt that he could indeed use the stool in other areas of the kitchen, so he thought of cooking, and to that extent his thoughts became more naturally attuned. He expected more motion of himself, even though walking specifically was not involved. That kind of stimulus, encouraged, and not forgotten or let go, will set up a new set of mental habits, and literally with no effort, as suddenly he finds enjoyment doing the dishes.

The mental patterns are all-important, yet you see you have initiated some new ones creatively, using both Frameworks 1 and 2. You are correct: the more activities of a natural kind that Ruburt performs, whether or not he can do them on his feet, the better off he is, and you are. This signals what you want into Framework 2, and those activities will indeed be done better. It was, you see— I am explaining simply—too great a leap, if you will forgive me, to expect him to walk easily up his dentist's steps at this point. His faith could not take that leap. What you have begun, however—if you keep to this frame of mind—will indeed accelerate his physical improvement, for his mind will already have made necessary changes.

(9:43.) He can help out with the cooking, or make special dishes or whatever *(as she did today)*. This makes him feel more a part of normal living, and sets his own creative mechanisms more vigorously into new directions. The suggestions you gave him are excellent.

There are no impediments in Framework 2, then, to desires that are natural, creative, and that promote life. It is far easier, basically speaking now, for the body to heal itself than for it not to. Only beliefs otherwise, constantly and steadily applied, can impede that progress.

I believe that you are <u>finally</u> beginning, both of you, the last few days how to get a hold of your natural creativity in connection with Ruburt's situation, and to <u>apply it</u> to that end. If you continue then you attract from Framework 2 everything that you possibly need, and other areas of your lives will also improve, for to whatever extent they are somewhat shadowed by your attitudes resulting from Ruburt's condition.

The mood, however, and the results that you achieved today, if sustained, draws to you from all of your experience and from the vast potential of Framework 2 those body events, healing situations, dreams, impulses, or whatever is needed to right Ruburt's condition.

Faith itself then becomes an active ingredient in your lives in that regard. That is why your suggestions of today are so vital, stating that you do have faith that Ruburt's condition is <u>now</u> in the process of being healed <u>in Framework 2</u>, and that the results will show in Framework 1. It is important that you realize that the healing is now taking place in Framework 2 <u>whether or not you see</u> immediate results in any given day or not. That is where faith comes in.

Three years ago there was no *Cézanne* or *James* books. There was no evidence of them—no stacks of paper, no contract. *James* had been thought of, but Ruburt certainly had no idea he would, or could, possibly write a book on painting.

Now the books exist, for no impediments were put in the way here, yet again there was no physical evidence. Ruburt had written books before—<u>but Ruburt has walked before also</u>.

Give us a moment.... I hope over a period of time to explain Framework 2 even more clearly—and still for now your touch with creativity is your best method, for it comes naturally to each of you. And used as you have just begun using it, it can show you through action some issues most difficult to describe. It sets into motion all kinds of not only possible but rousing sentiments that of themselves have a restoring quality.

If I try too specifically to help Ruburt become consciously aware of methods he uses naturally in his creative work, he is apt to get too detailed in his physical efforts, where the creative activity you have begun of itself can carry itself along in physical areas if you allow it to.

The body wants to move, to act, to perform, and Ruburt needs some physical sense of satisfaction and accomplishment. This also allows his mind to refresh itself. When you are enjoying yourself you are not worrying.

A day like today is now beneficial then from many standpoints. Once you allow your faith to take some root, then you yield far more than you sow in Framework 2, and in results in Framework 1. Positively, you see that kind of acceleration in Ruburt's work, and if you give yourselves a chance you will see it also as far as Ruburt's physical condition is concerned. The body tries. It continues its own processes toward healing. You have only to encourage these, and to have faith in the body's abilities and intents. Unless you have questions, that will be it for this evening.

("Well, I've got questions, but I don't know whether he wants to continue or not. Let's take a break.")

We will indeed.

(10:08—10:25.)

There is of course an important give-and-take between the two frameworks and between mental and physical action. Mental and physical actions each stimulate each other. You think of what you do. You visualize yourself at it <u>naturally</u> and effortlessly. Nobody has to tell you to do it.

As Ruburt tries more physical activity even in the house, the creative abilities will automatically trigger certain processes so that he finds himself mentally concerned for example with what he will cook, or what cupboard he will wash, or whatever. Those thoughts can trigger unconscious muscular activity that will indeed make physical performance easier.

The enjoyment, again, automatically means that for that time he is not worrying—and beside that, the physical activity gives his muscles more to do, and gives him a sense of physical accomplishment. These issues and processes then act as excellent feedback, and reverse the negative habits that before operated.

The peace of mind will enrich his creative abilities—and that will automatically minimize whatever fears he has that physical activity would cut down on his creativity.

Impulses toward action will be naturally rearoused, and desires toward spontaneous action will find more and more release. Driving now is good, for it represents one of Ruburt's few connections with the natural outside world, and as he <u>does</u> improve, his impulses, natural impulses, will begin to show themselves. He will think of wanting to go <u>into</u> a restaurant you pass, or whatever, whether or not he can, say, at that moment.

He should look over his clothes, for example, lay out his special ones, or whatever, so that he <u>can</u> begin to feel he is capable of choosing his own attire for the day. A small point, but important, that he started out the day with that kind of choice.

Your own creativity being applied in this new fashion will also show its results in your painting and writing, for it adds a new cast, not only to your understanding of creativity, but to its application.

Some of the material in this session is extremely valuable in the handling of health problems, because of its clues in rousing the creative abilities from one area of life to another. The great thrust of creative abilities, utilized in the health area, will automatically bring Ruburt flexibility. Before, his condition was the one area in which he was not creative, as far as his flexibility was concerned.

He has a strong constitution, for he left that alone. End of session, but I will have more to say concerning creativity and Frameworks 1 and 2. My heartiest regards, and a creative good evening.

("Thank you very much, Seth. Good night.")

(10:42 PM. Lately I've been suggesting to Jane that when she finds herself hassling something she reminds herself that she has "a simple, profound faith that whatever needs to be done for an improvement in my health can take place in Framework 2. There are no impediments in Framework 2. Its creative workings there can show themselves in Framework 1, in my improved physical condition. I need not be concerned with details in any way...."

(This emphasis on that simple profound faith seems to be the key, and using that approach Jane has already achieved some good results. Her vision was much better yesterday afternoon on our ride, and today as I type this she is working on a painting—the first one she's attempted in some weeks. Her ability to read has been remarkably improved today, even without glasses. Other changes continue to take place in her body also.

(She still has to understand her automatic reactions of panic and fear of lost working time when I suggest going out, as I did today about going to the bank and post office tomorrow. But at least now she's <u>conscious</u> of her reactions, as she said, and can do something about them from that position. It's a certainty that she can much improve that situation.)

DELETED SESSION
OCTOBER 24, 1977 9:21 PM MONDAY

(Jane told me as we sat for the session tonight that she'd had some hints from Seth that the session would be on faith. I mentioned two questions: 1. Some comments on my dream about Louise Stamp recently, and the series of connections Jane had made, based upon it. It sounded very much like another instance of the workings of Framework 2; 2. Some comments on my recent dream involving my meeting my parents in the great marble hall, as I called it. I thought it might represent psychic contact with them, as well as other things.

(Both dreams are on record in my own dream notebook. Jane herself wrote up the Stamp dream and its many connections. Most interesting... Now she told me that Seth's recent prediction that her eyes would show noticeable improvement shortly has evidently come to pass; she wanted me to note that here. Her vision, while not nor-

mal in all respects yet, has greatly improved. And consistently, to her delight. Jane is also recovering from the tooth challenges very well.)

Good evening.

("Good evening, Seth.")

Now: in the most basic manner, each person and creature possesses faith, whatever its degree or nature.

Without it, there would be no family groups, animal or human, or civilizations or governments. It may seem that the retribution of law holds societies together and keeps, for example, criminal elements down, so that you have operating processes that insure more or less stable living conditions. The laws, however, are necessarily based upon man's faith that those laws will indeed be largely followed. Otherwise the laws would be useless.

You go on faith that there will be a tomorrow. You operate on faith constantly, so that it becomes indeed an almost invisible element in each life. It is the fiber behind all organizations and relationships, and it is based upon the innate, natural knowledge possessed by each new creature—the knowledge that it springs from a sustaining source, that its birth is cushioned by all the resources of nature, and that nature itself is sustained by the greater source that gave *it* birth.

You cannot be alive without faith, yet faith can be distorted. There is faith in good, but there is also faith in "evil." In usual terms faith takes it for granted that a certain desired end will be achieved, even though the means may not be known. In usual terms, again, there is no direct evidence, otherwise you would have no need for faith.

When you fear the worst will happen, you often are showing quite real faith in a backwards fashion, for with no direct evidence before your eyes of disaster, you heartily believe it will occur—you have faith in it *(with emphasis and irony)*. That is, indeed, misplaced faith.

The young woman, Frances *(Gardella)*, who wrote Ruburt, with no evidence was certain she would be followed—tomorrow if not today. I want to point out that faith is not all that unusual, but a prime element in your life. You can have faith that you will be ill. This should be obvious, because for example there are healthy people also, with no evidence of any disease, who have utter faith that disease is hidden within them, or swiftly approaching.

It is, therefore, quite to everyone's advantage that Framework 2 is not neutral. Faith in a creative, fulfilling, desired end, sustained faith, literally draws from Framework 2 all of the necessary ingredients, all of the elements however staggering in number, arranges all the details, and then inserts into Framework 1 the impulses, dreams, chance meetings, motivations, or whatever is necessary so that the desired end then falls into place as a completed pattern.

(9:40 in an intent delivery.) You must begin somewhere, so you state your purpose clearly in Framework 1. Then you have the faith that the event will be brought to pass.

Your own creative, abilities are instantly mobilized in that direction. Your behavior in Framework 1 must automatically change. The ways and the means, however, cannot be questioned, for they will come about from a greater source of knowledge than you consciously possess.

I am trying to give you some kind of an overall picture so that you can make your own helpful comparisons, and understand more thoroughly what is involved. Often I will use examples that do not involve health, for you can apply them to health yourselves even more effectively, for you will make your <u>own</u> connections.

Someone may plan an airplane trip. Everything will be arranged—the last detail taken care of. The person may take great precautions to see that the plane is not missed. Persons may have been contacted to care for the house during the time of absence. Children may have been sent to camp, neighbors assigned to care for pets, and every logical situation cared for.

Let us say that this particular plane may well crash, and in fact does. After all of this person's planning, hard work and effort, at the last moment everything seems to go wrong. Nothing seems right. The children do not leave for camp in time. One of the animals runs away. A ticket is lost. Our individual comes down with indigestion, or a headache. Lo and behold—for while everything seems so poorly, our friend's life is being saved, for he misses his plane.

Later he wonders what happened, that his life was saved, and his plans altered at the last moment. Our friend wanted to live and had faith that he would. In spite of his own conscious lack of knowledge, he was brought to operate according to the information available in Framework 2, though he was not aware of it. He lost his ticket—a stupid error, it seemed. The lives and events of all those involved with his trip—the neighbors, the children, and so forth—all of those issues were arranged in Framework 2, so that while the events seemed most unpleasant, they were highly beneficial.

If our friend learned of the plane crash, he saw this only too well. If he never learned of the plane crash, and did not have faith in the beneficial nature of events, then he might simply remember the entire affair as highly unpleasant, stupid, and even think that it was another example that he could do nothing right.

The entire pattern of your lives is taken into consideration in Framework 2. There is no need for bargaining. Ruburt does not have to fear that he must give up some creativity for physical freedom, <u>for the two go hand in hand</u>.

(9:58.) Give us a moment.... Framework 2 contains all the dreams, plans, and thoughts of all human beings of any time. <u>There</u>, the spacious present is operative. <u>There</u>, it makes no difference if you have had an undesirable physical condition for a day or a lifetime. <u>There</u>, you are not impeded by the past.

If your beliefs in Framework 1 make you assign great power to the past, then you impede your progress. I have said many times that spontaneity knows its own order, and I am speaking of true spontaneity. I say this because often anger, for example, may seem spontaneous—and may be—but is more often the explosive, finally forced expression of reactions long withheld or repressed.

True spontaneity however comes directly from Framework 2, and behind it are endless patterns of orderliness and complexity that are beyond your conscious Framework 1 comprehension. The small instance of Ruburt's doing the dishes this morning is a case in point – and <u>that</u> emerged as the result of those abilities mentioned in our last session.

(This morning, for the first time in well over a year, at the very least, Jane spontaneously decided to do the dishes after breakfast <u>while standing up at the sink</u>.)

Such an impulse, followed, will lead to its own performance the means will be given. Before, Ruburt's fear prevented him from even acknowledging many such impulses to act. Ruburt's assessment of your dream and its conditions is another case in point. The inner organizations immediately trigger all the necessary actions required, from Framework 2. This applies to any issue – but again, your creative abilities, used on behalf of Ruburt's physical condition will give him a normally cooperating body.

(Intently:) Each improvement is to be considered as a significant piece of a puzzle being put together, even though you may not see any connection between one improvement or another. Again, you should not double check at every moment. As Ruburt's *Cézanne* simply came out of nowhere, so will his complete flexibility.

Now take your break.

(10:11—10:43.)

It is not simply that in Framework 2 there is no resistance to creative, fulfilling, natural, life-seeking desires, but that the medium of. Framework 2 itself automatically adds its own <u>magnification</u> to them, so that <u>once you get rolling</u>, so to speak, the acceleration is spectacular, in whatever issue is involved.

(We've already had hints of this.)

The entire *Cézanne* book was inherent in the first page. Ruburt's faith and habits allowed the initial impulse its freedom, and that impulse, expressed, carried within it the means of its own fulfillment, and the book unfolded.

What you have seen lately are just beginning sentences in Ruburt's condition. The body <u>intends to</u> follow through. In the past you put into Framework 2 your intent, individually and jointly. It was ill-formed, not certain, cluttered by questions like "If I am well, should I go on tour or shouldn't I?" Or "Will I lose working time?" or whatever. It was not clear intent, <u>really</u>, on either of your parts.

It was constantly questioned. At best, it got you a status quo. *(Long pause.)* I do not want you to blame yourselves for the following, but I do want to point out that in the past, when Ruburt began to show improvements of a significant nature, you fell back into old habits. The status quo meant, with your attitudes, that you could not trust improvements.

Since you did not clearly state your intents for, say, normal walking and flexibility, and had little faith in it, then you feared that improvements could not be trusted, for in your experience they went so far and no further. Yet any poor performance was taken by Ruburt, particularly, as evidence in the other direction. You were caught between the ideal and a very poor performance, one contrasting with the other.

I hope, as you understand how Framework 2 operates, that you can clearly state your intent: Ruburt's normal flexibility and good health, and that you will be able to see each improvement as a step in that stated direction. Indeed, you <u>do</u> change your psychic organization, and hence attract the significant events you want. They fall into place.

Again, it is imperative that Ruburt realize there is absolutely no conflict, and that his creative work will fulfill itself in certain ways that would be most difficult to achieve otherwise, if not impossible, practically speaking.

Any conflicts, however, can automatically be absolved in Framework 2, whatever they are. No bargaining, again, is necessary.

The material of mine that Ruburt read tonight can help him again now. His creative abilities work, no matter what he is doing, and they will work better and reach further when his body is normally flexible, able to relax normally as it should. Speaking in the vernacular, you get extra bursts of energy with greater and greater acceleration the longer you keep at it.

Other examples should be appearing in your lives. Look out for them. Beside stating your clear intent, having faith in the processes as given, leaving the means and details in Framework 2, you have simply to refrain from worrying as much as possible – and <u>that</u> becomes easier and easier as you go along, for the events themselves, and the added enjoyment from life will minimize worry.

(11:30.) Give us a moment.... You were aware of your parents in Framework 2 *(in my dream of Oct 19, 1977)* with the hall as your symbol.

Basically speaking, these were your parents as you knew them. I believe there is a connection with the man from Sayre—he is not dead that might very well appear in your normal life as a contact. There may also have been a connection with the house in Sayre.

To you the hall was a neutral-enough meeting place, but not one of intimacy, and to some extent at least it symbolized the relationship—at least as far as you were concerned—in that while you were a child of your parents you felt to some degree a stranger, and the hall lacked intimacy. The dream was a statement of those particular feelings.

The meeting itself was quite legitimate. You were like people who visited the same building for different reasons. Now that is the end of the session unless you have questions.

("No, it's been very interesting.")

Then I wish you a good evening.

("Thank you, Seth. Good night." 11:10 PM.

(The following may be one of those incidents from Framework 2 that Seth advised being on the lookout for: Last week I rather seriously thought of ordering a copy of The Origin of Ccs In the Breakdown of the Bicameral Mind *by Jaynes. I saw the book listed in a catalog from which I was ordering some other books, and nearly included it in the order. I've been curious about it ever since it was published —last year, I believe—for from the reviews printed of it I believe it contains some material that may be a distorted version of Seth's "sleepwalker" material in Volume 2 of* "Unknown" Reality.

(The book is rather expensive—about $15.00—and I passed up the chance to order. I did think that I'd like to have it, or at least see a copy. Today, then, the mail brought a copy of the book from a fan that sent it as a gesture, remarking about certain similarities it contains with some of Seth's material. As far as I know, we've not heard from this particular fan before.

(A note: As Seth said, the Framework 2 concepts, once initiated, do seem to accelerate almost of their own volition. Since I personally have begun working with it, new applications for its use seem to pop up from everywhere—natural enough, I suppose, yet I feel an impetus there as though I've finally found something that will be of immense use in daily life. It will be interesting to see what develops. Last night as we were retiring, I thought of a good use for the Framework 2 data: to use it to insure that the books reach the greatest audience possible—this without worrying about the number of copies sold, the money involved, etc. All those things should follow naturally from the original idea. After all, I told Jane, getting the books distributed is *our main goal; now it would be great to see that happen without the impediments we've put in the way all this time.*

(Since she began sitting down in the bathroom, Jane has done so once a day each day. I can see her confidence and ease of performance increase each day.)

ROB'S SUGGESTIONS ABOUT
FRAMEWORK 2

(I have the simple, profound faith that anything I desire in this life can come to me from Framework 2. There are no impediments in Framework 2. Framework 2 can creatively produce everything I desire to have in Framework 1—my excellent health, painting, and writing, my excellent relationship with Jane, Jane's own spontaneous and glowing physical flexibility and creativity, the greater and greater sales of all of her books. I knew that all of these positive goals are worked out in Framework 2, regardless of their seeming complexity, and that they can then show themselves in Framework 1. I have the simple, profound faith that everything I desire in life can come to me from the miraculous workings of Framework 2. I do not need to be concerned with details of any kind, knowing that Framework 2 possesses the infinite creative capacity to handle and produce everything I can possibly ask of it. My simple, profound faith in the creative goodness of Framework 2 is all that is necessary.)

DELETED SESSION
OCTOBER 29, 1977 9:54 PM SATURDAY

(Several times during the last week I'd mentioned to Jane that we should get more information from Seth on her eyes—insisting upon more specific reasons why they were so protuberant. Most of the time we felt that her eyes were healing themselves, since often now she would be able to see with great clarity at various distances even better than with her glasses. Tonight I found out that Jane too had been dunning Seth—but mentally—about more on her eyes. Now she became rather upset as we both voiced our opinions just before the session, and this probably contributed to the later start of the session. But I still thought it very strange for the eyes to cause problems if the body was in the process of healing itself, as Seth has so often said recently is the case. Why should another part suffer? I was ready to admit that the body could repair itself in ways that might be mysterious to us, but at the same time I certainly wanted additional reassurances from Seth that we were doing the right thing in going along with his information. I also realized that Jane's quite unique set of symptoms might lead to effects as they released that we'd certainly be unprepared

for.

(*Last Thursday afternoon as I lay down for my customary nap before supper, I had an experience that was new for me: I've been meaning to write it up, so this place will serve as a record. As Jane and I have decided to do lately, I began giving myself suggestions about increased sales of her books. I was very comfortably ensconced on our couch. As I gave the suggestions I abruptly realized that they seemed to be penetrating—what?—some sort of barrier or limit that I'd usually assumed marked the limits of ordinary conscious awareness. Rooms ordinarily alien or unknown to me seemed to open up, although in a very concentrated focus, as say from the beam of a flashlight. But I knew that the suggestions had penetrated as never before, and I thought they had reached their goal in Framework 2 in a way that I could be aware of. The sensation was brief but unmistakable, and very enjoyable. It happened again a few moments later. Then I fell asleep.*

(*Attached to this session [see page 76] is the carbon of the suggestions I wrote up recently about reaching Framework 2 through suggestion and faith.*

(*Today we received from the Museum of Modern Art an acknowledgment that William Rubin had received the* Cézanne *book I'd mailed him on October 17. In a note dated Oct 25 his assistant implied that Mr. Rubin would get in touch later, after the affairs connected with the Cézanne show there had subsided. He hasn't looked through the book yet, however. I mentioned to Jane that it would be fun if Seth could give us a little bit on Rubin's reaction when he saw the book on Cézanne—not on its contents.*)

Good evening.

("Good evening, Seth.")

Now, give us a moment.... Let me try again to explain a few points, mainly concerning Ruburt's condition.

Until the very recent past, his body in a way was overdisciplined, so that it maintained a fairly stable but rigid framework. Certain postures were allowed, certain motions, and not others, <u>as if</u> Ruburt operated his body as though it were a puppet, keeping it in certain ritualized motions by holding the strings too tightly.

In this case the strings would be the muscles and tendons. The body is not a puppet, however, so the tightened ligaments and muscles restrained the joints to some extent—all of them. Little by little they demanded less lubrication, for use did not stimulate it.

Each muscle, ligament, and joint was to some extent affected, drawn too tightly. The head could move, and the neck, in certain positions. The eyes looked forward, moving with the head's motion. The eyes did not roll easily, but since no attempt was made to roll them, the restriction was not noticed, except when Ruburt tried to roll his eyes when they were closed, for an exercise once or twice.

The eyes were not held rigid. They moved sideways, but in very limited fashions. The rigidity was <u>largely</u> set up in the head and neck regions—arms and shoulders, thus necessitating the bending of the knees and so forth.

Improvements could occur, and did, but at one time or another the portions of the body had to begin to break away from the overall blocked picture. Spontaneity had to be allowed if any normality of motion was to occur. You did not want a body in the same position, simply moving faster, for example. Therefore in the late months the various ligaments and muscles, and tendons began to loosen.

As you know, the overall dependability of the old posture could not be relied upon anymore. That in itself was a definite step forward. Our friend Frank Longwell verified the loosening of the ligaments in the knees. They move now constantly, trying out their new freedoms and as they do they stimulate other positions of the body to one extent or another. The same applies to the right foot particularly as new ligaments loosen.

The neck ligaments, as mentioned, and the jaw area were particularly involved. Ruburt had some habits he was only vaguely aware of. He used to close his eyes tightly, often, when he sat down, tensing the knee ligaments and the eyes at the same time. This was because the knees hurt. In another learned response he did not look sideways. When he reached for something to the side he reached like this: his eyes did not follow the motion.

(With gestures, Seth simulated Jane reaching to one side while keeping her head and eyes facing straight forward.)

In other ways he did not use his eyes to follow sideward motions, and often tensed the entire head area when he executed any movement he felt was difficult. As the knee and neck areas began—as they are—spontaneous motions, unused activities of the eyes also began to show. They have not been synchronized. Part of this is because all the small ligaments in both the head and knee areas are released, or are being released. They are constantly exercising themselves, but are not themselves working smoothly.

(10:17.) Added to this is the fact that joints now require lubrication. His head feels fuller, and other portions of the body also. These changes mean that the pressure in his ears and head changes. The lubrication allows more spontaneous actions on the part of the joints, ligaments, and muscles. To <u>some</u> extent the changing pressure accounts for the eyes' protuberance, so that they have plenty of moisture and do not become dry as the eye muscles and other portions of the eyes exercise their new activity.

Give us a moment.... *(Long pause.)* To some extent this has allowed the eyes to read now and then without glasses. The alterations in Ruburt's knees, however, send various messages to the brain, for as he walks, due to the present activity, his position is not constant. He is not always so many feet, for example, from the floor. As the ligaments and muscles in the legs activate, they are learning to work together under entirely different conditions.

The messages do not all agree, then, as they would in a smooth locomotion—even a <u>rigid</u> smooth locomotion.

The varying pressure in the joints is also involved here, and all of these issues are connected with depth perception. The body of course knows your situations, and the demands put upon it. If Ruburt were a traffic cop, other methods would have been taken so that he would not get run down, for example. I understand your concern, and perhaps I should not comment, but if some of my suggestions had been followed, you would have had quicker results with the eyes. I know you both fairly well, however, so I usually give you a number of suggestions toward action, so that at least some of them *(dryly)* will be followed.

In your joint creativity, you sustained each other's faith through the years. You gave your <u>desire</u> freedom, and you believed in it. That belief dissolved impediments that lay in your way—even some you did not recognize—attitudes, for example, that you had but did not see were detrimental. You were not driven by fear, but desire, not by doubts but by hope and faith. You did not project failure into the future, but success. Overall, these last few weeks you have done well. Ruburt has noted sometimes a worry and lack of faith, and so have you. But those times are <u>now</u> becoming—<u>becoming</u> the exception rather than the rule, and before them the opposite applied.

On occasions that you barely recognize, one of you has been in a doubting mood while the other was in a mood of faith, picked this up, and was able to change the situation also for the one who felt doubtful. Both of you at different times operated that way for the other, scarcely noticing.

It is Ruburt of course whose moods are more noticeable, but he still should feel free to discuss his fears with you <u>when he is</u> in a poor mood. For even if you are not filled with faith at such times, you can usually recognize that <u>his</u> fears are exaggerated rather than realistic, even in those terms.

Your statements *(of suggestion re Frameworks 1 and 2)* are excellent, and should be read over.

(10:41.) If your goals fit in with overall natural purposes, you can do anything at all with your consciousness, while still maintaining ordinary contact in Framework 1. *(Whispering:)* I suggest that perhaps once a day in as creatively playful a way as possible, without trying too hard, in naps or when you are read-

ing your statements, or anytime, to simply try to get the feeling of Framework 2.

When you were working with sales the other day, you felt that contact *(as described)*. You felt motion happening. Sometimes, perhaps, when Ruburt is listening to music he likes on his radio, let him try to get the feeling of Framework 2 again, without trying too hard, and imagine himself dancing, anyway he likes. This does not have to be long or involved.

Give us a moment.... If his knees could see, they would also be disoriented. *(A great line.)* The fear of the situation does not help, of course, for any such tension holds back the relaxing process—and the eyes are relaxing, and the neck and tendons, for example, letting go. Often at times when his vision is disorienting, that activity however also results in the better focus in reading that is coming about. Usually it is changes in focus that are involved. He will be reading fairly well, then perhaps look up at the television set, following motion of the screen, and then it will take time again—a few moments, perhaps before he reads well again. Or he will be reading well and look up, eyes roaming about the room, and then become disoriented visually.

Hot water on the knees will help, as does his new practice of hot water on the forehead. Sitting on the stool, he could apply hot water on the knees while letting them drop down.

You are <u>beginning</u> to awaken your faith, but still afraid to believe. Ruburt has had some excellent moments of such faith, however, and those moments add up. It is highly important that you continue thinking creatively in terms of his condition, of not being afraid to believe that he can indeed walk normally.

He must avoid contradictions, while at the same time not putting his normal walking into some distant future. You must believe that in Framework 2 all of the necessary procedures involved in his normal walking are now happening, and believe that improvements and obvious <u>states</u> of that process will occur in Framework 1. The evidence will appear in Framework 1 as you believe it. At the same time, however, you must not be ever-checking Ruburt's condition for the evidence.

(Very intensely:) the inspiration for a book can come in a moment, though for months nothing may appear. So Ruburt's condition may show no physical improvements of the kind you are looking for—may not—while suddenly the work that has been done unconsciously during that period can suddenly emerge, seemingly from nowhere, as a spectacular improvement. If you do not have faith in the meantime, however, you hamper that kind of development.

On the other hand, improvements may be gradual, but steady. The whole point is to trust that they will come, in whatever fashion, but in a reasonable time, without making other qualifications.

Any other ways that Ruburt can increase his daily enjoyment will also help. The cooking efforts, the dishes, have benefits that do not show beside those you are familiar with. If you do follow my suggestions concerning Framework 2, given this evening, your own experiences will lead to other creative ideas involving Ruburt's condition, sales, and creative activity.

I will end the session, or take a break as you prefer.

("We'll take the break, thank you."

(11:02. During break Jane said she knew that either she or Seth could tune into the situation at the Museum of Modern Art, but that she could "feel resistance" to the idea. Resume at 11:30.)

As a child, you are immersed in Framework 2. Along the way you are taught that it is unrealistic to have any kind of faith unless physical evidence is behind it, but then, of course, you are not working with faith at all.

You have both been afraid that Ruburt would not return to normal flexibility, to have faith in that situation, for fear your hopes would be aroused then dashed. You did not <u>free</u> that desire. You gave it no expression. You did talk of improvements, <u>but you saw them going toward no completed direction</u>. Again, because your fears did not allow you to express or release that desire.

Again, the more normal activities, as with the dishes, et cetera, that Ruburt tries, the more he states his intent to do normal things. The more his attitude changes, the more flexible he becomes, the more freedom he allows himself. You must not be afraid to hope, for hope always leads to faith.

The fact that you even sent books to artists and art institutions shows that you have changed your attitudes in Framework 1, thereby opening resources in Framework 2 that did not exist, practically speaking, earlier. Many artists have strong psychic leanings, whether or not they admit them. The *Cézanne* book will have more effect on the people that you sent it to than they realize, or may be apparent at this time, because you are uniting two strong forces—the artistic and creative ones. You should get some excellent responses, though some people will not want their names used.

(Odd that Seth would say that; as far as I know, neither of us have any conscious idea of trying to use the names of people who respond to the Cézanne *books.)*

You have made your first strong impression in Framework 2, however, in certain fashions, for it is the first time you have personally contacted people about these books in any concerted manner. <u>That </u>change of attitude is vastly important.

The exercise I told Ruburt to do about dancing can also trigger responses on his part in ways now impossible to expect. All of the resources, the endless resources on Framework 2 are available to you, and you will use them in many areas, but you must trigger them through desire and intent, with the faith and belief that they are indeed available at your command, in the area in which you are interested.

Before, for whatever reasons, already given, you were each content with the status quo. You did not trigger the complete response, then. That is the secret.

End of session, except that you can also suggest that you become acquainted with, or visit, Framework 2 while in the dream state, and remember the event. With your focus now, you should have decent results. Remember applying the creativity to Ruburt's condition, and to increasing daily enjoyment. A small note: you did not free your desire in terms of sales, either. You wanted the books to go so far and no further, because you did not trust your own abilities to handle the situation if the books did really well. My heartiest regards and a fond good evening.

(*"Thank you, Seth, and good night." 11:48 PM. I told Jane that I now had full confidence that we could handle anything that arose as a result of greatly increased sales.)*

DELETED SESSION
OCTOBER 31, 1977 9:40 PM MONDAY

(*At the end of last Saturday's session, I thought of two questions for Seth. They were based upon his discussion of the* Cézanne *book, and our changed attitudes, as demonstrated by our sending the books out. Jane suggested I write them down for tonight.*

(*1. Was there any connection between Jane's* Cézanne, *and the New York City Cézanne show appearing at practically the same time? Did this have Framework 2 connotations? Both projects had been underway for a long time before surfacing to the public. See the note about William Rubin and the Museum of Modern Art, at the start of the last session.*

(*2. Did Cézanne "himself" have any sense of awareness, or of completion, connected with Jane's book and the New York City show happening at the same time? Seth had said that William James did, in connection with Jane's book about him, and his interest in gifted mediums. My own thought at the moment was that something different, or at least not the same, was involved with the Cézanne events—less personal.*

(*Last night we watched on television Alan Neuman's show on the paranormal.*

SESSION 10/31/77 83

We liked most of it quite a bit. See the clipping on file. His secretary wrote Jane on October 13. After the show, Jane wondered about Framework 2 immediately responding to the efforts shown by some of the gifted people on the show—those doing the firewalking, moving objects, fogging film, etc. The results were obtained without delay, evidently from Framework 2. Of course, Jane wanted these results for herself, also. She wondered if Seth might comment on this question, as well as the show itself. She wrote Alan Neuman a letter; this morning I mailed him a copy of Cézanne.

(Instances of the operation of Framework 2 keep cropping up. Two happened today, or at least I felt that one happened today, and we heard about the other one today. Frank Longwell cited a case whereby his brother Waldo obtained encouraging answers to a set of business problems that had been bugging the Longwells for some time. The setting was a restaurant Waldo had never been in before; the urban renewal director came up to Waldo and <u>offered</u> just the help needed, without being asked or previously contacted, etc. This is a simplified version.

(The second instance involved the hassle we've been involved in with Elmira Video over mistakes in our billing. Has been dragging on since July. All the details are on file if needed for reference. Friday afternoon, when we received another erroneous bill, Jane called Elmira Video; the bookkeeper, Mrs. Trafzer, promised to call Monday to tell us what we owed. Over the weekend I found myself stewing about the silliness of the whole thing several times. I thought of legal action, among other things. Monday morning as I painted, I found myself doing the same thing. Rather irritably I told myself that I was throwing the whole thing into Framework 2, and that I wanted it taken care of.

(At breakfast I'd even considered paying the whole bill demanded of us—I told Jane—just to be rid of the entire affair. Late this afternoon Mrs. Trafzer called, as promised to tell us that we were to forget the bill and to send in the regular monthly payment of $15.94, instead of the $33.00 we were charged with. Something about her not being able to trace the skein of payments and errors through their computer, she said. We expected to pay more, of course. It took me a while to realize that I had received an answer from Framework 2, and that for us it couldn't have been better.

("But keep your fingers crossed," I told Jane, "until we get next month's bill." Mrs. Trafzer has promised to personally put the proper figures into the computer, thus ending the billing confusion. I mailed her payment this morning, Tuesday.)

Good evening.

("Good evening, Seth.")

Now: this analogy holds only so far, yet the firewalker's performance can in a way be compared with Ruburt's writing and psychic performance.

The man not only walks, but he walks on fire—to most, a seeming impossibility. It seems to Ruburt that the firewalker must have an instant rapport with Framework 2, that Ruburt does not possess. Ruburt is in fact in constant rapport with Framework 2 when he is writing or psychically involved, and often he has contacts with other frameworks also.

If he is considering his own personal situation, however, let him remember that the firewalker utterly believes in his ability. He does not worry that he will be burned. He walks on coals as automatically as Ruburt writes, or speaks for me. His feet are not burned simply because he has faith that they will not be. The performance is evidence of the fact that beliefs have a far greater effect upon the body and its capacities than is anywhere seriously considered. The man's focus is <u>there</u>, as Ruburt focuses in his work. He has learned to focus faith in a highly specialized fashion, and has built up a backlog in that area.

It is difficult to explain some of these issues, for in doing so I have to watch your attitudes, to avoid any concentration upon seeming contradictions. *(Long pause.)* The fact is that the processes necessary to the desired end are instantly put into action in Framework 2. There <u>is</u> immediate response in Framework 1, though it may not be apparent because the conscious mind is not always equipped to recognize significances that are outside its usual context.

The firewalker's performance involves one overall clear-cut performance, in which faith has already been achieved, as in Ruburt's writing, say. In the case of Ruburt's physical situation, the response from Framework 2 <u>has</u> been immediate. The conscious mind is not able to follow the pieces of the puzzle, so to speak, as it is being put together. A sensation here, another one there, a pull of tendons, a sudden softening of tissue—such matters cannot be consciously interpreted. The response has not been complete, but it has been immediate.

(9:58.) Give us a moment.... I do not want Ruburt to try too hard, but I do want to explain the characteristics of Framework 2 as they interwork with your world.

It is possible, then, to have a sudden complete healing. In most such instance, however, the inner work has been progressing in Framework 2, and suddenly emerges in Framework 1. Desire, faith, and beliefs are the keys.

Frank's experience concerning his brother is a case in point. His brother did not know that the urban renewal gentleman was in that particular restaurant where the two might meet, and until the meeting did occur nothing showed in Framework 1, though much was occurring in Framework 2. The creative potential knows exactly what changes must occur in Ruburt's body so that he can walk normally. It also knows what changes must occur in his mind—what conflicts must be resolved, and all of this is being taken care of. The process of his complete recovery includes body events and <u>other</u> events that may seem to have no connection—events perhaps that will change an attitude here or a belief there.

Your lack of knowledge can lead you to insist upon your own ideas of what must occur, or how or when. All of those people who might in any way help Ruburt change certain beliefs, for example, are notified in Framework 2, so that the most auspicious psychological events occur, triggering further body releases.

The timing of such events is outside of your time, but the results appear within it. The intent is to walk normally—not just to improve. Then the improvements lead to that desired end.

Give us a moment.... Ruburt, you see, does not say "I must have a certain new book next week." He is so sure of his ability that he produces far more books in any given time than the majority of writers. Only his doubts lead him to worry that recovery might take too long. The recovery is taking place now in Framework 2. The now is important.

The *Cézanne* book, the show, your own interest in Cézanne, and your own painting abilities are also connected in Framework 2, along with the fact that Cézanne himself had a secondary interest in writing, that fell by the board, so to speak. Your own art interests have always attracted artists to our books in general, through Framework 2's constant communication. There are individuals who go through many lifetimes with one main interest or desire, attaining finally a culmination that they have sought for. Cézanne was such a one. In those terms, his interests are now the same, but he no longer looks upon his historically known works, but considers them as background pieces, so to speak. He paints in another reality to which his own intent has led him, except that his creativity has opened up so that he no longer feels the same need for isolation.

His inspiration comes now from all of history, and from that larger reservoir he forms the new focus of his art. It was his secondary interest in writing, largely unexpressed in life, that formed some connective between he and Ruburt.

Take your break.

(*10:25. Jane said that she didn't feel that she was "quite with it, tonight," for some reason, although I thought her material was as good as ever. Not that she didn't feel like having a session, she added. She was speaking with a number of long pauses interspersed. Resume at 10:35.*)

All portions of Ruburt's body are gently and almost constantly being stretched and then exercised in the best possible order. He is able to walk in the meantime. The constant activity however prepares the body for normal walking, and exercises necessary portions, <u>then stretches them further</u>, so that while

Ruburt is not walking more noticeably upright, he is indeed taller, particularly when standing; different portions are exercised when he is sitting or standing, so that each change can be counted upon for the next alteration in posture.

The upper portions of the body, particularly important, are also lengthening the arms and releasing shoulder ligaments for greater motion. Balance is also being maintained, with the eyes learning to roam in a more ordinary fashion. Little of this shows, although he is aware of the sensations, which are signs of the healing processes.

The thighs are being worked on considerably. Following these procedures, the body posture can gradually right itself, and the necessary muscles will already have been activated and strengthened. Again, concentration should be on his creative activities, though he should read his statement, as he has been doing. The process also includes psychic insights and experiences, and all of these patterns fit together in ways that will be quite apparent after he has recovered.

Remember that the organizations in Framework 2 are different than your own, so you cannot know the means, but trust they will be taken care of. The statement and release of desire is all-important, and some psychological activity on Ruburt's part has already occurred lately, that will be very important here.

You are also being treated, so to speak, with a variety of examples of how Framework 2 operates, and you will learn to recognize when you are making excellent contact there. Framework 2 includes all of the creative work behind the scenes, and your desire brings all of the necessary events together.

Ruburt's desire to walk normally for that matter comes from Framework 2, for it is a natural desire, in harmony with his basic being, that would flow into actuality on its own—had *he* not put impeding beliefs and contradictions in the way, so that the desire itself was buried beneath, say, debris.

Now he removes debris, and desire is free to follow the natural lines of its own fulfillment.

I will end the session for the sake of his mouth now—

("Okay." Since her recent tooth extractions, Jane has noticed an increased mouth dryness after she's spoken for a while.)

—but you should have further experiences yourselves with Framework 2 before our next session. I believe you can count upon it.

My heartiest regards, and a fond good evening.

("Thank you, Seth. Good night.")

A note: at one time I had wooden teeth, put in with glue that never stuck correctly.

(10:51 PM. I was tempted to ask Seth what life he was referring to, but that

would have kept Jane talking longer.)

DELETED SESSION
NOVEMBER 5, 1977 9:42 PM SATURDAY

(Last Wednesday Jane had the last of her extractions done; she is recovering very well indeed. This week she has experienced many more small but important physical improvements throughout her body, all adding up to a considerable change in her physical condition as far as sitting, walking, etc. This is all very encouraging; her improvements to date of course mark by far the longest period of sustained improvements that she's shown in many years. I seem to feel an unaccustomed excitement about it all; this hovers offstage, one might say, at the chance that she'll make it after all.

(Before the session we talked about the firewalker's performance on the recent Alan Neuman show. I remarked that the seeming violation of physical laws posed serious challenges to science, and so forth. We've been educated to believe that if the flesh is touched by fire as hot as that in the pit, that flesh will inevitably be burned; yet it wasn't.)

Good evening.

("Good evening, Seth.")

Now: apropos of your firewalker, fire of that temperature would indeed burn the flesh if it touched it in your practical reality.

<u>In a manner of speaking</u>, the man's feet touch the ground but they do not touch the fire. The man believes his feet will not be burned. That belief generates certain actions or events, so that practically speaking, while he sees the flames, and perhaps smells the smoke, the heat of the fire will have no effect—because <u>for him</u> its character is changed. He ignores the evidences of his senses.

For him, the area taken up by the fire becomes "dimensionally neutral." For the time of his walk that space is empty. In a manner of speaking, again, he erases the fire's practicality, <u>so that it can have no effect</u>.

If you have a light bulb lit, it is bright and hot. If you turn the light off, the bulb is still there. Its light and heat become latent, but <u>practically</u> nonexistent. To your hand a light bulb that is not turned on will be cool. To your eyes it will not be bright. The bulb is still there, but its power is neutralized.

Our firewalker turns off the fire—for himself, however, though its form, like the turned-off light bulb, remains. His faith is the power that neutralizes the fire.

You live in a world of root assumptions, to which all agree. They are the ground rules of your reality—but not the ground rules of all realities or of all probabilities. Your firewalker inserts another probability, and hence reacts to and with that reality of the fire in ways that are not considered normal. I have said his feet touch the ground but not the flames. Actually, what I can only call an invisible shield protects him from the flames, so that his feet and ankles are surrounded by an aura that repels the fire actively. This is a definite force, a psychic force field, if you will. This ability is quite ancient, though little known.

(9:59.) Give is a moment.... In very ancient times, medicine men had to perform such acts as part of their initiation ceremonies. I am not sure how to explain the process, however. The belief triggers body chemicals in a certain fashion, though the process itself involves an interaction between the air and the chemicals of the body, which form together a protective shield that repels the action of the fire.

What you actually have is a case of cold flame. Stories of walking on water give you the same kind of proposition, where you have to all effects and purposes dry water, or solid water.

You do not seem to understand the importance of your organizations, particularly your habitual biological ones, for they dictate the ways in which you examine your reality, and they program also your biological reaction in very practical ways.

They program the interactions within the body, so that certain effects always appear inevitable, when such in basic terms is not always the case, necessarily. You can intrinsically walk on fire, or thrust your hands into the flames, and be unburned. I would not suggest that too many try it, however. The mind and its beliefs are the basic determinants. That firewalker shares his reality with nonfirewalkers, in general terms, but in this one instance the firewalker superimposes a strong counterbelief, and it works

The rules of physics are no more than gentlemen's rules of the game but the firewalker plays a different game, with different rules, and they work also.

Give us a moment.... In Framework 2, as mentioned, existence is also organized in a completely different fashion than you are used to. In that Framework, the best possible overall conditions for growth are available. Your firewalker seems to be breaking a natural law. He is simply acting according to another belief, but he is being true to his nature, which in this case led him to the desire for such an achievement. In Framework 2, therefore, the nature of each individual actively seeks out its own greatest potential, in the world of Framework 1, practically speaking, in the world where time and space are realities.

Ruburt was correct: your spontaneous creative self dwells in Framework

2. There, your nature is intimately known, with all of its unique characteristics and capabilities. There, automatically, computations are made so that you will meet, in Framework 1, with the necessary opportunities, situations, or whatever it is that your circumstances require.

Those desires of yours, <u>that are fitting to your nature</u>, will automatically come to pass, unless you block them through disadvantageous beliefs. They cannot be blocked by others. If they <u>seem</u> to be blocked by others, that assumption is incorrect, based on ignorance.

Imagine, say, a young woman named Sally. She deals with people very well, exceptionally well. She has a mediocre voice, though pleasant enough. For whatever reasons, she decides that she wants to be an opera star. The desire is not in keeping with her own abilities. It may have been triggered by envy of another person, or for the sake of fame, but it does not fit her abilities. She may ignore the fact that her talents lie in having an excellent rapport with others. She puts into Framework 2 a desire that is not in keeping with her own best development. She may train her voice, take lessons, while yet she is thwarted at auditions, until it seems people are against her.

All of this is known in Framework 2. Even then, events will be arranged for her own good. She might, for example, through a series of seemingly chance encounters, end up in another branch of singing, less formal, where she also deals with her contemporaries, as in a music company.

Those desires that are in keeping with your nature meet no resistance. They are in fact promoted automatically. Ruburt's walking is a case in point. The idea about the seminars in an example of Framework 2's creativity, as it begins to provide goals that automatically imply physical flexibility and confidence.

(10:29.) He is beginning to release the desire to walk normally, rather just to ask for improvements—for before, he was not sure where he wanted those improvements to lead. The seminar idea means that he is changing in his mind, and that is where the changes must occur. The physical changes follow automatically. The desire to walk, released and expressed, again automatically triggers in Framework 2 all of the necessary conditions. The hints and clues then appear in Framework 1, and you build upon those significances.

Before too long, <u>naturally</u>, without effort, Ruburt will find himself visualizing himself outdoors, or in a restaurant, and the physical facts will follow. Before, his mental horizons did not include that activity. Already, at least mentally, he sees it can be easier to sit down in the bathroom, and that activity will follow naturally, without effort. Mental and physical events, then, form new organizations, and the interactions between Frameworks 1 and 2 become quicker, and, again, you have an accelerating activity.

That accelerating activity is natural, as it appears in Ruburt's writing. You form your reality through various mental and physical cues to action that you recognize, through the significances that you habitually accept. Left alone now, Ruburt's thoughts are more positive, and the worries not as frequent. The significances change.

Take your break.

(10:39–10:54.)

The way of least resistance is always followed for desires that are fulfilling and fitting to your nature.

The only impediments are those you impose through your negative beliefs. Because the organization is so different, however, in a way you must forget cause and effect, for things fall into place almost in a circular fashion.

Even when nothing shows in Framework 1, if you have properly inserted your desire there, then all the proper circumstances and conditions are being brought together. Again, they may suddenly appear, or they may not appear in the order in which you think they should, because your vision must be limited in comparison to that available in Framework 2.

I want to mention again that all kinds of events are involved with Ruburt, for example—physical, psychological, and even social. His improvements of late are excellent, and highly significant. They are the result of the faith you have built up thus far. Do not try to program the improvements. The descriptions given by James in the later part of the book actually apply very well to the creative medium of Framework 2, for your needs are anticipated and automatically provided for, if, again, you do not impede them through contrary beliefs.

Ruburt will shortly feel more and more energetic, and even be provided with greater wealth of creative material, as the energy that has been used to maintain symptoms is automatically freed, transformed into those vital areas of his interest.

In many cases of health problems, energy is actually being applied to block the body's normal healing processes. This is almost always the result of beliefs that do not fit in with the person's own best interests. Your social beliefs are of course important here, mass medical beliefs. In a vast number of cases this represents a dilemma of a psychological or psychic nature. It is the body's attempt to cope in the face of the mind's confusion.

I hope to go into the ways in which computations are made in Framework 2, and how they interact with your world. The body of course exists in Framework 2 also, or it could not exist in Framework 1 at all. You are in constant touch with Framework 2, then. It gives you your life.

(11:10.) I do not want you to put Ruburt's normal walking in some indistinct distant future. On the other hand, I do not want to tell you it can happen tomorrow, because I do not want you to concentrate upon it. It can indeed, however, happen overnight.

Your faith is the answer, and the use to which you put your creativity, for the more you apply it to Ruburt's condition the quicker the results.

You must not be concerned with time, yet you must have the faith <u>that in your terms of time</u> Ruburt's normal walking will come in an immediate rather than distant future.

(To me, in answer, evidently, to some of our conversation before the session:) You are already writing a book—<u>you</u>— in Framework 2. It simply waits for the proper conditions here. I do not want to overstress, yet again it is important that Ruburt use the words "normal walking" without comparing that desire to his present locomotion. But it must be the goal, clear and distinct.

My heartiest good wishes, and a fond good evening unless you have questions.

("I, guess not. Thank you, Seth. Good night."
(11:15 PM.)

DELETED SESSION
NOVEMBER 7, 1977 9:43 PM MONDAY

(Jane had no special questions, beyond saying she hoped Seth would continue with material on Frameworks 1 and 2. She was very relaxed, and expressed qualifications about having s session; she did want to try, though.

(Before the session we discussed the one séance we've ever tried, and which is described in Chapter 3 of The Seth Material. *I said that the spectacular results obtained had seemed to come straight out of Framework 2. We also discussed the long essay on early man in* Time *for November 7, and I remarked that I'd like to ask Seth some questions about the state of our present "knowledge" about our heritage.*

(Once again I note that Jane's physical improvements continue as described in recent sessions. She now sits down much more easily than in the past, with more ease even than she did last week. She sat down three times today in the bathroom, for instance, the most she's done so since a little over four years ago, as we figured it. Jane laughed that she'd have made it four times in a row if Willy hadn't interfered.

(Incidentally, Willy One died on November 5, last year.)
Good evening.
("Good evening, Seth.")

Now: in Ruburt's story of *Emir*, he presents a theoretical new earth, yet in the truest meaning of that term, earth is ever-new, for fresh energy comes into the exterior world from an interior source.

Framework 2 is a source of ever-renewing energy. Now generally you believe that the body must wear down, become slower, that you are given so much energy at birth—a hypothetical but definite amount, which is then used up heartbeat by heartbeat. Those beliefs of course program your emotions, and bring about their own evidence.

Each creature in its way is born with great expectations, and attempts to use whatever abilities it has to the fullest, to exercise them, and simply to thrill in their use. The day before Willy *(One)* died, his <u>expectations</u> were no different than they were when he was a kitten. His illness made performance more difficult, and yet in periods of rest he would start out again expecting to make the same leaps, and so often he did.

He did not wear himself out with worry, and so he lived a long life. The body must die. There are many means and methods, but it must not necessarily slow down for need of energy. Framework 2 provides an energy as vital as any given you at birth, and that energy constantly <u>renews</u> the body. I want you to understand that renewal. Literally, portions of your physical being are as new as at your birth. You have new skin. Within the framework of physical reality, then, granting the necessity for death, the body has renewing qualities that come to it from Framework 2. The cells of your body are immersed in Framework 2's reality. Your cells have great expectations on their own, and rejoice to use their abilities and perform their functions.

The spontaneous self, the creative self, is also immersed in Framework 2, and the creative conscious mind springs from there also, even though its focus must of necessity be in Framework 1's world of space and time.

When for whatever reason you feel unsafe over a long period of time, or when you begin to retreat, in a <u>frightened</u> fashion—for there are many kinds of retreat—then you cut down your options to whatever degree, and you must of necessity cut down your expectations also. Under certain conditions in one area or another, or sometimes in many, you have dire expectations. There are too many people who expect the worst from you, yet even then the creative self will try from Framework 2 to bring <u>all</u> resources possible, through dreams and intuitions, to alter that pessimistic progress.

To that degree people are saved from themselves, so to speak, far more often than they realize. In Framework 2 <u>all</u> resources and knowledge are available. The position of everyone on the planet is known. The plans of each person are registered, with all of their probable variations. Dreams events are not only registered there, but their possible effects upon daily life on an individual and mass basis.

Look at Ruburt's Turkish dream. It was as real in Framework 2 as a dish or an apple. An apple rolls if it is on sloping ground, and you can watch its progress. Ruburt's dream had motion also, rolling, say, off the edge of Framework 2 into Framework 1, where lo and behold it changes its form and becomes a book.

Now: in somewhat the same way, Ruburt's more or less newly optimistic thoughts are inserted, say, in the opposite direction, into Framework 2, where then they find their best creative form: in this case they roll into Framework 1 as increased mobility.

As I mentioned, a desire that is fitting to your nature automatically in Framework 2 collects all of the resources necessary to bring about its fulfillment in Framework 1. Because the desire is one fitting to an individual nature, it is also fitting in with the overall purposes of nature in general, so that the desire also attracts the limitless resources that are behind nature's own majesty and power.

The individual is working with his nature, and with nature in general, rather than against it. This causes a transforming reorganization of energy, thought, and creativity—a vast transforming process, for behind the individual is the entire good intent of nature, which springs from the resources of Framework 2.

Take your break.

(10:10. Jane now felt so relaxed that she didn't know whether she could continue the session, or would even want to. We sat waiting to see what would happen. Resume at 10:20.)

In a basic manner, physical events are formed originally in Framework 2, where all the necessary computations are done in terms of probabilities, so that physical events then mesh properly in space and time.

In a manner of speaking, and to a certain extent, one level of dreaming almost always involves a probable event that may or may not be actualized. That portion is taken into consideration, <u>along with the same portion of all other dreams</u>, so that the raw material for future events is processed. This occurs on a global basis, and is an everchanging process, for free will always operates, and the field of probabilities constantly changes.

In this way private and mass events click together.

This will be a brief session. All of Ruburt's improvements, however, spring directly from the fact that he is freeing his desire to walk, stating it in Framework 2, where it is being brought to pass.

You will indeed continue to have other experiences with Framework 2, some of a most significant and quite noticeable nature. Remember that such a clear intent is like a key, opening in Framework 2 all the resources necessary. There, however, the desire is "magnified." It grows in that nutritious creative medium, so that everything falls into place.

Remind me, however, of your question about early man, and I will give you some material for it at our next session.

I want Ruburt to relax now, and will utilize part of the energy for this session in my own way to further his psychic faith and physical improvements.

His interpretation of your dream *(about my father; see my notebook)* was correct.

My heartiest regards and a fond good evening to you, and *(pointing to Willy Two, who was jammed up against my left leg and elbow as I tried to write)* to your friend there.

("Okay, Seth. Thank you."

(10:32. Jane was very relaxed. She said she could have continued the session, yet decided not to.

(I'll note here a small sign of the workings of Framework 2. Today I received a letter from the secretary of the British Psychic Society, Eleanor O'Keefe, thanking us for sending her an autographed copy of Cézanne *a couple of weeks ago. She remarked upon something that at first escaped us both: her interest in art. Hence, I'd decided to send her a book on art, derived through Jane's trance abilities. At the same time, I told Jane, we shouldn't attach too much significance to this, since we've been sending out* only *Cézanne books—that is, anyone we send a book to gets one on art.*

(It's of further interest to note that no sooner had I mailed a letter to Ms. O'Keefe this morning, asking her help in locating an address in London, than her letter was delivered at our door upon our return from the post office. I asked her help re the address of a physicist in London, to whom I thought of sending a copy of "Unknown" Reality. *We'll see what turn this little story takes next. Incidentally, Ms. O'Keefe wrote us that Jane's* Cézanne *would be in the library of the British Psychic Society. Who knows what might happen?*

(Ms. O'Keefe also noted that she knew of the Seth books, and would now start reading them.)

DELETED SESSION
NOVEMBER 12, 1977 9:28 PM SATURDAY

(Once again Jane was so relaxed that I suggested she forget the session. She

wanted to have it, though, especially to get more information re Framework 2. Her entire right side, especially in the head-neck area, has been undergoing profound changes, today and during previous days. Things are much looser in certain parts, so much so that at times she feels disoriented because of the unaccustomed changes in posture, etc. Her legs seem longer when she sits, also. These notes don't really do justice to the extent of her bodily changes, improvements, that she's been undergoing. Her subjective changes in feeling have been especially deep. She has periods when her eyes coordinate well; she has learned now that the eye difficulties are deeply involved with the other muscular changes taking place.

(In the last deleted session Seth had promised us some data on early man, but I told Jane to forget that for now. She replied that she'd see how she felt as the session progressed.)

Now, good evening.

("Good evening, Seth.")

Some time ago, I said something to the effect that seeming miracles were simply caused by nature unimpeded.

Nature's source, in the terms in which we have been speaking, comes from Framework 2. There, all of nature's true potentials lie ready to be actualized according to the circumstances and conditions, the needs and desires, of the natural creature in Framework 1. The true potentials of nature are hardly suspected in most areas.

Since the nature of Framework 1 constantly flows into it from Framework 2, then Framework 2 is responsible for the shapes, forms, the behavior, the potentials of nature as you know it. When you are working with Framework 2 you are indeed working with nature in the most basic way. In childhood you do this automatically. You do not question the gifts of the gods, so to speak.

Ruburt's physical condition was the result of nature impeded. You cannot really know your neighbor's subjective reality. Some people throughout their lives merge the two Frameworks unconsciously in a childlike manner. Others begin early to concentrate in Framework 1, so that Framework 2 goes more and more out of focus. Because you <u>are</u> natural, however, your existence is couched in Framework 2, and to some extent you are even saved at times from your own beliefs because additional insights or solutions are directly inserted into your mind in the dream state, or in other moments of the day.

Often such information will be given time and time again, in different ways, until its importance is finally impressed upon your mind. You may have a series of dreams, all in one way or another stating the message. Whether or not you remember the dreams, or can interpret them, they will be, in a dream-drama series, painting the reality of the world in a new fashion, giving the significant clues, and to some extent altering habitual psychic organization.

In <u>a manner of speaking</u>, now, such dreams can operate as, say, posthypnotic suggestion, so that you begin to react in a new way, without perhaps knowing why.

The kind of dream Ruburt interpreted for you, about the Cézanne exhibition, is an example of an excellent message dream, important enough to come to consciousness because you were ready. Then, you consciously assimilate the information, and add the strength and power of the conscious mind, and conscious intent, to the power of the dream's message.

(The dream Seth refers to happened on Wednesday morning, November 9, 1977, and Jane did an excellent job of interpreting it. The dream actually reviews the whole of Jane's and my life together, our motives and actions, fears and beliefs, etc.)

Once you begin consciously working with Framework 2, help, support, solutions, all begin to come, for you line up your conscious faculties with your unconscious ones, in the most beneficial way, and your conscious goals fit in with your unconscious natural goals—the primary ones given you at birth. You are set right with yourself again.

Again, this process automatically brings about powerful beneficial changes. Any misconceptions, contradictions, seeming dilemmas, are resolved, for now you are not going against your own nature but with it, and from Framework 2 you draw out the greatest natural potentials that are uniquely yours.

(9:48.) You are both doing very well. In a way, as Ruburt mentally changes his significances, so does the body. It responds to even physical data in a new way. Vast inner changes have occurred this week, that will make the actual normal locomotion possible. Your suggestion about elimination was a great help, for this automatically means that the body is exercised more in walking, and that bodily wastes are eliminated much more readily, hastening recovery. The body will feel less sluggish.

Ruburt's <u>response</u> to the suggestion means that his attitudes are indeed changing for the better. Your intent is specific, and should be stated as such, as Ruburt is doing, but that specific intent draws multitudinous areas into actualization, and Ruburt will feel himself more and more supported in both his physical and creative endeavors.

Framework 2, again, in a way magnifies your intent. The work done there is out of all proportion to the effort expended once your intent is clear, and the clear desire stated. Framework 2 is a powerhouse from which physical energy springs. It flows, that energy, to you automatically. Only when you say "I do not want it in this area," do you cut down on that energy flow.

Give us a moment.... Very briefly now, for this will be a short session. In your terms of history, man appeared in several different stages, or ages is a better word. Not from an animal ancestor in the way generally supposed. There <u>were</u> men-animals, but they were not your stock. They did not lead to anything. They were species in their own right.

There were animal-men. The terms are for your convenience. In some species the animallike tendencies predominated, in others the manlike tendencies predominated. Some were more like men, some more like animals.

The Russian steppes had a particular giant-sized species. Some also I believe in Spain—that area.

There is considerable confusion, for that matter, as to the geological ages as they are understood. Such species existed in many of these ages. Man, as you think of him, shared the earth with the other creatures just mentioned. In those terms so-called modern man, with your skull structure and so forth, existed alongside of the creatures now supposed to be his ancestors.

(10:06.) Give us a moment.... There was some rivalry between these groups, some cooperation. Several species, say, of modern man died out. There was some mating between these groups—that is, of all of the groups—at various times.

The brain capacities of your particular species were always the same. Give us a moment.... *(Long pause.)* Many of the man-animal groups had their own communities. They might seem limited to you, yet they combined animal and human characteristics beautifully, and they used tools quite well. In a manner of speaking they had the earth to themselves for many centuries, in that modern man did not compete with them.

Both the men-animals and the animal-men were born with stronger instincts. They did not need long periods of protection as infants, but in an animal fashion were physically more agile at younger ages than, say, the human infant.

The earth has gone through entire cycles unsuspected by your scientists. <u>Modern</u> man, then, existed with other manlike species, and appeared in many different places on the earth, <u>and at different ages</u>.

Give us a moment.... There were then also animal-man and man-animal civilizations of their kinds, and there were complete civilizations of modern man, existing before the ages now given for, say, the birth of writing. *(3100 BC.)*

Take your break, or end the session.

("We'll take the break.")

(10:20–10:32.)

Now: this will be brief.

You are indeed affecting sales for the better, through Framework 2, because you intent has become clearer. Before, that intent was diminished as far as its effect was concerned, by your fears, your concern about details, your worries about too many visitors, or demands.

(Evidently our concentration on increased sales is working. Tam wrote us this week that he thinks so, and that "sales have never been better. There are also no returns." The lack of returns lately, I told Jane, might be the best sign of all. Naturally we want to see much more evidence of our concentration; this should automatically come if we are indeed on the right track.

(At the very least, the fact that we're even concentrating on greater sales marks a great improvement for us, a great change of attitude.)

Framework 2 brings about your desire, but also considers it in the light of your entire life situation, so that it comes about in the best way possible, fitting in with your natures. The clear intent, then, takes it for granted that the results will indeed be highly beneficial, and not cause detriments.

Your growing faith in Framework 2 about Ruburt's condition has also helped free your intent about selling books. Before, you tied Ruburt's physical problems in with the selling of the books. Several important joint areas are clearing in Ruburt's body. New tendons and muscles are stretching, and the large forehead area is now being relieved.

He is working well then with his methods. You should read a few of the later sessions, however, to keep the characteristics of Framework 2 in mind.

("Can I ask a question?")

You may.

("Our sales have increased but our mail has dropped off quite a bit. It seems like the two things have taken place together. I'm wondering whether there's any connection, or whether the mail thing has taken place for other reasons.")

For one thing, Ruburt sent out messages that he had enough mail for a while. This fits in with Framework 2, because it was known he needed the weekends right now to relax. The time of the year had something to do with it, for many people are already spending spare time Christmas shopping.

Some of the people most influenced by the books, however, particularly *"Unknown" Reality* and *Cézanne*, are the kind of people who will take time to digest the books before writing. There will most probably be an increase in mail. You are setting forces working for you in Framework 2. Some of the results show and some do not as yet.

It is important that you keep your intent with Ruburt clear, that he will walk properly, that the books will sell well in a second instance, and then trust that the pieces of the completed pattern will all fall into place in Framework 1, as indeed they shall.

End of session.

("Thank you.")

Look to your dreams, then, and keep your eyes open for further connections in Framework 2. And a fond good evening.

("Okay. Thank you very much. Good night."

(10:45 PM. The session had lasted longer than I thought it would. Seth's news about the reasons for the slackening mail fit in with some of our own speculations. I suggested to Jane that we try an experiment: we'd start concentrating on more mail reaching us, as we are doing now on her physical condition and increased sales, and see what happens.

(I thought this would be an interesting experiment to try because we could turn it on and off at will. This would also give us a great chance to check it out over a longer period of time. Jane agreed to try it.)

DELETED SESSION
NOVEMBER 14, 1977 9:37 PM MONDAY

(This evening I finished Appendix 18 for Volume 2 of "Unknown" Reality, *and Jane read it. At the same time she was experiencing rather profound physical changes in both her legs and feet, as she demonstrated for me. Her hips were also more flexible. Once again she felt somewhat disoriented, and once again I suggested that she forego the session. But as before, she wanted to try having it.*

(Today we received an acknowledgement from the artist, Raphael Soyer, to whom I'd sent a copy of Cézanne *a week or so ago. He told us he was reading the book.*

Now: good evening—

("Good evening, Seth.")

—and a few remarks to clear up some issues in our last session.

There were "modern," or highly sophisticated civilizations, utilizing some technology, long before the dates given for the invention of writing *(about 3100 BC).* Writing was invented and reinvented the art lost, then reemerging.

There were languages then long before your earliest evidence of them, and in written form. Your civilization is organized around science and technology, and <u>generally speaking</u>, now, the arts and other schools of knowledge have been <u>largely</u> subsidiary. Long before the time of the Egyptians, now, there were sophisticated societies, utilizing some technologies and advanced in the arts of writing. But these civilizations were not organized around technology, so that the technological advances, while highly sophisticated, were not pursued with the same diligence as in your time, and they were considered novelties—playthings for the wealthy, advanced toys, but not considered in a serious light.

There were several such civilizations, some mainly agriculturally oriented, and in those technology was applied, but generally only for that purpose—to increase agricultural yield. Some were religiously oriented. Some were socially oriented, enjoying a kind of comradeship that would find, for example, television's impersonal communications a mockery of the give-and-take that they enjoyed in personal contacts.

The evidence of much of the writing, the records and so forth, vanished, for some of these civilizations did indeed have paper, of a kind, and printing presses of a kind. As a result, your evidence shows the much later reemergence of writing on more durable objects.

Unfortunately, the evidence for the existence of modernlike societies does not physically remain, for buildings, for example, were not constructed to last. As people lose the kind of ancestral roots that exist in "less advanced" societies, so many sophisticated civilizations, with rapid overturn of goods and products, with printing presses and writing upon fragile paper, are lost to history.

One or two societies had microfilm, but microfilm needs another technological society for its interpretation, where scrawls upon a rock endure physically, to be interpreted by any onlooker.

I said that your conventional geological ages were faulty, along with your theories of the age of the earth, for it is far older than is supposed. Obviously it has changed geographically—that you know. There were vast civilizations, however, where now there is only the endless expanse of the ocean waves, and ruins that most likely will never be discovered, for they are obliterated in the very life of the planet itself.

There <u>were</u> electric batteries *(as we've read lately; see my files)*. There <u>were</u> airplanes *(files)*. There was not a technological organization however as you know it, so that the technological achievements were considered somewhat in a fashion that your society now considers fine art—esthetic, to be collected by the wealthy, delightful, good for collectors but not particularly practical. The aura of the mind of man simply had a different cast.

In a way mental organization itself was different—psychic priorities, if you prefer. Religious ideas of course held their own sway then as they do now. The earth was felt to be a more lively participator, it was personified. Some of this is impossible to explain. People felt that the sun and the moon would be <u>offended</u> if electric lights were used, for example, that in retaliation they might refuse to shine.

Reading was generally accepted. Books were numerous, but reading was done in the daytime. Technology was considered a plaything. Airplanes were not generally used. They were novelties. People identified so with the earth, they could see no reason for <u>fast travel</u>. There were automobiles, again considered as fanciful, technological art.

(10:04.) In one way or another, the race played with technology through the ages, in a subsidiary manner. Almost any of your modern inventions at one time or another existed on the face of the earth in the past, in your terms. Sometimes in a developed manner, or simply in plan form, but never in the same organized domineering fashion.

Your ideas of the history of your species, then, are largely distorted versions of the latest chapter, <u>in those terms</u>.

The poles at one time were reversed. The earth has formed and reformed and reformed. The inner psychic organizations always determine the kind of challenges and civilizations that emerge. There have been civilizations devoted mainly to art, in which all other endeavors were considered subsidiary, and the quality of workmanship was everything, no matter what the product. Mass production was inconceivable, because the originality of each piece of art, or furniture, or bowl, held its value in that manner, and the idea of producing a copy of anything would have been considered ludicrous, or considered an act without reason.

Give us a moment.... Beside all of that, there were cultures advanced enough for space travel, before the numbering of your geological ages. But even those did not organize life about technology in the way that you do. In the tangled areas of time, in one way or another, messages were left from one group of civilizations to another, whether they could be read at once, or not for centuries.

Take your break.

(10:15. No matter what her feelings may have been before tonight's session began, Jane's pace and delivery had been much more animated and energetic than it usually has lately. She felt better at break, also. The material that had come through was quite unexpected. Evidently it had been inspired by our conversation after the last deleted session, about Seth's material on animal-man and man-animal. Now I speculated about trying some drawings or paintings of man-animal, animal-man. Resume at 10:25.)

Now: Ruburt's improvements are accelerating.

If you could see the body with x-ray eyes, or could perceive its activity, you would observe an almost constant reactivation and revitalization of all those parts devoted to motion and locomotion—increased circulation—precisely the amount required: not too much or too little, and overall adjustments, so that all parts of the body are prepared and exercised, so that the final stages of the pattern will then easily seem to fall into place because of the work being done now.

This will be another brief session. The reason for the brief sessions, relatively speaking, has to do with the exercise of the jaw areas, which is being executed in precisely the best fashion, but not being overdone.

As far as your sales are concerned, trust Framework 2 to know exactly where and when the sales should be accelerated, and in what fashions, and do not specify particular books. Be clear in your intent, however, and clear in your faith that the sales increase will benefit all portions of your life, and not cause any problems.

In that instance also, your natures are known, so that the sales increase will happen in a way that beneficially suits all of your other goals, and in no way defeats them.

You can, however, think of what you will do with the money—how you can use it to increase life's enjoyment, which will in turn benefit your work, and others.

Such imaginings can be quite helpful, for you must also take Ruburt's future condition in mind at the same time—a sneaky remark that I threw in, for you do understand what I mean.

Someday you may want to leave money to insure that our books continue to be printed after your deaths. If Ruburt seriously gives seminars, you may want more room, or a different kind of establishment. A vacation. There have been many expectations held in abeyance because you did not feel sure that Ruburt would recover, so your mental attitudes will change.

Continue to do your Framework 2 approaches. You build up interest there, as you do with money in a bank, and you will collect that interest. Ruburt's approach with the phone call *(to Tam)* today was excellent, and that approach can be used in many other areas of your activities by both of you. He felt the contact taking hold, as you did one *(recently)*, working with sales.

You, Joseph, try that with Ruburt's condition, also.

(10:40.) Give us a moment.... In the bathroom procedures, remind Ruburt of spontaneity. That will help, when he spontaneously follows the impulse to go to the bathroom, rather than think he must, for example.

There is a connection on your part between your own interest in the Jewish past, and your art, and the gentleman *(Raphael Soyer)* who is an artist and a twin, to whom you sent *Cézanne*.

I want to emphasize that Framework 2 keeps track of connections beyond your conscious knowledge, and can make computations in the twinkling of an eye. I would also I like him to give suggestions before sleep that in one way or another during the dream state your knowledge of Framework 2 will be increased. That is the end of our session. You can expect further improvements with Ruburt. My heartiest regards and a fond good evening.

("Thank you very much, Seth. Good night." 10:44 PM.)

DELETED SESSION
NOVEMBER 19, 1977 10:07 PM SATURDAY

(The session began later than usual because we watched a television movie on the idea of cloning. Jane had no questions for Seth other than her usual desire that he continue his material on Frameworks 1 and 2. I didn't either, not having taken the time to focus on any.

(I think that some of the material in tonight's session is a reflection, or answer, to an article that Jane read this afternoon, in the British Journal for Psychical Research, September 1977. The piece was written by John Beloff: Psi Phenomena: Causal Versus Acausal Interpretation. *Beloff is one to whom I want to send a copy of* "Unknown" Reality *when we receive copies from Prentice-Hall.*

(Theodore Reff, a professor of art history at Columbia University, to whom I sent a copy of Cézanne *not long ago, sent us his acknowledgment this week, although he has yet to read the book. I told Jane that I was somewhat surprised to hear from him so quickly, and by his evident interest.*

(Jane was again very relaxed before the session. Her improvements continue, although earlier this week both of us fell off our newfound faith in faith to some degree.)

Now, good evening.

(Good evening, Seth.")

It is a meaningful universe. You are known by the universe. In a manner of speaking, some portion of your mental, physical, or spiritual reality is in correspondence with a "like" portion of the universe.

This is difficult to explain. Give us a moment.... It is not just that the universe knows you as you, but that you carry within yourself a knowledge of the universe also, and an innate, intimate, though unconscious, feeling of relationship, and a certain sense of identity with that cosmic heritage. In a manner of speaking, again underlined, and in the terms of this discussion, you bear a correspondence with portions of the universe that you will never visit personally, physically. You carry within you the innate knowledge of other galaxies from which your earth was born.

There is nothing in the universe that does not have meaning, that is not meaningful. That meaningfulness is not only of good intent, but of <u>superlative</u> intent, seeking the greatest possible development and fulfillment of all of its parts. Each creature has its own meaning within it, and that personal meaning fits in with the greatest good of all others.

Following one's own nature, therefore, would ideally lead to the greater fulfillment of the species and the world. When you are thinking in terms of cause and effect you cannot glimpse that greater meaning. It is beyond all questions of beginning and ending, for out of its framework spring such concepts and realities.

Your world is full, however, of hints and clues that are relatively invisible simply because you do not look for them, since they do not fit the overall view of reality that currently rules the civilization.

Scientists look for the objective most of all, and clear-cut cause and effect. They examine what they think of as an impersonal universe. The universe is however personal most of all. It is filled with intimate relationships. It has a subjective rather than an objective basis.

Civilizations do not rise and fall because of weapons, or economics, or technologies. They rise and fall because of the great sway of emotion and belief.

People do not die of disease. They die because of emotion and belief, and because there is a subjective rather than an objective time for dying. You live then in a personal universe, in which each being of whatever degree comes personally in contact with space and time, alive with meaning, alive as a portion of reality that no other being could or can replace.

All of your exterior communication, your physical events, national affairs, and private gatherings, are the result of the interrelationship of subjective realities, whose very basis is not physical at all. The power that moves the world does not come from the world, but at each moment comes <u>into</u> the world. The ordinary events of each day are overloaded with coincidences and significances that are nearly invisible because they are so taken for granted, and they are so multitudinous in number, and fit so perfectly into the framework of the days.

These coincidences do indeed hint at another kind of organization, and throw a different perspective indeed on the nature of events. Those coincidences and significances are indeed giving hints of the actual organization behind the facts of your world. This organization is personally, intimately tuned, in that it gives evidence of a spectacular psychology on another scale that organizes events in a manner that is for each individual personally significant.

It hints at the most precise and powerful focus, so that amid an infinity of data, events can be arranged at times so that two particular people, for example, separated in childhood, could, 30 years later, find themselves living next door to each other. In the meantime, they might have hired detectives, and all objective avenues may have yielded no results, until by chance they meet at the corner grocery.

Before that meeting, while consciously doing what they thought should be done—hiring detectives, searching down clues—they each followed inner directions without knowing it, because you are not taught to think of such things.

(10:40.) Their conscious decisions for making numberless moves, for example, changing jobs perhaps, and the literally numberless decisions involved, were all made consciously for different reasons. They hired detectives to find each other—a clear-cut motive that seemingly had little to do with their own separate personal lives, their jobs, or their families. They could not then see the entire picture, or understand for example that a seemingly innocuous, or even a seemingly unfortunate event, that led from a move to one place from another, had anything to do with the search.

Certainly, when finally the two moved to the same street, neither thought of looking <u>there</u>, consciously. When they met, therefore our hypothetical people, they could only gasp with amazement at the ways of coincidence, and the strange fashion of chance or fate.

You take it for granted that you are alive in a universe that has no feelings, much less any feeling for, or knowledge of, your own desires or intents. You think that it is organized along mechanical lines, or absolute lines, or objective lines, and that any intents that you have exist almost <u>in spite of</u> the organization of the universe.

Science's eyes, at least, have been largely closed, because it does not know how to read the personal script that is written everywhere in the passages of the chromosomes, or in the passages of a poem. The chromosomes above all bear a personal message. They are not hypothetical, <u>generalized</u> plans of an objective species to its offspring, but a genetic message carried tenderly to each specific individual of that species *(intently)*—so uniquely couched that none of those individuals are the same.

Your organized patterns of thought cause you to look in all the wrong places, usually for the wrong reasons.

Ruburt's desire to walk properly and see normally is his own, yet it is also the desire of that greater nature from which his existence springs. He is beginning to release that desire, after being afraid of doing so for fear that his full attempts would not work. In your present circumstances, it was more or less inevitable, generally speaking, that when he began to release that desire, the fears that had earlier impeded its release would also come to the fore.

He began to creatively consider what he would do, and then out of habit projected, at times, his present circumstances, so that they seemed to contradict his hopes. Both of you to some extent did the same thing for the same reasons. Until our hypothetical friends met each other at the corner grocery, it seemed that all of their efforts and searches brought no success. They might even have been living on the same street for a year before the meeting. They had no idea of faith in the terms of which we are speaking, yet in Framework 2 their desires came about—and not as a result of detective work.

In Framework 2 Ruburt's normal walking is coming about in the same fashion, only you have far more clues to which still to some extent you close your eyes, as our hypothetical friends did when they lived on the same street without knowing it.

Ruburt almost every day speaks of a muscle releasing here or there, a new motion, however slight. He reports feelings of certainty, yet overall you have a tendency, shall I say *(with irony)* not to focus upon those new significances, those new coincidences, for you think still "in terms of the evidence." Yet <u>now</u> in so doing you are not being true to the evidence.

(11:03.) You are at times ignoring the significant clues, and seeing them instead as insignificant, in the light of the completed normal picture. Now that causes an additional tension, and impediments in Framework 1 that slow down the process to whatever degree, which is exactly what you want to avoid.

You certainly know consciously the importance of those significant clues, or the body's reasoning or processes. It is not releasing itself with no purpose. It is a meaningful universe. Almost all of your doubts come directly to that point. Either that or you doubt your ability to impress the universe.

You have agreed that Framework 2 exists, that it is helpful. Your faith has been achieved on that point. Ruburt fears at times he cannot impress Framework 2 properly, and becomes impatient with himself. Your faith is not secure there either. You have, however, the clues, and again, begin to organize your reality along those lines—to take each release or new motion, however small, as one part of the puzzle that is falling into place, in line with the greater pattern.

Your conversations, your drives, your mail, the television programs you watch—all of these are involved—involved in that you will be led to watch programs, for example, that in one way or another help the entire picture. The power of the universe is a personal one. When your intent is clear, events fall into place in your lives, from the most minute to the most momentous, that bring that desire to pass.

Thousands of books could be written, showing how such patterns work in individual lives, and in mass encounters. In the most mundane of terms, try to maintain your good spirits. Help each other in that way. Remind Ruburt to think of ideas in his writing. Anything that increases his enjoyment increases his work—in your situation, now—and increases the healing process and his spontaneity.

The worry about the time element is the result of your present concern over whether or not you <u>are</u> affecting Framework 2 properly. You <u>are</u> affecting it properly, but your worry causes impediments.

Ruburt's playing with the cat was of great benefit. Your Tom and Jerry shows are another. A good drama on television helps. Riding is excellent now. You need, both of you, that change of scenery, and familiarity with the countryside, and touch of your world's bustle. Driving downtown is stimulating to Ruburt, but he should not feel out of it at such times, or concentrate upon the comparison between his present and the desired state. Have him tell you his fantasy today of the motel, and his thoughts about it. You must begin to change your mode of thinking, but it will automatically change as you remember what I said about creativity, and stop worrying, both of you. Creative thought is the mode of thought that most clearly approximates Framework 2's mode of organization, and the nature of the universe.

<u>Now</u>—read this session together tomorrow. Take it to heart. My heartiest regards, and a fond good evening, and happy coincidences.

("Okay, Seth.")
<u>Allow them</u>.
("All right. Good night."
(11:25 PM.)

DELETED SESSION
NOVEMBER 21, 1977 9:30 PM MONDAY

(Jane was very relaxed as session time approached; she had been for quite a while. I suggested that she forego the session, but once again she said she wanted to get something on Framework 2, etc. The changes continue to take place in her body, including a periodic trembling in the muscles of her legs [entire body]. Her eyes, generally speaking, are improved—quite a bit at certain distances, and are "holding" the improvements.)

Now: this will indeed be a brief session, for it is an evening of body events, as far as Ruburt is concerned. The last session should be read whenever you feel yourselves falling out of balance with these new ideas. The body was freed to some extent following the session because Ruburt was reassured. The actual transition itself to normal walking is being assured by those changes that are occurring now, making the correct positions finally possible.

Ruburt's brief experiments with the relaxation and energy exercises helped further. The trembling was felt as the result of a spontaneous, sudden increase in motor activity and circulation. It was brief, but enough to reawaken certain motor responses, which will then show themselves in normal rather than exaggerated activity.

His heart action was also quickened, and certain pressures put upon the capillaries and blood vessels, that are needed for normal activity. The feelings of relaxation naturally followed.

When he feels like exerting himself he should do so, and when his body seems to want relaxation, then he should follow that line. The latest series, so to speak, of necessary adjustments are occurring, so that again the relationship between neck and shoulders, with the hips and knees, are beneficially altered.

The important neck areas are being further improved. Without getting involved in contradictions, have him remind himself that the entire process <u>can</u> be easy, and relatively effortless, and will be more so as his faith grows.

The body has its own plan. It knows what it is doing, so try not to second-guess it. I want to point out the efficiency of faith when you feel it, so take advantage of those moments when you feel faith strong in yourself, for at such times you connect with Framework 2 most securely.

Your doubts and fears have their effect, but they do not connect with Framework 2 as securely as faith does, for they do not fit in with the overall, curious and open, courageous elements characteristic of Framework 2's activities. Comparatively speaking, a small number of clearly felt connections with Framework 2 <u>can</u> undo a year's doubts. Your confidence will continue to grow, and Ruburt's inner improvements are accelerating.

Your own faith is also beginning to arouse new confidence in your work, in your painting. Faith does not restrict itself to one area, but shows it effects in all portions of your life.

Your individual and joint psychic activities should also begin a new expansion for the same reasons. The idea of a personal universe is highly important, and I will have more to say in that regard.

Ruburt should relax for the rest of the evening, however, and once again I will add energy that would otherwise have been used for the session. You have heard of time pills. Therefore I will give you some of the energy now from the session, and some when you are in the dream state. Before you sleep remind yourself that extra energy will be available, and that you can use it for a beneficial dream experience of your choice.

End of a brief session, and my heartiest regards.

("Thank you, Seth. Good night.")

(9:49 PM.

(Jane—I did have 3 very hopeful dreams—see dream notebook.)

DELETED SESSION
NOVEMBER 26, 1977 9:44 PM SATURDAY

(Before the session I told Jane I'd like Seth to say more about her eyes. Her vision was somewhat better, but still I was concerned. Then I asked her if she had any questions for Seth. She didn't. I answered that she seldom did because it probably saved her from dealing with certain problems; and as expected, my remarks got a quick reaction.

(Jane repeated several times that she had no questions, except to wonder why "it was taking so long to get over the whole thing," and so forth. "You can put those in." She added that she hoped that in each session "he'll just come up with something that I can use to blaze right through with, that's all." Her physical improvements continued in general terms, although it had seemed to be a slower week.)

Good evening.

("Good evening, Seth.")

Now: you know generally how associations work in your own mind, seemingly bringing memories or images to you out of context—that is, not following the usual patterns of time or cause and effect.

You know also that your own previous memories in this life are all available to you at other than conscious levels. You read without remembering learning to do so. The days or hours spent in school are consciously forgotten. The experiences are utilized constantly, however. Your performance as you read is the result of that forgotten learning process.

Associations are highly personal, bringing together in thought and in dreams highly individualistic constructs in which actual events and fantasized ones come together. In Framework 2 those freer associative patterns are everywhere potent. The associative processes of the world, with their literally infinite capacities for creative constructs, are there available. Your world is first of all a mental one. The organization of Framework 2 is then highly associative.

If you try to get a feeling for the vast sweep apparent in your own private associative processes, you might perhaps gain a slight glimpse of the interworkings that occur when those associations mix and merge with the associations of other individuals. The potential for the creation of events is so staggering in number and yet out of those highly personal charged associations spring the specific concrete events of experience.

The connections among such associations cannot be followed from the standpoint of intellectual logic, for those associations are first of all emotional. Some are more charged than others. Because of culture and religion, an apple may remind many people of the Garden of Eden, or sin. The apple can be used as a general symbol in that way. In deeper terms, however, an apple might be associated with a cellar, a kitchen, a still life, a death, a birth, or with a million other items or events, according to a given individual's own chain of associations.

All of that is known in Framework 2. There, personal and world associations form their own kinds of patterns. There, your thoughts are as actual as physical events, for the physical events could not occur without that inner activity. You have conscious intents. These act as your directional signals. They automatically pull to you what you need from Framework 2, drawing out all of the associations that you need in order to have certain events occur.

Your intents in Framework 2 will automatically attract those whose own intents will correspond with your own plans in whatever way. The same is obviously true for others from their standpoints—loose lines, so to speak, or loose maps for action, or patterns for action, begin to form. This kind of interweaving occurs constantly, so that no relationship of the minutest kind exists without it.

You were quite correct: it was not coincidence, for example, that you heard from Bill Macdonnel just after the Burt Ryerson story. The Spain connection with your friend the traveler, Carlos *(Smith)*, and with the question of foreign translation of the books. There are obviously many patterns—some prominent and some subordinate, but they all work, often invisibly, adding up to seeming coincidences.

(A brief account for possible future use: Around November 17 we received a postcard from Carlos from his winter mooring berth in Alicante, Spain; card dated November 10. On Thanksgiving day, November 24, Carroll Stamp called us to tell us that she'd met Burt Ryerson, who had just returned from Spain. She didn't know where; but Ryerson told her that while over there he'd heard that Jane and I had bought a house in Spain and were moving over there. I found this all quite unbelievable. We don't know whether Carroll's story is distorted, whether Ryerson may have things confused, or what. Evidently Ryerson was in Spain at the same time Carlos was, [and is, of course]. If Ryerson met anyone over there who knows us, we are quite unaware of it. I note these items in case something further develops out of Framework 2.

SESSION 11/26/77 111

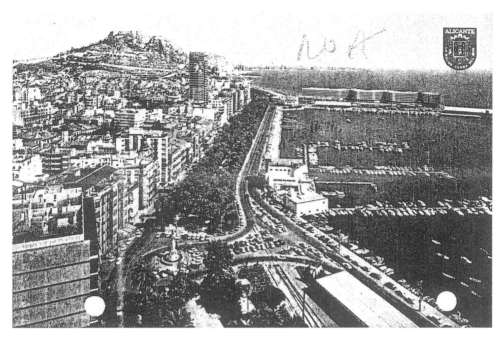

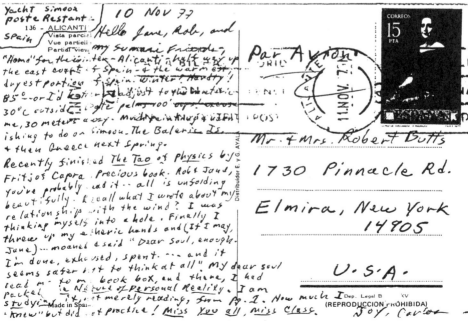

(Carlos Smith's card from Alcanti, Spain.)

(The next day, November 25, Bill Macdonnel called. I told him the Ryerson story. Bill knows Ryerson, and sees him rather often. Bill, Ryerson, and I are artists, of course. Jane also knows Ryerson, much better than I do. Ryerson lives within a couple of blocks of us.... I did think it a Framework 2 operation when Bill called us the day after Carroll told us the Ryerson news, but Jane didn't credit the events like I did, for whatever reasons on her part.

(I didn't think of any foreign book-publishing rights being involved, though, as Seth indicates. Last month we were informed through Tam and personal letter from Switzerland that a foreign translation of Seth Speaks *may be in the works, but nothing concerning Spain that we know of. Tam wrote that Prentice-Hall wouldn't notify us of such deals unless they go through, usually, so perhaps a Spanish publisher has expressed interest? We don't know....*

(It may simply be that Seth was referring to a foreign publisher in any *European country, as one of the ingredients in this story of the workings of Framework 2. Card from Carlos attached to this session for reference if needed.)*

Ruburt discarded that instance, you see. I want to make the point, however, again and again, that physical events spring from mental events.

(10:10.) Ruburt has been worrying, rather than concentrating upon his creative work. Neither of you have moved mentally, even playfully, ahead in terms of imagining what you will do. Ruburt's fantasy that I mentioned—that was an attempt. The imagined motel trip a beginning, a mental move. I suggested you imagine a vacation. Neither of you have done so, though Ruburt did make a few attempts. You must move mentally, and you will move physically.

Ruburt thought of the seminar, or at least of seeing some such people, but then became discouraged. Nor have you helped in that kind of creative endeavor, Joseph, though you have of course in other areas.

You have faith in your work. You use Framework 2 beautifully, both of you, in that regard. Your intents insert plans for action in Framework 2. Ruburt has had some results. The difficulty with walking, <u>physically now</u>, is caused by the head and neck areas, which are being released. Physically now, tension causes the head and neck difficulty. The eye problems are, as I gave them, related.

Let me give you something perhaps more specific. Your remark about doing the dishes, and Ruburt's subsequent use of the stool, led to the breaking up of associations earlier connected with dishes. It allowed earlier <u>pleasant</u> associations to rise to the surface instead. That made possible some further physical relaxation, more pleasant thoughts, and gave him some breathing space.

As you begin to make mental plans for a freer future, the same kind of events happen. Events that before seemed impossible first of all seem <u>perhaps</u> possible, or you can see that they can indeed be carried out right now to some extent, in perhaps a limited fashion. Your mental world becomes freer. That freedom induces physical improvements. You must be free in your imagination. You must learn to reinforce each other's faith in

Ruburt's constant improvements, as you have encouraged each other's faith in your own and each other's creative abilities.

When Ruburt feels blue he does of course show it, yet he is still worried that such moods will weaken your own faith, and the same applies to you. Your thoughts are far more important than any physical act in terms of changing a situation, for <u>only</u> your thoughts will allow you to do so.

I would like Ruburt to make a red star each time during the day he finds himself thinking pleasant or optimistic thoughts, and a large one each day or time he feels a strong surge of faith or exuberance. The game, of course, is to get as many stars as possible, and to improve in that respect from day to day. He is not to count the negative thoughts, for that is not the kind of concentration we want.

(10:28.) This session is highly important. You make mental plans for your creative work. You are both highly reluctant to change your mental habits, much less your physical ones. You have no idea of the creative potential you are missing. The idea of a night in a motel, easily accessible on the ground floor, even with dinner in your room, is a beginning, out of all proportion to any events involved. That particular event or fantasy, nipped in the bud, is simply an example of the way that you nip such possibilities even in your imagination.

I mentioned hypnosis before. A concerted, enthusiastic, united response from both of you did not of course occur. Simple self-hypnosis on Ruburt's part, just to induce physical relaxation, would also be of excellent benefit, <u>because it would mean he was willing</u> to induce relaxation.

Now for all of that, Ruburt does have his intent clear. The body is responding, but not in the ways that you necessarily think it should. You recognize improvements, but you do not see him walking better, and you are not pleased, either of you, with his vision; though it shows that great activity is going on, and that there have been improvements there also.

If you have faith you will not question the means, or the process. The questions of course add to further tension, and inhibit your mental creativity about the condition. I want you to become enthusiastic about my red star exercise. I feel that I must explain to you from A to Z my reasons for initiating it. I must tell you that it can help in a new organization mentally, break down some negative associations, and so forth.

As you allow your mental creativity reign in this direction you automatically bring into play exactly what is necessary to make such creativity practical. You have been afraid of the enthusiasm that you have both felt at different times. When you do feel that way, immediately tell the other. Concentrate, remember those feelings of faith, and encourage them in the other.

Your upbringings have made you think that pessimism is a more practical response—and it is indeed, if trouble is what you are after.

Take your break or end the session if you prefer.
("We'll take the break."
(10:43 —10:51.)
Physically there is nothing wrong with Ruburt's body, except constantly applied tension, partially caused by negative habits of thought.

Loving massage can be of excellent benefit because of what it implies on your part, because of touch, which is important, and because of a certain assurance or reassurance that you can indeed give on another level on such occasions. In such an atmosphere you bypass, or can bypass, conscious layers that are anxious, and communicate a biological and spiritual comfort.

Before, you did not have sufficient faith to be of much help there. You do have latent healing abilities, however, as per a probable self, and in connection with your medical drawings. This will be helpful at your present stages, where earlier both of your attitudes would have stood in the way.

You have been united in so many pursuits, however, and used your creativity together, there is no reason why you cannot do so in this regard. You definitely double your benefits when you add any united moments of faith together. Your Framework 1 exercises, however you do them, done at the same time, increase your effects.

Reading your statements together in the morning is a case in point.

End of session—and use it. My heartiest good wishes to you, and a fond good evening.

("Okay, Seth. Thank you."
(11:00 PM.

(A note: I don't really understand why any sort of Framework 2 connection should arise involving us and Spain, however—the question arose as I typed the rest of the session after writing the notes on page 110-111. Strange, it seems, on the surface at least, that events involving us and Spain should arise, seemingly without our conscious participation or awareness at all. Neither of us is very interested in Spain, per se, or events connected with it. We haven't seen Ryerson in years, and see Bill M. seldom. So what brings all this about? Why is Framework 2 offering us these events?)

DELETED SESSION
NOVEMBER 28, 1977 9:37 PM MONDAY

(Jane has been employing to good effect Seth's suggestion about using the red star, as he gave that idea in the last deleted session. Various changes continue to take place throughout her body. For myself, I wanted Seth's comments on the Spanish Framework 2 connections that he detailed last session, re Ryerson, Macdonnel, our books being translated, and the card from

Carlos Smith; I wondered what had initiated any Framework 2 connections for us via Spain, since we had no interests of note there.

(Last August Jane received a letter from Nelson Hayes, who was one of her professors at Skidmore. Actually, it was a note from him to Prentice-Hall, asking for review copies of the Seth books, and that his note be forwarded to Jane. He wanted her to write him. I kept the letter, finding it after it had been initially misplaced, feeling for some reason that Jane shouldn't answer it at the time: I trusted my intuitions, then. This was before Seth began the Frameworks 1 and 2 material, I believe. Jane mentioned the note at various times, wondering what had happened to it.

(I gave her the note finally on Sunday, and she answered it, so we'll see what develops, if anything. I now felt that it was okay to answer it. She agreed that perhaps originally she wasn't ready to handle it, for whatever reasons. I give this information here because it crops up in the session tonight.

(After supper we discussed various attitudes about work, art, writing, and other subjects that we'd held over the years. Time, money, and so forth. These subjects also show up in the session.

(A note: This noon, Tuesday, I mailed to P/H Jane's manuscript for* James*. She is now working on the epilogue.)

Good evening.

("Good evening, Seth.")

Comments and commentaries.

The Protestant work ethics give you great technology sometimes. Sometimes they provide a backbone, an impetus, a direction, a framework, in which people not specifically gifted can find a place, sometimes. Protestant work ethics do not produce great art, and they can finally undo the good that they have done, by turning all work into a meaningless performance in which the product itself becomes a means to an end, and loses any esthetic value.

The Protestant work ethics lack exuberance. The men who have succeeded within it, the inventors for example, never really fit within its confines. To a certain extent, of course, the impetus in an industrial society is upon throwaway achievement and mass-produced goods. A certain amount of time spent assembling a certain product, performing the same motions over and over on an assembly line, will at the end of a certain period give you a certain number of assembled items. Creativity is the one thing not needed, for the products are to be put together in a fairly regimented fashion.

There are variations, and actually James has explained the natural background there, for it is all tied in with religious, psychological, and scientific beliefs.

In that framework, you each found yourselves artistically gifted. While you went to art school, you recognized that in larger terms art cannot be taught, merely basic techniques. Ruburt recognized that no one can teach you to write. You could not therefore count on a series of well-known steps to bring you to your own, as a carpenter or a doctor, or a dentist *(humorously)* can.

You had no social or cultural framework, then, ready-made for you to follow. Nor did you have any certainty that any self-imposed period of training and learning would succeed in leading you to your goals. In practical terms your goals were nebulous enough, in that there would be no degrees granted you, to say you had achieved them. You also had to survive economically.

Ruburt's reading in college, and his friends there, led him to believe that the artistically gifted were not too well equipped to handle normal living. He thought they were fascinating, charming, self-destructive, and wasted most of their time in emotional and sexual excursions leading nowhere. He was determined not to fall into that trap. He did not realize that the people he knew — Nelson Hayes, for example, and Mauzet—were not basically artists, in this case writers. They would never write the books they talked about. But he made his judgment.

You had highly conflicting ideas about "the world of working people" and the world of the artist. You both made many artificial divisions there, but over the years you became determined, both of you, to spend as much or more time at your work as our hypothetical working man in the factory.

In a manner of speaking, and in the terms of this discussion, you adapted the methods of the Protestant work ethics to your creative endeavors. Lest people decide that you were lax or lazy or irresponsible, you were determined to show that you not only worked as hard as they did, but harder. They might have vacations, but not you. They might quit at five, but not you. I am speaking here of you both. To some degree, you squeezed your exuberance into a tight fit, and tried to make a creative productivity regulate itself, to fit the industrial time clock: so many hours bringing a feeling of virtue, even if the attitude itself cut down on the exuberance of inspiration.

Ruburt as a woman took all precautions so that he would not be considered frivolous. The creative abilities do follow your conscious intents to some degree. One portion of you is not blind to the needs of other portions. The creative abilities are quite capable of helping your physical survival, economically speaking, when they are freely followed. To some degree you both decided that you would ration your freedom. You cannot ration freedom—you have it or you give it up.

What attitudes do you have that still linger? How do you communicate them to each other? You both want Ruburt to walk normally now, and you are seeing results in terms of body releases and improvements. In the past you have been in the habit of putting off "distractions" until this or that book was finished until you were sure that you could cope with freedom. If Ruburt were better completely tomorrow, would he suddenly want to disrupt the whole applecart before *"Unknown"* was finished, and go to Florida?

(If he was, and did, I'd go.)

That question, with its implications, for I have simply taken one example of your fears, is to some extent in each of your minds. Can you handle the possibility of normal activity?—and I tell you that you can. The change of beliefs and feelings, the acceptance of freedom mentally, will vastly accelerate both of your creative abilities, releasing on both of your parts energy that has been withheld.

(10:13.) It has been withheld because you have not understood your creative natures. Your own are obviously not limited to art, per se, or art would have satisfied you so completely, and taken your attention so completely, that you would not have looked in other areas at all, so there is a place meant for you, in which your artistic—meaning painting—writing, and intellectual capacities form a synthesis in which all those abilities take part, and <u>are</u> fulfilled. Spontaneity knows its own order.

In Framework 2 your abilities from birth seek their fulfillment, not at your <u>expense</u>, not despite your own best interests. Your biology, your abilities, your mind and your emotions, are not conflicting elements, one battling the others so that you must fight to attain <u>your</u> goals. In Framework 2, effortlessly all patterns are set into motion at your birth, opening up innumerable probable pathways, each leading to the best fulfillment of your potential, so that events, chance encounters, everything works together.

You both believed you had to fight to survive—particularly as artists—against the society; and Ruburt believed he must fight his own biology.

Your purposes merged. You felt that you had to isolate yourselves <u>to some extent</u> from the world not because you wanted to, which would be all right; and to some extent you wanted to, but because you felt you must. You did not grant that others would understand your pursuits. Or if they did, you felt, they would not honor your intent.

Creativity has its own ebbs and flows. It uses time, but is not used by it. It is not regular as clockwork. It takes time to paint or write, but the great <u>inspirations</u> of painting and writing transcend time, and the feeling of freedom and exuberance can give you in a few hours creative inspirations that have nothing to do with the time involved.

The Spanish connection is important not because of Spain, but because of its international implications: the newer, broader field of your own thought. A small clue in a larger pattern, that your name and works are beginning to <u>pop up</u> more and more in other countries a ripple in an ever-increasing area of activity.

The instances of Framework 2 activity as you become aware of them will show you the true nature of creativity, and acquaint you with the mental feeling of freedom and spontaneity. You have not understood the connections between your work and your life. A problem in a painting or in a book might be solved through an hour's lovemaking, for often what might seem to be a problem of technique is, as you are beginning to understand, an emotional equation instead. None of your impulses are meaningless. You cannot separate your work from your life. Spontaneity <u>as you understand it now</u>, in the light of your knowledge, can only add to your work, for it is not meaningless license, nor is it composed of impulses contrary to your work.

Spontaneity as you are aware of it represents the force of your being, with a full knowledge of your work and intents. It is the voice of inspiration, whether or not you recognize it as such. End of session, or take a break as you prefer.

("We'll take the break."

(10:35–11:05.) If you are born into a time that does not seem conducive to your talents, it is because that society offers needed counterpoints to questions that concern you, or because it provides a particular kind of framework that will color your abilities in a certain direction, bringing out nuances or accomplishments not possible otherwise.

If you are a creator in those terms, you will use any society as a part of your medium. You think of a work of art as composed, say, of a theme or overall design, of various techniques and personal idiosyncrasies; and yet works of art, while transcending time, are indelibly impressed by the times also. A Rembrandt living today would be an entirely different Rembrandt, granted that he used his gifts fully.

You have used your own abilities, both of you, and done well with them despite your overly protective attitudes toward them, and despite methods you used, Ruburt in particular, to insure their use. You cannot cut down physical freedom without inhibiting creative freedom, so to some extent Ruburt's methods have inhibited his creativity. You cannot inhibit spontaneity in one area and not in another, but he did not get it properly through his head that spontaneity did not mean license, or that spontaneity was going to work against his work if he gave it half a chance. *(Very intently.)*

His intent in Framework 2 was so clear that his creative spontaneity was retained to a large degree despite the blankets he threw upon it. He equated, again, the writer or poet as highly gifted but emotionally not stable, so that he <u>thought</u> he had to set himself against his own nature in order to produce.

This is bound to inhibit creative inspiration to some degree. He felt he needed financial freedom in order to work, but in those terms work was equated with the Protestant work ethics, where spontaneity was frowned upon. Artistic work will show its own regularity. It will find its own schedules, but your joint ideas of work hours were meant to fit in with a time-clock puncher's mentality, and not your own.

Left alone, you would both work many hours, but under completely different mental conditions. Left alone, you would both have altered your schedules simply because <u>creative</u> work enjoys variety. You would each have had periods where you worked nights for a while, and then days, or whatever, or when you began work at eight and worked until one in the morning. But you would have felt free to follow the inner scheduling.

In Framework 2, your writing abilities were also known, of course, and they continue to develop, continue to seek for outlet, continue to search for a pattern; despite your relative abandonment of them, they came to the fore. It may not seem so, but only your ideas of time, and not time itself, relatively closes your mind to the idea of a book of your own. For once stated, that desire —which is a desire—would lead to insights and inspirations that would collect in odd hours, scribbled down in a few moments, that would lead quite easily to a finished product.

I want Ruburt, again, to encourage spontaneity in all areas, and to trust that the spontaneity is the result of quite orderly sequences in Framework 2, and of larger patterns of creativity that are not yet consciously apparent. I want him to allow for greater physical spontaneity, to perform a physical act when he feels like it, and for greater psychic and creative spontaneity, both in his working hours and outside them; to concentrate on creativity, not time; for then you use time and it does not use you.

(11:29.) If he feels like a nap, there is a reason for it. He may not be relaxed enough of mind so that that particular nap yields what it is supposed to; then he becomes angry for the lost time. He is afraid that if he trusts himself he will not work the proper number of hours. That is what you have taught each other, as if your natural drives and abilities would not automatically seek their own expression within time, but must be forced to do so.

You began all of this out of natural intent, natural characteristics, natural leanings, because that is the way you are, naturally. Those abilities will naturally work in and through time, without force. You are not going to be interrupted that much. Your worries interrupt you far more, and those interruptions that do occur are often gift horses, providing in another form precisely what you need in your work at that time.

End of session. Read it together. Use it creatively, in time and out of it. My heartiest regards.

("Thank you, Seth. Good night."
(11:35 PM.)

DELETED SESSION
DECEMBER 3, 1977 9:41 PM SATURDAY

("I haven't done spectacularly with those red stars Seth suggested," Jane said, "but as far as the week is concerned I've done pretty good. I had some lapses, especially that one day—Thursday—after I finished the Epilogue for James. I'd get down other times, too, but not for long...."

(At my suggestion Jane has started a notebook in which to record experiences with her "beam of energy," a concept I personally find most interesting, and with out-of-body trips, and other such adventures. She's already added several episodes to her notes.

(She had no idea what Seth would talk about tonight. Neither of us asked any

questions.)

Good evening.

("Good evening, Seth.")

Now: in basic terms you form your reality, privately and en masse—through your beliefs, of course, and those beliefs cause you to organize your psychic world in certain fashions.

You use such belief organizations to concentrate upon certain data and ignore other, so that consciously and unconsciously you organize inner and outer stimuli so that it makes sense according to your beliefs, and forms therefore a more or less dependable framework in which action and response are possible.

History is written according to the present beliefs of a historian in <u>his</u> time. As you know, your western world followed its own mixture of Christianity, Darwinism, and Freudian psychology. Because those ideas still are largely in the mainstream of your society, your television news, newspapers, and magazines are invisibly slanted. <u>The news is invisibly organized to fit certain patterns</u>, so that when you read or hear it, it carries the seemingly indelible mark, confirming the basic beliefs of the culture.

I am not speaking strictly of political parties or political newspapers, or of any specialized journals or magazines, but of the overall pattern displayed by all of your mass communications. You can see easily, however, the highly specialized, intensified view of the world that is apparent in scientific journals. These are in sharp conflict with, for example, religious journals. If you look you can easily become aware of these specialized worlds.

Regardless of these differences, the overall picture is largely the same: you cannot trust yourself, your body, the natural world. You are everywhere presented with the evidence. The headlines speak of problems between nations, mass and private crime, illness. The misuse of animals, man's stupidity and cruelty, so it seems that the species is nearly insane.

Let us look at the invisible organization behind such material, however. I do not want to shock you, but there are quite as many cases of honest heroism as there are crimes committed. There are patterns of highly constructive change that never show, as far as your media is concerned. There are as many people recovering from diseases, even by themselves, as those who succumb. There are compensating, creative earth patterns occurring in terms of energy, but these do not show.

If you do not understand this, then you will take your newspapers and other news unthinkingly, thinking that a fairly adequate picture of world events is being portrayed—a picture that only deepens the negative feelings that are behind the invisible organization of such data. In such a way you miss any significant evidence to the contrary.

Privately, then, you will to some extent or another have to take up defenses against that reality. As long as you think that your physical information about the world, through newspapers and so forth, presents a fairly adequate, objective view of events, then all of the evidence to the contrary will literally be invisible, for you will continue to organize your view of the world in the old way. You will think, for example, when a story about misuse of political power is concerned "That's only <u>one</u> story. How many more politicians do the same thing?"

For the newspapers also act in a <u>suggestive</u> fashion, further programming your expectations. In a way you organize your physical experience as you do your inner life, through association, through emotional association. I am not simple speaking of sensationalism in newspapers or on TV. When you read the news or hear it, however, because of cultural beliefs you are programmed to behave in a certain fashion, in a fashion that validates, seemingly, the concepts of Freud and Darwin, and the most unfortunate aspects of Christian pessimism.

This is not done with any ill intent. Individuals collect the news and write it. To many people, some kind of organization, even one that is wobbly, is far better than facing the task of setting up an entirely new view of reality. The inner structure of most of your organizations and institutions are based on those old precepts. Individual lives have been constructed along those frameworks.

(With gentle irony:) You made a remark earlier this evening to the effect that the individual could do nothing in the face of such organized behavior—a remark that by now I'm sure you regret voicing. *(I laughed.)* Those ideas to begin with began with individuals. The people who make and report the news are individuals. The people who read or view the news are individuals. To some extent through the books you are helping people alter their psychic organizations, to look at the world in a different fashion, and therefore to view a <u>different</u> world—a world in which their experiences are different than they would have been otherwise.

(10:14.) Many people are already beginning to alter their picture of the world, but they are afraid of trusting their own intuitions. Consider the lengthy letter from the young English gentleman. In a large measure, the world in which he now lives is a highly more enjoyable and productive one than it was before.

His experiences are entirely different than they would have been. In terms of probability, he took a new probable road, which means that his individual impact upon the world, and everyone he meets, will also be different and more creative than it would have been before.

Unless Ruburt does, no one will remark about this young man. No one will trace the beneficial change in his life, and their effects upon others.

People generally have been taught to play down their own heroism, and to concentrate upon man's weaknesses, and so your newspapers contain categorized fact upon fact, emphasizing man's errors and stupidities. It has become virtuous to keep track of these, as if concentrating upon errors will do anything but compound them.

I am, again, not telling you to be blind to physical events, but to realize that the news media, and your organizations, are not giving you an "objective" view of the world, but a view compounded and composed by Freudian and Darwinian beliefs. I would also like to remind you both of the difference between direct experience and second-handed tales. Examine your own personal experience with physical reality now and then when you have a moment *(with irony)*, relying only upon your own experience. It is impossible, I know, and not really beneficial, to try to separate yourselves entirely from the cultural world, but you should understand the makeup of that world, and be able now and then at least to separate your private experiences from it, even though they must occur in its context.

How many crimes have you each <u>personally</u> encountered? How many people have been generally well-disposed toward you? How many have been actively vicious? What has actually been your own experience with war, with prejudice, with hatred? How much of your view of reality has been formed by direct experience, and now much has been formed through secondary sources, such as communications media, or tales brought to you by others?

This is an excellent exercise because it puts you in touch with your own experience, and at least gives you a point from which you can make judgments of your own.

Your neighbor, Joe, had pneumonia, or a cold, or the snivels *(upon returning from Florida last week)*. To Margaret he had pneumonia, because she organizes reality in a certain fashion, and by slightly exaggerating certain data, she then uses it to reinforce certain beliefs. She then must take steps of course to protect herself against illness, and she is in fear of robbers for the same reason.

She does not trust her body nor her fellow men. She watches news for stories of illnesses and robbers.

Take your break.

(10:33—10:40.)

Those ideas do not exist alone. They have an emotional effect.

<u>To some extent</u>, it is because you have accepted the newspapers' view of reality as real, that you have allowed yourselves to dwell upon certain attitudes about your fellows—so that for example sometimes the world does not seem to deserve great art; or that you even feel you do not want to share your work with the stupid bastards *(Seth said, staring at me. I laughed again)*.

I am trying to induce Ruburt to drop his muscular armor. In the world of his experience he does not need it. His direct experience has not included it, the cruel adult world that he must protect himself against. It certainly does not include a frightening psychic world, actually or otherwise. Any fears he had there he picked up through reading, or through the reports of others, so let him also separate his private experience in that respect.

Collecting such distorted data about inner or outer worlds can only make an individual build up defenses, or want to. The newspaper world is, then, highly distorted, organized in such a manner that its data reinforce negative beliefs, and constantly give evidence only of negative patterns. These then are taken as an objective picture of the fact world.

All of the heroism, the private and even mass triumph, and the good intent, have been left out. The world is seen as a patient, sick in body, insane of mind, a thing that needs treatment, a Freudian and Darwinian monster. Even with your own changed beliefs, the two of you still see that mirror when you read a newspaper, and do not realize the invisible organizations behind the news. It makes it seem foolhardy to relax, doesn't it? *(Ironically, leaning forward for emphasis.)*

All of these things to some extent stand in the way of Ruburt's recovery. They point precisely to those areas in which both of you heartily agreed, though Ruburt's way of getting work done was not yours. This session must be taken into consideration with other ones, for I am making certain points here that are important, but that do not of course stand alone.

You can if you prefer forget terms like hypnosis, but between tonight's and next Saturday night's session, I strongly advise that you take a half-hour: it can be nap time. Or any time. Have Ruburt lie of the bed comfortably. You sit beside him or lie on the bed as you prefer—but verbally reassure him. Tell his body that the muscles can relax, that you are there, and it is <u>safe</u> for him to let go.

Use relaxation techniques, as in hypnotic techniques, if you want. I have mentioned this before. Often I do not state the reasons for such suggestions. <u>To some extent</u> —underlined and qualified —you hypnotized yourselves into your view of reality. You helped Ruburt form his. You have not taken my suggestion before for a very simple reason: part of you, Joseph, was not ready to reassure Ruburt in such a fashion, for you were not certain that it <u>was</u> safe to relax in such a world, and you did not want to lie to Ruburt because you believed the newspaper world so thoroughly—with all, now, of its implications, as Ruburt did.

Such an event represents an intent on both of your parts, you see, a joint effect, a changing of bodily response to a situation.

(11:01.) The newspapers act as hypnotic suggestion of a potent kind. There is no one present who can confirm the newspaper's evidence. You cannot ask questions of a newspaper, or of a news program. The entire pattern of these latest sessions deals with your inner reactions to your beliefs about yourselves and the world. Tonight I am dealing

with a specific area. To some extent, however, these newspaper beliefs shut you off from full utilization from Framework 2's potency.

Hopefully, I am teaching you to reorganize your inner lives, so that you attract the best to yourselves from inner and outer reality. Your suggestions to Ruburt along psychic lines were excellent—that he do more energy experiments. His own intention to try out-of-body experiments again is also excellent because it shows a change of intent.

I want you to encourage his bodily relaxation in the same manner, creatively. You do not take chances, creatively or any other way, unless you allow your curiosity and exuberance some free play.

If the world seems too unsafe, you set up projections often against shadows, because you have accepted those shadows unthinkingly as facts. Those ideas, mentioned earlier, even inhibit the free creative flow of our books into the world <u>to some extent</u>, for you do not have as clear a channel as possible.

Never compare the sale of our books to the sale of other books. Different realities are involved—and you can <u>then</u> get involved with cross purposes.

I have said what I intended to say. Again, these sessions are more packed than you realize. Each suggestion I give you is not only given for a reason, but has within it potentials that of course remain latent unless the suggestion is followed.

Do you have any questions?

("No, I guess not.")

There is a pattern to your own dream life, however, that is emerging, and the suggestion I gave you this evening, involving Ruburt's relaxation, is rather double-barreled in that regard. James had a rather good remark, that the hypnotist must first hypnotize himself—and that is also a double-barreled remark, for my suggestion will benefit both of you also in other areas.

Now what I want and what I get from you two is sometimes different. I want to establish a habit beginning with tonight's suggestions, with you reassuring Ruburt.

For a while I would like that done twice weekly. Then, however, I would like you each, for one-half hour twice a week, to use your own separate relaxation techniques. Such exercises state and reinforce your intent, reinforce it through physical action, and the relaxation will set you free in your psychic endeavors, bringing your nightly dreams into clearer focus, because you are setting up consciously a better relationship between your mind and your body.

I would prefer that those exercises not be forgotten, for I know their benefit.

<u>End of session</u>.
("Thank you, Seth.")
A fond good evening.

("The same to you."

(11:18 PM. Jane's trance delivery had marched right along through the evening. I thought the session an excellent one. I'm still surprised, I guess, that even after all his efforts, Seth can creatively come up with fresh approaches to try to help us—this time through our examining our worlds through our personal experiences. This may not be the first time he's ever mentioned this approach, but still it's presented tonight with a new twist. I can only partially put what I mean into words.

(For those reasons I got a charge out of the session. Yet at the same time in a way I feel sorry for Seth, for his unceasing efforts to help seem to usually fall on infertile ground. Perhaps his attempts to reach us are often like battering at a brick wall. Although I liked the ideas in the session, then, in another way I found it discouraging, for it's also saying that after all this time we're still left to struggle with the old challenges; it hardly seems that we've moved very far off dead center, I guess. I often wonder at the great difference between Seth's thinking and ours, yet fully agree that the three of us are closely involved. Is it possible then that although we may be closely linked, we're also quite separate in vital ways? This seemingly contradictory state of affairs may be the best evidence of all that Seth is truly what he says he is—"a personality energy essence, no longer focused in physical reality.")

DELETED SESSION
DECEMBER 5, 1977 9:25 PM MONDAY

(This afternoon, as Seth suggested I do in the last session, I gave Jane beneficial suggestions for 15 minutes or so at naptime, until my voice became tired. I didn't try outright to hypnotize her, although certainly hypnotic factors must have been involved. I stressed her general relaxation, mentioning each part of her body often. I used the word "heavy" several times also, meaning that she could be aware of the normal weight of her body, but later wondered if it was a good word to use. Jane enjoyed the experience; she lay on her right side with her face covered, and I sat beside the bed. After I'd finished Jane said that although the experience was enjoyable she didn't feel "anything great." Then we slept.

(When we woke up from our naps, however, we were considerably surprised, for it appeared that the suggestions had taken rather deep effect after all. Jane was so relaxed that she could hardly walk. She yawned again and again, and finally made it out to the couch for supper. Her head rolled, her limbs seemed to behave on their own at times. Her body had spells of shivering, although she said she wasn't cold in the usual sense. I got her a sweater. The expression Jane used to describe her

state was that she felt "more physically content" than she had for a long time.

(*I was really pleased. As we talked Jane said Seth was around, and she gave me a capsule summary of what he'd have said had we held a session. It had to do with the power of suggestion, our reluctance to use it, and so forth. It's explored more fully in the session below, yet I also feel, from the description Jane gave me at the time, that Seth explores the whole thing from a different angle, too.*

(*Jane did want to try the session, even though she was so content. She's also going to write her own account for her energy notebook. Even now I'm aware of how to proceed with future episodes of suggestion, and will try to implement the ideas. I also forgot to mention anything about Jane's eyes, which should have been done. I also didn't ask Seth about Jane's delayed reaction to the suggestions, so am making a note of that for next Saturday's session, at Jane's request. All in all, the affair was a great success, we feel, and most encouraging. We may have learned a great lesson.*)

Good evening.

("*Good evening, Seth.*")

Now: you use suggestion very well. Everyone does. People use words somewhat in the way that you might use dream images. One word carries many meanings, and no matter how spontaneously it seems you speak, even the most mundane remark is carefully chosen so that it serves as the spoken symbol for many unspoken ones.

Animals not only enjoy the sounds that they make, they are to some extent enchanted by them. The animals' interior world is silent. The sound of an animal's hoof upon the ground fills it with a sense of power and affirmation. The cat's meow *(amused)* is as enchanting to the cat as to its owner—meaningful sounds that communicate feeling. These are enjoyed by all such species. Man's language, and the sound of the words, brings the greatest sense of accomplishment, biologically and psychically. The infant's discovery that it can communicate in such a way is indeed magical to it. No matter how wasteful with words a person might seem to be, each one contains an amazing economy, and is chosen precisely because it is a perfect carrier for certain intents or feelings that are all organized by that word. There are many obvious simple examples, such as the word "home," which can automatically organize psychic, emotional, geographical, natural, and time information.

In your daily lives, then, you use words so easily that you often overlook their power. You do not understand their implications, or the great inner organization that is behind the most simple utterance.

(*9:30. The telephone began to ring.*) Do as you wish.

("*Maybe it'll stop,*" *I said. We waited. Then:*)

Now: you use words and their suggestive elements to reinforce and communicate your own purposes, beliefs, and intents. There are all kinds of verbal and body signs that tell you which words are to be attended to more than others, so that the quality of the words is strengthened or qualified. In a family, certain phrases are spoken over and over again through the years. The power of those communications rides upon the same kind of symbolism as dream images, in which each image is actually tightly organized.

You both have had this kind of communication through the years. I am simply stating a few examples. Years ago, when walking down the street with Ruburt, he exuberantly ahead of you, you often said "Slow down." A simple remark. Yet it did contain indeed, at the time, sexual, social, and work implications, and it was carefully chosen. It meant "Don't be so unconventional in public." It meant "Don't be ahead of me sexually," further meaning "Don't want sex when we are involved in other issues." At that time, long past, you were worried and somewhat jealous of Ruburt's work progress. You both knew what that remark meant. That is an example of the kind of remark that acts as potent suggestion on many levels.

Nothing would make Ruburt comply, of course, to the suggestion unless it met with his own acceptance, because of his own fears.

Now look at another remark, made far more often. "You must use your abilities. I know you are highly gifted." That meant "You are highly gifted as a writer." Ruburt did not have to follow that suggestion either, but it also fitted in with his intents. He had his reasons for following it. The most careless remark in any situation is not careless. That is the nature of communication.

Both of you use suggestion individually and together to suit your purposes and your beliefs. You yourselves, had you the time and inclination, could trace such issues as they operated in any area through the years. You felt Ruburt's psychic abilities, particularly in the beginning, so extraordinary, once you accepted them, that you each felt they must be protected—not only from himself, until you understood the abilities, but particularly from anyone who might scoff, ridicule, or attack. You felt in any case to some extent that those with any creative abilities had to so protect themselves.

Your daily conversation over the years has carried a steady stream of suggestion, in which your time must be protected almost at any cost. You have tempered many of those ideas. Suggestion has served you both well in many ways. Years ago you learned how potent suggestion could be when Ruburt used hypnosis with you, and you promptly dropped it. You did not use it with Ruburt, nor did Ruburt make any serious attempts to use it himself. You tried on a role for size, and did not like the fit. Moreover, Ruburt would simply not go to work, and lose writing time to support you so you could paint.

(9:56.) You did not exactly change roles, you modified them. It would be Ruburt who would stay home. He would accept the financial burden gladly, if he could <u>combine</u> it with his writing, and in return you would do much of the household chores. You would have financial security at least so that you could paint without money worries.

You would have a kind of isolation from the world. You did not like galleries, nor the give-and-take with the world. You waned a situation where you could each write and paint relatively undisturbed. Ruburt's relative <u>fame</u> almost upset the applecart, so further measures were taken by both of you. I want it understood that I am using you both as examples here, for such conditions operate in any situation. You began to accept more physical responsibility for the house, and Ruburt let you. In a manner of speaking, you encouraged him to become more dependent in that way, while encouraging him to use his mental and psychic abilities. For these he received verbal reward. He went along, you see, for it suited his purposes also.

As you learned, you went through periods where you tried out alterations. Sometimes you did this together, but as explained some time ago, one or the other would cut the affair short because you were not jointly ready. The suggestions you were each using were invisible to you, while in your creative lives suggestion was quite apparent. Many people have such invisible areas, because it suits their purposes.

Any attempts on Ruburt's part to help more in the kitchen or wherever, will for example now take time, in that you could perform the same chore far quicker —so you will run up against your old beliefs about the value and use of time.

The exercise this evening, and its results, gave you a small preliminary example of the potency of suggestion when you decide to use it jointly for such a purpose.

The actual words you use, again, no matter how spontaneously chosen, have meanings on many levels, and speak of your own intent, Joseph, as much as Ruburt's. Before, you see, when I brought up such issues, you would become defensive, thinking "Must I watch every word I speak?" or "How can suggestion be that important?" Ruburt would react the same.

Yet, in those areas in which you are so proficient such issues would never arise. I do not need to tell you not to tell Ruburt that he is an untalented dumb ox. I do not need to tell Ruburt not to tell you that you are an untalented painter. Such things do not enter your heads. You do not have to watch yourselves every moment, so that you do not give negative suggestions in those areas.

Ruburt constantly tells himself he cannot walk properly. It is reasonable for him to say that now he is <u>not</u> walking properly. The <u>ability</u> to walk properly is his, however. He <u>can</u> walk properly. He has hypnotized himself into believing that he cannot. You have helped reinforce that suggestion, for reasons that should now be obvious.

Now, you take a person gifted as a writer and constantly apply the suggestion that to the contrary the person cannot write. That person will soon stop his efforts. He will do no writing at all after a while. He may write his name on a check, or scrawl an inadequate letter to a relative, and his very handwriting might even deteriorate. The writing ability is still there, though his performance is as impeded as Ruburt's is in his walking.

When you were discussing the letter from the young English gentleman, Ruburt was impressed with his progress. You said "But he was walking," meaning that Ruburt was not. Ruburt is walking—as poorly as our hypothetical writer is writing. His walking is impaired, but the ability is there. Your world <u>is</u> a world of suggestion, for suggestion implies directions, communications to act or not act in certain directions.

No one accepts suggestion against their will, but <u>few people know their will</u>. You are so used to believing that there is a conscious mind that you call the will, and an unconscious mind whose intents are unknown to you, and seemingly not yours, that you, meaning people in general, are unaware of your own will, your own desire, your own intent. You are unaware as a people of your entire consciousness, and I am speaking now in pragmatic terms, not in esoteric ones.

(10:24.) An exercise such as this evening's simply allows you to unify your will with your body, and bridge the gap of separation artificially formed, to quiet the panic, to unify the so-called conscious and unconscious, and such exercises will release energy, not only for Ruburt's recovery, but will automatically revive your psychic lives. You are taking conscious control of the magic of words, in order to use them for new intents, and to dramatically change the old ones.

Unknowingly you went through the same process, when you initiated what you are now trying to get out of. There were no formal sessions, but there were impediments, for at that time you were momentarily convinced of your own physical difficulties. You had to suggest yourself out of those, with Ruburt's help. You had to convince yourself that you were not only capable, but physically capable enough to take over for Ruburt—and this at a time when he was carrying the heavy packages up the stairs.

He was not even making any money at his writing. In the face of that, you became the physically agile one. All of this was accomplished through suggestion. In a variety of ways, Ruburt was rewarded for mental and psychic spontaneity. You were rewarded for physical agility, and for your painting. He was discouraged from physical activity, and social spontaneity. This served for many years. Ruburt's strong constitution is amazing. Even his overall moods remained exuberant for years. There was no need to change for some time.

Your growing understanding, however, began to threaten that framework, for you saw that life itself was an art. In a way, much of what I told you threatened your framework, for my ideas of spontaneity clashed with your beliefs and the need for discipline above all. Your beliefs about time would prevent taking time out for relaxation exercises or for suggestion, as of this evening. You knew how well hypnosis worked, though the term is meaningless.

I would simply like you both, without stressing the issue overduly, to be more aware of your conversations, without <u>monitoring</u> them. See how you use suggestion naturally to reinforce and encourage your creative activities, and how you use it otherwise. You <u>mean</u> what you say. Your words are literal and symbolic at the same time.

It hurts Ruburt to walk. He is convinced of it, he has told himself that so often. One man who wrote you said he got sick to his stomach when he tried to write, and Ruburt could see easily the suggestion operating. Try reversing the suggestion.

Can you write a little longer?

("Yes ")

About Ruburt's predictions *(about yesterday's mail; very successful)*: many people feel such a performance impossible. You know everything there is to know about those issues that concern your lives. That reviewer *(Donald Newlove)* has connections with Ruburt in Framework 2, because of Ruburt's old intents when he published in the male magazines.

He was relaxed this morning to some extent, allowing his abilities to flow, and any psychic experiments he tries now will be beneficial from many standpoints. "Hypnosis" experiments, again, will free your energy flows, both of you. Suggestion operates as an organizer, bringing you from Framework 2 exactly what you want. Your purposes have changed. You now want Ruburt to be flexible physically, to be physically agile. You must alter the suggestion, then, that Ruburt primarily, and you secondarily, have been giving. I will have more to say about suggestion Saturday. For it applies in other than verbal terms, of course.

Objects have suggestive value. For example, I would like one of your badminton rackets, and a birdie, around in sight, for its suggestive value. You need not touch the items for now. I will have some remarks Saturday also about the psychic horror story in the *Enquirer*, stressing the power of suggestion in another area.

End of session, and a hearty suggestive good evening.

("Thank you very much, Seth."

(10:51 PM. As soon as the session ended Jane went right back into her extremely relaxed state. During the session she had been as active and animated as usual, however, her delivery good, etc. But now as she sat on the couch she once more had trouble coordinating. She yawned repeatedly, and so forth.)

DELETED SESSION
DECEMBER 10, 1977 9:55 PM SATURDAY

(Jane wanted to know about the delayed reaction she experienced to my suggestions last Monday, after our first such episode, following Seth's instructions. The effects she felt are described in the notes for the December 5th session. They showed themselves after her nap. I've given Jane suggestions twice since then, the last one being at naptime yesterday. as far as we can tell, her reactions to the first suggestion episode have been the deepest so far. Jane has also given herself one such period of suggestion.

(Today Jane's right leg "definitely felt straighter this afternoon," on two occasions, one of them being after her nap. She'd also noticed similar effects after our first suggestion period. Today her left side of the head, neck and jaw released further, quite a bit more than usual, she said. Her eyes have been generally better. Jane doesn't know which suggestion session —or all of them, say —brought about what effects. Overall, her moods have been better, her walking doesn't hurt as much.

(For Seth tonight she had questions about inoculations of humans and animals. If we create our reality, how come an inoculation will work, even if we don't want it, or don't believe in it? Why would it work even if it could be given to us without our knowing it? And why would an animal respond to an inoculation when it could know nothing about our belief systems, etc? There are a number of questions growing out of the original question.)

Good evening.

("Good evening, Seth.")

Now: you had a delayed reaction in the first session to some degree. This was the result of your own suggestions, for you said that Ruburt's body would continue to relax as he slept.

It is a good idea to use after-suggestions, continuing the benefits during later portions of the day or evening. Some of the relaxation was not apparent, either, until Ruburt began to use his body. You can generally expect two kinds of response—one dealing with relaxation, and the other with better functioning or performance.

The response of relaxation after the first session in fact helped set the stage for the better functioning that Ruburt noticed in various areas of the body this evening. While these may appear together or separately, the relaxation and the functioning continue. In the second session you were tired at the time—tired rather than, say, relaxed yourself. Nevertheless the suggestions you gave at that session allowed particular muscles a further but unnoticed relaxation—also contributing to the neck release Ruburt felt this evening.

The right leg has been preparing for some time to straighten itself further. The process was only noticed today. The late difficulty of the last two weeks or so coming up the garage step has simply been the result of changes in both legs —quite beneficial, although in certain positions, whenever weight must be placed <u>exclusively</u> on one leg, then inequalities come into play. Those inequalities however also cause him to draw upon muscular reserves, and trigger greater strength than he has had.

Coming up the step today, though difficult, actually helped the right leg in its release. You reminded Ruburt of suggestions you gave yourself once. He altered them. Your remarks, however, and his use of them, became an example of creative suggestive behavior, for he seized upon the idea of the luxury of motion, and realized that relaxation <u>is</u> motion. This should be stressed also in your suggestion sessions.

The sessions in a way will be cumulative. There is no need for either of you to fear that the body is suddenly going to relax into a helpless mass. That is hardly any real danger, and represents simply old fears about the nature of relaxation. Ruburt asks you to add suggestions for inspiration. Do so, for this reassures him that relaxation and inspiration do indeed go hand-in-hand.

Watch the suggestions you give yourself about your own writing and *"Unknown"*. Simply be conscious and aware of your own thoughts, for they serve as suggestion.

Your love-making last night was highly beneficial for both of you. The physical activity itself is excellent. It allows the organism to release tensions in a pleasurable manner, beside all of the other benefits I have more than once mentioned.

You did indeed come into good rapport with Framework 2 yourself on the occasion you mentioned *(December 1981; see my dream notebook)*. You can try, gently enough, imagining Framework 2 in your sessions with Ruburt. You fall asleep quickly, yet the simple mental image you use for Framework 2 can be an excellent suggestive tool before sleep.

(10:15.) It is quite true to say that Ruburt has hypnotized himself into his physical condition, because in the past to some extent he believed it necessary. To some extent, a lesser one, and with qualifications, you also believed the same thing, and so the suggestions you gave each other tallied. The fact that you are willing to consciously make an effort to change those suggestions is highly vital. <u>That is the change neither of you were willing to make before</u>.

Ruburt thought of wearing shoes, and when you came home he wore them until nap time. I suggest that he make this more of a habit, for the shoes have a suggestive value, as he well knows. Actually, <u>for now</u>, wearing shoes a good portion of the day is sufficient. For him the change of walking barefooted to wearing shoes and back again, allows the body beneficial alteration of posture.

Try to forget all notions that Ruburt might relax so suddenly that he would be in difficulty —not able to get about, say. He might be too relaxed to get up for an hour or so, or need your help at the moment, but the body is simply not going to collapse if it relaxes, and those ideas could impede your progress. That is exactly what Ruburt has feared, relaxing, so such ideas seem to confirm such needless worries to some degree.

The body is a responsive organism. Your life is dependent upon that intimate relationship between body and mind. You cannot compel a body to be <u>ideally</u> healthy—meaning never indisposed in any way, shape or manner, freed from the slightest ill.

<u>In a way</u>, illnesses are definitely a part of health, for life itself consists of a fine alignment, of imbalances. One disease may actually protect you from a stronger one, or from a detrimental course of action that you might otherwise follow. In the greater realm of activity—I am trying to put this simply—a poor marriage, for example, is on the same level as a chronic but not life-threatening disease. It is not simply that disease is disease, and relationships are relationships, but that the individual generally tries to achieve the best possible conditions for a satisfying spiritual, emotional and physical existence according to beliefs and intents.

At different times in life certain areas may become prerogatives, while other just-as-important areas are largely ignored, or downplayed, in which case they suffer. It is quite useless to say that people's decisions in such matters are right or wrong. They <u>are</u>. The same applies, for example, to national conditions, until finally the ignored areas become so obvious that something must be done.

There is no separation between body and mind, so that the body has emotional considerations to take into consideration also. It has mental reasons for its actions, then, as the mind has physical ones. A poor marriage, for example, bringing years of loneliness or bitterness is, again, the same thing in its way as, say, chronic kidney stones. Such a person <u>may</u>, however, according to intents and beliefs and focus, be in fairly decent physical health —because health may be a prerogative.

The entire life situation may be unpleasant. But I am trying to show that all ills are not necessarily physical ones. There will be changes, I imagine, in your sessions as you mutually move ahead to even greater resolution, so that you <u>dare</u> make suggestions that you might not think of right now.

I am going to end our session. I suggest the following, however. Watch television or whatever, but imagine—lightly, now—a pyramid with each of you at its base, going upward into Framework 2. The energy you sense in whatever program you watch imagine almost like a generator, as energy here drawing power from Framework 2 into the room, into Ruburt's body and your own, activating both your physical and psychic existences.

I have a reason for this, and as I have for everything. I am aware of your questions. Save them for our next session, and do your imagery briefly before bed also.

My heartiest regards, and a fond good evening.

("Thank you, Seth. Good night."

(We were surprised by the session's early conclusion. Jane said she was willing to continue, but.... Both of us tried Seth's energy suggestions as we watched television. We also tried it after we went to bed, but as usual I fell asleep too quickly. So did Jane.)

DELETED SESSION
DECEMBER 12, 1977 9:45 PM MONDAY

(We were preparing to have a suggestion session this afternoon at naptime, when I became upset as a result of our conversation. We didn't carry through, but slept instead. As we waited for tonight's session Jane said she "got sort of down" because of this, yet added that there was no doubt her right leg was doing good things about straightening more. She also had more freedom in that she could swing her arms up and down, further out from her ribs.

(I'd forgotten Jane's questions in the last session, about the inoculation of humans and animals.)

Good Evening.

("Good evening, Seth.")

Now: in large part inoculation, and that type of preventative medicine, is the result of your particular methods of dealing with the world.

Give us a moment.... In historical times as you think of them, pre-industrial man had no need of those particular devices. He dealt with reality differently. It is not necessary to say his way was better, but it was vastly different. Some of this is most difficult to explain in any terms that will make sense, because the entire belief system of your times bears physical evidence of course, that such inoculations work.

The belief has been in the miraculous quality of science, under whose banner such inoculations began. There are, as I told you, literally endless ways of relating to the body and to the world; each one will work—at least enough so that the system seems to hold.

Specific inoculations are given under various conditions. They are bound to affect the biological system. The people who take such inoculations within your own culture, now, usually do so because they do not want the disease specified, and they believe that the inoculation will prevent it. It is impossible to tell ahead of time how many of those individuals would come down with the disease otherwise, yet diseases do come and go whether or not inoculations are given. The mechanisms operate in such a fashion that by now overall belief has come to such a point that the same results would almost be effected if an inoculation of no particular value were given instead. The mind *is* as effective against viruses as anything else—and in such hypothetical cases immune reactions would be set up biologically, through the mind's beliefs.

You cannot afford that kind of method now, because you do not believe that the mind itself can help protect the body against disease caused by bacteria or virus. In many cases, whenever your culture and so-called primitive ones have met, inoculations worked, whether or not the natives believed in a particular inoculation, because they do believe in the "white man's superior power," and were as hypnotized by the white doctor's mystique as they were by their medicine men.

Again, most difficult to explain—for if you believe that diseases are carried by viruses and by bacteria, then the evidence is overwhelming in that regard.

It seems that it is a fact that certain diseases are so transmitted. It seems the sheerest nonsense, on the other hand, to believe that illnesses are caused by spirits or demons. In each system of belief, the evidence however is overwhelming, and in the vast nature of reality both notions are equally beside the point, and one is no truer or more false than the other—a hard pill to swallow for modern man.

The same applies in your treatment of animals. Animals respond to your feeling, your intent. You do not assign beliefs to animals. It seems inconceivable to grant to them anything approaching opinion or belief. It seems they are innocent of both. Animals in fact suffer greatly, for they often become so terrified of modern methods of medicine that an inoculation against one disease promptly brings about the occurrence of another.

Diseases have been wiped out through the use of inoculations. In past cultures, diseases have been wiped out through the intercession of <u>good spirits</u>. The specific nature of inoculations, however, means that more and more become necessary in that system, for the fear of each newly discovered disease becomes paramount—and no time is given, in your terms, now, for the body to respond naturally to those natural conditions, and therefore build up a natural immunity, biologically speaking.

A child is quite aware of its parents' beliefs, and quite aware of the parents' and the doctor's authority. Inoculations have great magical effect upon children in that regard. Infants carry a strong telepathic connection with the mother, which is not severed for some time, so that inoculations given the infant can work in that regard, even as a child can also be protected in other systems when the mother calls upon the appropriate spirit.

You number viruses as people number demons. The cause of epidemics, say, is as I have given it in the early chapters of *Mass Reality*. It is considered to some extent superstitious to beware of preventative inoculations. And yet the body knows that all-in-all, <u>ideally</u>, it does not make sense to inflict even a minute infection or illness upon the body, to introduce foreign elements that have not naturally been <u>accepted</u> by the body in its own context. Therefore often such preventative inoculations—by inoculations I mean here any method of enforced introduction of disease—these methods often bring about other effects of an unfortunate nature.

(10:17.) The entire body biology is often not considered, and the particular individual body is often ignored, so that you have mass-produced potions, produced generally for "the body," and certainly not tailored for any individual body. This is highly disadvantageous, and the effects are impossible to explore as far as the medical profession is concerned.

Individual belief systems come into strong play, of course. You had difficulties yourself with the Salk *(polio)* vaccines. You were afraid to take the treatment and afraid not to. You each had complications. On another occasion you received inoculations—I believe a rabies treatment in California.

("It was for tetanus, after I stepped on a rusty nail," I said. Jane, as Seth, nodded.)

You would not have had difficulty without the inoculation. At the time you did suffer a state of shock initially, but the body could handle that. You need general inoculations now, in the society at large, with children's diseases and so forth, because the belief in the inoculations is so strong.

(*10:25.*) Give us a moment.... I am going carefully, because much of this could be misunderstood. In a way, modern medicine has brought about many of the complications that now assail it. When women had too many children in the past, many did not live to adulthood. In the larger scheme of reality, this provided a framework for individuals to taste infancy or childhood without growing to maturity. It seems like the most heartless lack of compassion to say that such a situation was the most natural, and in the long run for all, the most advantageous. And yet that can be said, for the framework worked, individually, and fit in with the goals of the species. The quality of life is all-important. There were fewer suicides, for those who survived, survived because of their own intent, their own desire, and the young died when it seemed natural to them. They died <u>naturally</u>, that is, and wholeheartedly, and were not torn between life and death.

Take your break.

(*10:32—10:45.*)

This session is somewhat of a potpourri. I wanted to say something, however, about your questions.

(*Recently I'd mentioned to Jane that it would be nice if Seth would say something about the speakers, and counterparts.*)

The speakers, for example, bring information into your system of reality, beyond that body of knowledge physically available to you. They put this into the structure of your times, however, for otherwise it would not be understood at all.

To some degree everyone is a speaker. In deeper terms there are Speakers, with a capital, who specialize. Almost always the arts are involved, and serve as a medium as far as the physical expression is concerned. Beside using such expression, however, the speakers become the voices in people's dreams.

The speakers operate in individual capacity, and yet they affect mass life conditions, for they can point out needed alterations in, say, a political system long before this is apparent. The speakers use language, yet stretch it beyond its means. They are natural communicators, gifted so that their works affect not only the conscious lives of others, but also change and alter dream patterns.

People dream of our books, for instance. They dream of the three of us. We become important symbols, both in their waking and dream lives.

You may not realize how important that is. You are not effecting top-level changes only, meaning surface realities, but the books are reaching into that creative medium of individual and mass dreaming—<u>where all important change must begin</u>.

I will not quibble with either of you, and I am not by any means justifying any of Ruburt's methods, in the unfortunate restraint he has placed upon his body. I would like to make one remark: you do have many lives. Each person knows this on an unconscious basis. Some know it consciously. Any decisions made are made with that in mind.

You might decide, for example, to put all of your eggs in one basket in one life, knowing full well that in another you are taking a seemingly appropriate course of action. This is not the only life <u>you</u> will know. Any challenges, triumphs, or problems must be considered in that light.

If you had but one life to live, it would surely be a tragedy if you made any important errors. It would even be a tragedy if you made none—for whatever road you took would seem to be taken at the expense of numberless, perhaps more promising ones.

(10:59.) Ruburt's body is also a method of communication. It <u>is</u> communication. I want him to give another suggestion for a Turkish reincarnational dream, and I want him to suggest that he see his life in context with others that are equally his own—for from them he can draw greater understanding, energy, and the knowledge that physical vitality, and mental and psychic vitality, go quite well hand in hand. Both last sentences are important.

When he made his earlier choices, leading to his difficulty, he did so in a smaller context, and when he considers his condition, he still does so in the light of one life alone, therefore depriving himself of other knowledge, quite personal, that is available. You will note, if you keep track, that your high and low periods largely correspond, as this afternoon, and the period on Sunday.

I am saying all of this gently. Ruburt became overly concerned, trying too hard. You both let Framework 2 slide in your thoughts—generally speaking. Faith went out the window. If you both read your statements in the morning, and you and Ruburt read his together, that will help you program the day. You can each remind the other when you feel low, at least to read those statements, for the work is easily done there, in Framework 2.

Ruburt's right leg is in the process of stretching and lengthening. The jaw and shoulders are further releasing, but he compared those improvements—which he is aware of—negatively with the completed state of agility he now so desires.

You speed up the process of recovery by relaxing and trusting it. He tried to speed it up by negatively projecting present problems into the future, hoping to scare himself enough so that he would recover more quickly. The main methods, again, for him—one: read the statements in the morning, and when needed otherwise. Two: Ruburt should think of ideas and his writing in those hours devoted to it. He should allow himself creative freedom then. Three: he should remind himself that his desire and intent are impressing Framework 2, and that as much as possible he should relax his efforts here.

Try to do your mutual suggestions when you feel you have a good rapport with Framework 2. You were wise not to do so today. Ruburt did try self-hypnosis then, but he was so overly concerned whether or not he would meet with results that for a while he simply exhausted himself with worry and concern. He held the session regardless, however, and allowed himself breathing space.

It is no tragedy, it is of no matter if on a particular day he thinks from the feeling of his legs he does not want to go out. There are periods of stability, as he knows, when he forgets the issue, and other periods when one leg is "working" more than the other.

It is an error to worry in <u>anticipation</u>. When you are doing well, it is when you are keeping Framework 2 in mind, and when you make an effort to reinforce each other's faith. That is the only effort you need make.

Your own late dreams gave you the message. The creature that disappeared or wilted when you attacked it was doubt. You triumphed when you refused to be at the mercy of your doubts. There is a passage Ruburt read somewhere: "Do not take counsel from your fears"—an excellent piece of advice.

Your own difficulties after shoveling become exaggerated because you also make a division between what you think of as your own mental life as opposed to the world's physical orientation, as if in some way mental life makes you unfit for physical activity. The emphasis upon exercise is vastly overrated. And the most expert athlete can die in his tracks. The body is a mental expression, yet thoughts are physically expressed. There is no physical tremor that is not first a mental one.

(11:24.) As a speaker, I bring into your world information not generally a part of it, and in other terms as speakers yourselves, you contribute your knowledge of the world as it is in your time, along with that vaster knowledge that is a part of your heritage. You are aware of the books we write and of the sessions we hold. You are not aware of the larger ramifications, the communications that continue both while you sleep and while you wake. You are not aware of those greater dimensions of activity that go on as you work at your notes, or familiar with the millions of people who will respond to them in their conscious life, and in the multiconscious level of their dreams. It will help if you keep that in mind.

End of session.

("Very good.")

When you have moments of faith, run and tell the other, no matter what you are doing.

My fond good wishes.

("Thank you, Seth. Good night."

(11:28 PM. Jane's pace had been good throughout, and I thought the material excellent. It is after supper the next day as I type these notes. Jane wants me to add here that she has had many improvements today, in the eyes as well as other parts of the body. We went driving and shopping today, for Christmas, and she enjoyed the trip very much. After supper, sitting on the couch, she experienced what she called a "profound" relaxation—a term, she said, that she seldom used in relation to her condition. She was obviously extremely relaxed, yet did manage to get to the john, then out to her writing room.

(She told me it was hard to describe, but she has a different sensation of weight in her body, as though she's relating better to the floor. The feeling is much like that she experienced following our first suggestion period, she added, where my suggestions produced a different, better sense of bodily weight, even in the soles of her feet. It appears this evening that those suggestions are still operating—or Jane has simply learned from them, and her body is responding accordingly.)

SESSION 815 (DELETED PORTION)
DECEMBER 17, 1977 9:22 PM SATURDAY

(The following material is from the 815th session.

(10:48.) Framework 2—this is not dictation—has been the basis for white and black magic, for example. Both stress the importance of imagery and desire. Your mental images are therefore of course very important, and two of Ruburt's of a negative nature have been broken down. Very important: he got up from the bed quite easily in comparison with earlier behavior last night—surprising himself. That was the result of some of his <u>good work</u> in Framework 2.

He has not had nearly as much difficulty with his trousers in the bathroom, and the old image has been largely altered. He saw himself trying to walk without the table the other morning, spontaneously, and before breakfast—a sign of future physical motion of that nature. He stood at the same time while you put his jacket on, something to him unthinkable a while ago. Those were of considerable importance, yet they were not significantly considered. They were forgotten, generally speaking; not entirely, of course.

He did somewhat better on the garage steps today—because he is, as I said, in a period of transition, and now is able to pull his body higher. The stool was no longer comfortable simply because his muscles were stretching further, but his fear at the seeming poor performance previously led him to some negative projections. Then he had to deal with them, which he did, but they were not necessary.

Mental images are vital. They are more effectively used when playfully executed, and when no contradictions are involved. Ruburt hit on an idea yesterday, and forgot it: he mentally pretended that he was skiing. This is excellent. He doesn't plan to ski. No contradictions are involved, but the imagery involves the assumption of physical mobility.

When you use suggestions, together they should largely be playful, or relaxing, or authoritative. If you give the suggestions then to Ruburt, they must be suggestions you believe in. If you are in a blue mood, or indisposed, of course that is communicated telepathically and otherwise. The same applies to suggestions you give yourself, for example. If you want to relax and you are tense, it is often simpler to bypass the issue, and tell yourself instead to imagine a peaceful scene, in which case you will relax without ordering your muscles to do so. You react to images as well as to words.

Familiar images become imprinted, as your television games can be imprinted upon your TV screen.

I am speaking rather generally right here to make certain rather specific points, however. When you change details of any kind in your life, to some extent you change your mental images. When you change your routine however slightly, you do the same thing. When you change the furniture in the room the same applies. You can use such knowledge often, so that such changes stand for their symbolic inner alterations.

Take the last few sentences and apply them creatively. Such innocent suggestions of mine are usually quite important. Think of unaccustomed physical images, and mentally try them on for size. Some of these will "take," bringing into your experience opportunities that have lain latent. For reasons I will not go into now, and speaking simply, you are coming into a fertile period, each of you—in part because of changed beliefs, so that your relationship with Framework 2 is more intimate, practically speaking, now—and I would like you to take advantage of that.

It will take little extra effort on your part to remind yourself of the significance of your dreams again, and to bring those into a more workable, practical focus.

(*Heartily:*) That is the end of the session unless you have questions.

(*"No, I guess not."*)

Then I will bid you a hearty good evening.
("Thank you very much, Seth. Good night."
(11:12 PM.)

SESSION 816 (DELETED PORTION)
DECEMBER 26, 1977 9:24 PM MONDAY

(The following material is from the 816th session.
(10:22.) I have a few remarks—not new. I want you to keep the difference between the two frameworks in mind, however, in line with what I am saying.

You are both quite in the habit of asking what is wrong—not only in terms of Ruburt's difficulties, but generally speaking. It is difficult to explain what I want to because of your own beliefs and significances that you sometimes form. The young man *(see the 816th session proper)* was really comparing his life and the earth unfavorably with an idealized imagined world, to which he could never return. Just about everything in his experience seemed wrong, and his experience seemed thrust upon him—an exaggerated case, of course.

Yet in a way you each do the same thing, taking it for granted as a fact of existence that there is something wrong with each of you. You should have produced much more and much better art than you have. This seems to be a fact, so that you find yourself blaming yourself at times. There is definitely something wrong with Ruburt. Otherwise he would be walking properly. Ruburt would be walking properly if he did not believe there was something wrong with him.

Much of your mental experience daily is based upon the proposition that there is something wrong with each of you, for one reason or another. Again, it is difficult to say what I want to while still trying to avoid contradictions at your end—and yet it seldom occurs to you that you might just possibly be doing exactly what you were meant to do, or that you are in exactly the right place and time and circumstances.

It seldom occurs to you that you might be fulfilling your purposes quite beautifully despite all of your convictions—for they are indeed convictions—that you are not doing so, or that in some way or another each of you should be different in important ways than you are.

(10:32.) Your young man, your visitor, does indeed suffer torments because he is so thoroughly convinced he is in the wrong place at the wrong time, and all of his unfortunate experiences follow that conviction, which so far he has refused to give up. Incidentally, you both handled that affair very well. You avoided the kind of direct confrontation that would have resulted had you

said, for example "I do not believe your spirit," or "I do not believe he could do thus and so." Your whole attitude showed the young man, however, that he was the one who must examine his own beliefs, and without immediately panicking him you showed by inference your own belief that his delusion was doing him considerable harm.

In the terms in which I am speaking here and tonight, it is a delusion to believe that you should be other than you are in any important manners. Against that delusion you have no recourse, <u>for you cannot be different than you are</u>.

When you hold such a conviction you are always convinced that something is wrong, and your belief brings about a condition which gives you justification for feeling that. Ruburt can say "Of course there is something wrong with me. Look at my condition." But the condition began when he began to believe that he should be different than he is.

Your own chest feelings emerge when you feel you should be different than you are. We are not speaking of perfection, yet you are each perfectly yourselves. The feeling that there is something wrong then begins to become a strong significance in your lives. Without check, it begins to gain its own momentum, so that you become less and less aware of what is right, and more and more begin to focus looking for proof of your conviction.

The inherent rightness of your position cannot be underlined, but your <u>appreciation</u> of it, and your experience of that rightness <u>can</u> be underlined.

Almost in every instance, when you are upset in any way, this is a reflection of your feeling that you should be different than you are—your conviction that you have gone wrong in an important area. That conviction closes off your understanding, so that your own rightness is not apparent, so that a vital dimension is lost, <u>practically</u> speaking.

Often actions that are quite right for you then appear wrong, in the light of your misconceptions. I want you to keep all of this in mind, beginning the new year perhaps on better footing.

The understanding of your own rightness opens up from Framework 2 all kinds of creative opportunities that have been closed to you because your own set ideas have to some extent limited you. These ideas are extremely important. You have yourself, now, inhibited some Nebene material for that reason. Ruburt has inhibited some psychic information for the same reason.

There is a power in simplicity. To concentrate upon what is right opens up greater power than you can presently imagine.

Give us a moment.... The same applies to Ruburt's condition, of course, for he constantly concentrates on what is still wrong. But the material that I have just given should hopefully show him that he has been putting the cart before the horse.

If you have no more questions, I will end the session, and I would respectfully suggest that you take it to heart.

("Thank you very much, Seth.")

A fond good evening.

("The same to you. Good night."

(10:58 PM.)

DELETED SESSION
JANUARY 3, 1978 9:30 PM TUESDAY

(Jane and I have been very upset over the holidays about her eye condition, and my chest disturbances. Both have been very worrisome. I even talked about seeing a doctor on both counts. Our original understanding was that the eye condition would pass rather quickly once Jane began to loosen up—but now it appears to be another fixed state in the general scheme of our lives. We've had a number of discussions about the whole business, and what we can do about any of it. I'm afraid we felt little to cheer about. We planned for a session last night but it didn't develop.

(We haven't paid any attention to the last session, for December 26, 1977, yet it contains a line that I've thought of often since it came through: "Ruburt....constantly concentrates upon what is still wrong." Actually, this is true of both of us. For tonight, then, I wanted a session with answers in it, so that we could try again in spite of past failures. I still felt we didn't know the whole story about the eyes, as well as the other symptoms, and that Jane may have inhibited some material on those topics.

(I was also puzzled about our problems because, as I told Jane before the session, I couldn't see where as individuals we were doing anything so terribly wrong. I added that I wasn't trying to shift blame outside of ourselves—but still, why the extreme reactions we felt? I used the front page of the newspaper as an analogy, saying that it exhibited far worse behavior and beliefs than any we were responsible for, yet the news and world events seemed to be made by individuals who behaved much more badly than we did, and that further the people involved seemed not to suffer any consequences of note, beyond say losing a job or an election, etc. There was much more, which need not be repeated here. I concluded by saying that I did think we had plenty of insight into our own actions—far more than most people did—so why the extreme reactions?)

Now, good evening.

("Good evening. Seth.")

I will try again. Give me time to develop this in my own way.

Forget ideas of good and evil for our discussion. For one thing, men who perform seemingly evil acts but who believe those acts to be right and justified, can be carried along in relative safety for some time before their errors catch up with them, because the power of their own self-approval is so strong.

This does not mean that they will not face consequences, but their self-approval provides a sturdy rudder that holds them often aloft, where most men might perhaps be drowning in the same circumstances. I have given you much information that apparently has not sunken through, and I have couched information in various ways. I have given suggestions for you to follow, many of them, and any of them followed with a sense of purpose —any one of them— would lead you in the proper direction.

You even have some evidence that this is the case. The suggestions have not been followed with any overall sense of purpose or continuity. We will return to that later.

Beneath all of the other issues and reasons at any given time, and perhaps the answer to your earlier voiced question, is the act that, more important than you realize, that for some time in vital areas you have not approved of yourselves. You have not had your own approval. An animal approves of itself unthinkingly. It certainly does not judge itself against any other animal. It knows quite well that some are stronger and some weaker, but it approves of its own uniqueness—glories in it, without having any other picture in its mind of what it <u>should</u> be. It has its own approval.

Ruburt has not had his own approval. The physical symptoms are the physical materialization of that disapproval. They serve as a constant reminder of his imperfections—but <u>imperfections in relationship to what?</u> The same to a lesser extent applies to you.

Ruburt believes he <u>should be</u> a TV personality, a healer, a writer, an excellent psychic versed in all of the most esoteric traditions, a magnetic personality. He believes he should be objectively intellectual, cool and calm, and spontaneous at the same time. He should be in glowing health—<u>glowing</u>—and shine amid the multitude. A rather impossible task, that would make any individual feel quite inferior by contrast.

You expect yourself to be a <u>great</u> artist, lost in the intricacies of what you think of as an artistic emotional reality, innocent of any interfering intellectuality. You berate yourself on the one hand for an intellect <u>that it seems to you separates you</u> from immediate emotional contact with painting and with others. At the same time, of course, you would certainly berate a Van Gogh for his overly emotional behavior.

Your intellect operates beautifully in the notes and appendixes of *"Unknown,"* but instead of rejoicing in it, you wonder if your notes lack the very kind of emotionalism that would make that particular kind of clear intellectual objectivity most difficult. When you are writing you are pleased, finally at least, with the working of your mind—but angry that you are not painting. When you are painting you feel guilty not only because the painting does not bring in money—by now not that much of a concern, only a nagging accusation—but there also you haggle at your intellect. You wish for the intensified emotional preoccupation that would close your mind to all else but painting.

Physical exercise becomes the area between, taking you from both your painting and writing, and furthermore is a reminder, an angry one, that the physical working area—the chores—are largely yours to do.

Ruburt emulates your own work habits, and tries to regulate his creative life so that it bears a resemblance to yours. He tries to be disciplined, put in his time, temper his emotional nature, so neither of you approve of yourselves. *"Unknown"* simply became the platform. It shows the excellent ways in which your natures interact, and that is what the reader will perceive.

(10:00.) It also formed a platform for the ways in which you misunderstand each other, and therefore has served as a symbolic road of contention. The contention is one caused by riches, <u>creative riches</u>, and abundance.

Ruburt's creative work is highly spontaneous. It comes in bursts, in its own way outside of time. He is very impatient at the work involved in inserting it <u>into</u> time. The misunderstandings—and this has been covered—lead to over-reactions on both of your parts, and lead both of you to misinterpret your contributions, because initially you do not approve of yourselves.

You expect yourselves to be different people than you are—<u>not appreciating at all</u> the abilities and characteristics that you do possess, but forever weighing them against other abilities and characteristics that you have told yourselves you should possess.

You have written the equivalent of your own book from a unique standpoint in *"Unknown,"* but neither of you have really been able to recognize that. Ruburt, being true to his spontaneity, would forget publishing details. It is his attempt to try and match your individual methods of thought that confuse him. He is producing his books and mine—a double kind of production that entails almost two publishing schedules.

These books are more than the work of one personality. They cannot be anchored to conventional ideas of time. In a strange fashion, they go faster than your lives, so physically you do have "catch-up time."

Give me a moment.... You have, far more than you realize, utilized our ideas in your daily lives, both to insure financial comfort—but more, to achieve the satisfaction that you are indeed reaching others, helping to change their lives for the better. You have the knowledge that many do not possess—that you are indeed affecting your times.

Because you have that knowledge, you do not realize the frustration felt by those whose words have little if any—overall, now—impact, practically speaking. Your mental and emotional horizons have broadened, so that you now take for granted a mental world that others do indeed, and properly, look upon with wonder.

Your achievements, singly and together, have not brought you the joy they should, because you think indeed that your achievements should lie elsewhere—or that, in the face of the selves you <u>think</u> you should be, your realized selves are almost shoddy versions. This disapproval erodes your attempts to change, Ruburt's in particular.

Beside all that, you are trying to live your lives in a rather unique fashion, so that you are denied in large measure the comforts to which others flock. You see few people, so your moods can go unchecked by others, and you have found no measure to help break negative patterns effectively.

When you <u>do</u>, however, you see results. You pick up each other's negative moods, however, so you ride emotional storms. <u>Ruburt does not feel he can properly see his way out</u>. Your feelings of spontaneity and discipline go back and forth. Ruburt should stop telling himself that he does not want to see people. He may not want to have visitors at times. On other occasions he enjoys spontaneous encounters. The eye problem has to do, physically, with his present stance—the lack of balance between the two sides of his body, causing pressure on one side of the jaw, and the ear canal, which further aggravates the fullness in the sinus, hence affecting the eyes.

Beyond that, however, is the fact that you <u>allow</u> yourselves, and he allows himself, no rest. You know how often, Joseph, you think about Ruburt's condition, and it is not yours. So you can imagine how he is reminded of it with each step.

("Can I ask a question?")

You may.

("How is all of this hooked up with the walking difficulty?" By the question, I meant how has Jane's walking difficulties through the years resulted from her feeling that she should be all those things Seth recounted at the start of this session—a TV personality, a great psychic, writer, and so forth. I didn't make the question clear enough, so Seth answered it in more immediate terms—which is also valuable infor-

mation, of course, that we can act upon. However, the original question remains, and I explained it to Jane after the session; she suggested I ask it again next time.)

He favors <u>at this time</u> one side, and all his weight and emphasis and direction bears him to the right. The left leg is longer so that the stress is presently applied to the right side. Both the angle of his head and jaw, and the position of his arms, are involved. But the neck, those ligaments and muscles, largely bear the strain so that pressure is put upon the jaw on the right side, and this to some extent impedes sinus drainage in that area.

That entire situation however "ideally" should have passed some time ago. Ruburt's individual and your joint fears, however, prolong his tension, lengthening what should be a transitory period.

(10:28.) Give us a moment.... His feeling that his work pattern should be like yours makes him worry when he becomes very relaxed. The suggestions I gave you <u>about</u> suggestion fell short largely because at the same time you could not jointly find a position of calmness. It should be easy for you to see that when Ruburt was ready you were not, or vice versa.

His ommm exercises <u>can</u> serve a good purpose; they calm body and mind at once, that is at the same time, and they can serve you also. They allow a period of disengagement in which the benefits from Framework 2 have time to act. I have said before to apply your creative attitudes in this area—and when you have, again, you have seen results. You have not felt free to express your fears to each other, for fear one will upset the other, and so the fears simply grow and then explode.

Ruburt has not expressed those feelings of hope and faith when he has them, for fear they will lead nowhere, or mislead <u>you</u>. Your friend Bill Gallagher is highly sensitive about eyes because of his own condition. He picked up your joint fears like a sponge, and was highly frightened because of his own fear.

Your feelings of hopelessness must really be confronted when you feel them, otherwise they erode your position. You each have a tendency to over-idealize yourselves, and therefore to find yourselves wanting by contrast. The over-idealization is rigid. A true idealization involves loving thoughts of the development and fulfillment of your abilities to the best possible condition.

<u>It does not involve criticizing creative abilities of your own by comparing them to others that you think you should possess</u>.

My last session was largely ignored by both of you, and yet in it there were important clues. Your own painting is growing <u>despite</u> your own ideas of what you think it should be. *"Unknown"* is a creative triumph despite your joint ideas of what that book should be.

("Jane doesn't like it.")

Despite your joint ideas of what that book should be *(emphatically).*

All of Ruburt's concerns about that book have to do with his impatience in time terms. That has to do with his misunderstanding for he has not seen, really, that he is producing work for two personalities that cannot be squeezed into conventional publishing rhythms.

He quite understands the overall creative triumph. It is only when he tries to become overly literal that he becomes overly concerned with time. He has also reacted to your own doubts and fears about the book, and has picked up often your own ambiguity in that regard. Had he really been so against the idea of the book being produced as it was, he would have said so indeed.

Your feelings of hopelessness are your enemy. They must be encountered, not shoved under the rug. Often one could help the other, but when the feelings are not voiced they go underground. Ruburt should give himself so much time a day—an hour and a half, say—for free creative thought, writing or whatever that turns into poetry, painting? All right.

The work with predictions today, whatever the results, is creative, for it turns his mind into areas that will show results often in completely unpredictable psychic events. When you grab hold of your feelings of creativity, again, you have seen results, and you will see them. The ommm exercises can clear your minds. The freedom of communication will stop the erosion and buildup of fear.

Try those steadily, and give yourselves a chance. They will almost immediately help you with your chest difficulty.

Now I bid you a fond good evening—and I hope you will use this session, with all of its implications.

("Yes. Thank you, Seth. Good night."

(10:52 PM. At session's end Jane felt close to being physically sick, as she does when the material strikes close to home.)

DELETED SESSION
JANUARY 7, 1978 10:17 PM SATURDAY

(The session started at the above hour because of our later-than-usual supper. We'd spent a rather enjoyable day, sleeping a bit later than usual, shopping, doing various chores, roasting a chicken, making a cornbread and watching TV, etc. Jane's eye condition seemed to be better.

(Yesterday had been a different story, though. While at the bank yesterday noon I met Wanda, a nurse who worked in the office of a doctor I'd seen some years ago

for an ear problem. Since I'd been thinking of Wanda rather strongly last week, wondering whether the doctor in question could help Jane and her eye condition, I took our meeting as a clear case of the workings of Framework 2. On impulse I asked Wanda if she could arrange an appointment for Jane, and was surprised to hear that it could be set up for next Monday. Wanda was to call that afternoon and give Jane a time.

(Driving home, I had misgivings about my actions in making the appointment without consulting Jane, but told myself I trusted my impulse and the working of Framework 2. I also felt that Jane would never see a doctor on her own. I was very concerned about her condition, even though she'd recently embarked on a course of exercises and changing beliefs that was evidently beginning to help her. I thought Jane would be able to see the doctor and do her own thing without conflict. Jane, however, reacted strongly when I told her about the appointment. "How could you?—you've just destroyed all the confidence I've managed to build up in the last few days." She ended up in tears, and I felt that I'd made a rather considerable error.

(Note: Strange to say, but at the same time I felt that Jane was more concerned about trying to make it into the doctor's office—"Humiliating myself before all those people"—than she was about her symptoms themselves.

(When Wanda called, however, we learned that her doctor wasn't the kind of specialist Jane should see after all, so the situation was resolved seemingly without effort on our parts. Wanda recommended other doctors. We ended up with Jane more or less on a two-week test period to see if she could get results on her own—although in the light of tonight's session I doubt if the "deadline" matters. I don't envision her seeing a doctor at this time, now. Perhaps the session made me feel even more discouraged—this has happened before—or the evident errors in living on our parts that seemingly have been responsible for the whole situation over the years, certainly seemed beyond the reach of any medical treatment. We'll see what develops.

(Yesterday, also, Jane received the chair I'd ordered as a Christmas present early in December. We also expected Frank Longwell to drop in at noon or thereabouts, since he'd returned from vacation in Santa Marta, Colombia, South America. I mention these things because they too play a part in yesterday's events.)

Now: good evening—

("Good evening, Seth.")

—the Wanda saga.

You both comment often about Ruburt's literal mind, forgetting that it is most knowledgeable as far as symbolic content is concerned. His interpretation of your dreams should make that apparent. So he spoke of his new chair and the Wanda incident and the piece of jewelry *(from Frank)* in one breath. Quite acute.

Framework 2 was involved, and so was the chair and so was Frank's return. In the back of your mind you questioned whether giving him a new, more comfortable chair to work in was or was not a smart thing to do: would it encourage him to retreat to his room and his writing, and simply serve to intensify old conditions? Frank, who was away, had returned, and would visit that day. Your fears, brought to the forefront by the Gallagher episode the week earlier, again surfaced with the event of the chair and Frank's return. Would Ruburt then simply continue seeing Frank now, and the old, it seemed useless, rituals go on?

Furthermore, in the back of your mind, and somewhat at least as a result of the Gallaghers' well-meaning query, you also wondered if you were doing your duty should you not insist that Ruburt receive conventional but definite help? Better that this be set up, it seemed immediately, so that Frank was met with the accomplished fact of a set appointment.

You had indeed thought of Wanda somewhat earlier, quite aware of course of her employer. The episode jelled, however, and at lunch time, when the chair had already been delivered and was an accomplished fact also. Were you just making it more comfortable for Ruburt to continue in old ways?

(*We expected Frank to visit at noontime, as per his call the afternoon before. I quit painting at 11:30 and went to the bank in order to be back home by the time he called. However, Frank didn't see us until about 4:15 PM.*)

That fear led you to make, during your short drive, a quick and quite a desperate entreaty into Framework 2. Wanda had several errands, the bank merely one, and it was her lunch hour. She thought of making the bank trip after lunch—that is, after eating—and instead changed her mind so that you met. She never forgot the help you two gave her one night, when she was frightened, and that connects you to her in Framework 2.

Whenever anyone helps you, you keep track of them unconsciously in Framework 2.

You were unsure of yourself, however. Your fear was definite, and your uncertainty was next. You were quite aware of the fact, unconsciously, that Wanda's employer was in fact not going to work out. He deals with mechanics. He deals with them well. You also wanted Ruburt to be aware of your concern, hoping that the concern would serve to accelerate his own determination and ability, and to trigger his resources so that a medical visit would not indeed be necessary.

You felt guilty about the chair—*(amused:)* not that roller skates would have been a more suitable present. Wanda made sure you could have an appointment if you wanted it. This was arranged through ways impossible to tally, all taking place in Framework 2, with the juggling of appointments days earlier, involving appointments made and not made.

You pulled from Framework 2 exactly what you wanted. Wanda also wanted to repay your old kindness. Frank, who was expected at noon, did not come until later, because unconsciously he was also aware that something of that nature was occurring. He brought you gifts that were replicas of ancient power sources.

(10:37.) Give us a moment.... One or two out of every four or five sessions gets through to you, meaning both of you. Generally in your society, you grow up taught by many sources that self-disapproval is a virtue. Both religion and science, parents and schools, stress that idea, and it is one of the most important causes of mental alienation, spiritual and physical distress.

Behind all of my suggestions and attempts to help you lie realms of historical culture, or personal episodes, that go back to that main unfortunate habit of self-disapproval regarded as virtue. I do not see particularly a benefit to outlining the origin of the concepts throughout history, and you can for yourselves trace them in your personal lives. The intellect's function seems largely that of a critic.

You are taught to question your motives, your behavior, your feelings, and everything but your beliefs. When you really believe disapproval to be a virtue, and you believe in virtue, then you obviously find yourselves in a position where the more you disapprove of yourself the better person you think you are—a contradiction of the most insidious nature, for how can you approve of a self you disapprove of?

In such a quandary all you can do is add disapproval to disapproval, in some twisted hope that somehow some trust or love of the self will ensue.

You take it for granted that something is wrong with you personally. As soon as you buy that you are in trouble, for you will begin to form significances in your behavior to bear out the proposition. This area, hidden, of course, will find materialization, sometimes generally, so that all portions of life have a drab grayness in which the self can never shine.

Other people will refuse such a situation, and accept one mar, or one mar after another—an organ after organ. Another person will lose job after job. Another person will never find a compatible mate. The symptom or symptoms will follow the area in which the person most strongly disapproves of himself—will hide, distort, or exaggerate those tendencies about which the person feels such disapproval.

I have told you steadily that Ruburt has no disease. Diseases are simply groups of symptoms that you have categorized in certain orders to begin with. He approved of his mind. For many reasons given in earlier sessions, he related

SESSION 1/7/78

mentally. Nothing wrong in that. You both had exaggerated ideas, or distorted ones, about the nature of creativity, and about people who were creative, and you considered yourselves rightly as creative people.

Ruburt knew that spontaneity was the basis of his creativity, and of anyone else's. To that extent you disapproved of it. You felt it could be easily overdone, as say Bill Macdonnel or Van Gogh. Ruburt feared that spontaneity had to be tempered, because spontaneity meant unbridled, rampant, uncontrolled impulse. That belief is a basic one in your society—your religions and your sciences. So in feeling it you were both after all quite conventional.

Panicky, Ruburt began in his later 30's to check all impulses except those to work. Remember that <u>then</u>, back then, your circumstances were different. He found himself at that age not having as yet produced what he thought he should; because of other reasons given earlier he wanted that creativity to pay financially.

When he began to achieve some success, so that tours were offered, for example, he checked himself further against such "temptations" and to some extent, in theory if not in practice, you heartily concurred. The habits were set up. They were reflected in the body's motion, day by day, and by your joint patterns of thought and belief.

The effects added to the disapproval, for while one purpose was achieved, his stance and walking were affected. Lately he has realized that spontaneity cannot be treated in such a manner, and that he has given up too much. But your joint disapproval was still there. It makes you uncertain of your abilities, erodes your self-confidence, and prevents you from appreciating your accomplishments—for you feel you must in some way disapprove of them. It prevents you from seeing your individual selves as they are.

(11:05.) Recently I have helped you make some stand against that disapproval. The ommm exercises help, again, because they disengage you and put you in a free drive, relieving the body momentarily at least of stress, and reacquainting it with ease.

Ruburt rediscovered the rune book, hardly by accident. The ommm exercises, with his late understanding, relieved the body enough so that the excellent rune exercises began to work, on his mind as well as his body. He allowed his body, finally, to begin to demonstrate some action. This is because he suspended his self-disapproval for a while.

You did not trust your chair gift because of your own habit of disapproval. You dared to be spontaneous with Wanda. Whenever you suspend that disapproval body and mind automatically function better and together in a smoother fashion. Only your feelings and disapproval and the lack of confidence generat-

...opelessness about Ruburt's situation that frequently assails you

...rned to communicate your disapproval to each other far better as a rule than you communicated your approval. What Ruburt is doing now is excellent and should be continued. If continued it will pay more benefit than your present attitude allows you to imagine. The ommm exercises, or a version, should be followed by you also, Joseph.

I gave material on the eyes, and that stands as of our last session. That situation is being remedied now with the changes Ruburt has recently noted. End of session, unless you have questions.

("No, I guess not.")

Then use these sessions. My heartiest regards and a fond good evening.
("Thank you, Seth." 11:17 PM.)

DELETED SESSION
JANUARY 9, 1978 9:33 PM MONDAY

(Lately Jane has been going over her old notes. She told me that she'd often written that her vision was much improved when her symptoms were better: "The colors are great today," etc. Now she thought the correlations were obvious, especially since her seeing and reading ability today were much better when she felt better otherwise too. She thought Seth would discuss such relationships this evening.)

Good evening.

("Good evening, Seth.")

Now: the message of the Christ entity was, in religious terms "You are all children of God—the 'sinner' as well as the saint." Indeed, according to the original Christ thesis, while a man could sin, no man was identified as a sinner. He was not identified with his failures or limitations, but instead with his potential.

The Christ entity knew the vitality, power, and strength of myths. That vitality allows for different readings, of course, and through man's changing development he reads his myths differently, yet they serve as containers for intuitional knowledge.

Christ's thesis was inserted into a Jewish tradition dealing deeply with guilt, and the new thesis was meant to temper that tradition, and to spread beyond it. Instead, while carrying the belief in man's potential, Christianity smothered the thesis beneath a slag heap of old guilt. Guilt can be used to manipulate people, of course, and it is a fine tool in the hands of government, religion, science, or any large organization that wants to retain its power.

Christ dealt with myths, once again—potent ones that stood for inner realities. Christ clothed those realities in colorful stories geared to people's understanding. I am using the name here, Christ, as one person for the sake of discussion, for that entity touched many lives, each leaping into a kind of super-reality as it joyfully played its part in the religious drama.

(Just as I was about to ask....)

The message was "Do not condemn yourself or others," for Christ well knew that self-righteous condemnation of the self or of one's neighbors served to darken the door through which man might view his own potential and its greater source.

The Christian concept of heaven with its riches, God and his bounty, the source of nature itself—all of this in our terms was a symbolic structure describing in storybook terms the attributes and characteristics of Framework 2.

In our terms, All That Is exists in Framework 2 as elsewhere, but Framework 2 represents the source of your known physical reality. From it flow all of the known facts of your world. Christ hoped to show that you survived death psychically and spiritually—that you "returned" to the father in heaven. Literal minds, looking for evidential proof, would insist that the physical body itself must rise, ascending, hence the related stories, the misinterpretation of data. "Ask, and you shall receive." Christ well knew that that statement was indeed true, but men who condemned themselves, who considered themselves sinners, would not know what to ask for, except punishment to relieve their guilt. Hence he stressed time and time again that each person was a child of God.

He also stressed the importance of a childlike belief, knowing that the adult mind was apt to question "How, and when, and in what manner can my request be granted?"

The words "Let thy will be done," represented excellent psychological understanding, for according to Christ's teachings as originally given, God the father represented the source or parent of the self, who was by nature free from the self's ignorance or lack of understanding at any given time, and who would know better than the known self those experiences that would fulfill the self's hopes, dreams, and potentials.

In this way, with the words spoken "Let thy will be done," the self could free itself from its own misconceptions, and attract from Framework 2 benefits that it might otherwise not be knowledgeable enough to request. A portion of each person dwells in Framework 1 and Framework 2. Understand that Framework 2 is a psychic or spiritual or mental structure. In deepest terms, of course, it is not a place. It is, if you prefer, a spiritual landscape of far greater resources than the one you know. It brings forth the world of your experience in that world, and so it is your source also.

"Let thy will be done" meant "Let me follow those greater dictates of my inner nature." Even without all of the distortions, that formula worked for centuries in large measure. The God, the source, was put outside of nature, however, finally becoming at last too remote, and the story itself became frayed at the edges as man tried to tie intuitive truths to objective fact.

(10:06.) Give us a moment.... To be a child of God was to trust in your own worth. You could admit failings, transgressions of one kind or another without identifying yourself, say, with failure. The child of God would automatically find salvation, and everyone was a child of God. When Christ said "Believe in me, and you will be saved," he meant "Believe in your relationship to God, in that you are his son, as I am, and you will surely be saved." Again, he spoke in religious terms, for those were the terms of the times. This knowledge, however, of the innate goodness of the self literally gives the individual the inner support necessary for the exercise of man's fullest potentials.

In civil and governmental terms, such a policy could not be tolerated—nor has man yet learned how to deal with that basic principal. It is almost automatic, for example, to label a man a murderer, and identify him with his crime. The society never came to terms with the vast complications inherent with Christ's teachings, and so it abandoned them. Man's great exuberant spontaneity has never been allowed its full sweep as a result.

Do you want to rest your fingers?

("No.")

You both chafed against the belief of your times, that man was a natural aggressor, tainted from birth, that he was damned by his very nature, condemned by his early childhood background, by original sin, or by his genes. At the same time you were also tainted by those beliefs, and seemed to see evidence for them whenever you looked into your selves, or outward to the world of your fellows. Each person carried the brunt of that self-condemnation. Ruburt is hardly outstanding in having physical difficulties, and overall your lives and the work speak for more of the potential of personality than of personality's lacks. You set for yourselves a goal of shoving aside all of the beliefs and distortions for yourselves and for others.

Now: you went beyond your family's beliefs individually, searching for yourselves and trying various roads. You accomplished the quite difficult feat, in certain terms, of finding each other, so that you each had a mate who would aid you in your pursuits—and you tried as best you knew to encourage each other. You were still plagued by remnants of self-disapproval and self-condemnation, however, yet the spontaneous self in each of you managed to push here and there and blaze forth whenever you gave it a chance, with some quite outstanding results.

I always have to couch my material for you personally, just ahead *(emphatically)* of where you are at any given time. Overall, however, the main thrust of the material of course has always been way ahead of where you are, practically speaking, at any given time.

In terms of your lives, you are able to use certain portions of the material at different times. No one could put it all into working order at once in a given life. Ruburt then used and enjoyed his spontaneity, and has been developing it along the lines of his understanding. It is not, as it may seem, that he had something of spontaneity and lost it.

(10:28.) Give us a moment.... Spontaneity knows its own order, and freely comes into order. Years ago, before the psychic experience, he was not for example psychically spontaneous to any great degree. He used his writing to hold back and yet contain his innate psychic knowledge. He disapproved of his own dancing, sometimes even of his sexual yearnings. Now those disapprovals simply piled up, with resulting physical difficulties. He would through the years begin to approve of spontaneity in one more area—spontaneity in class, for example—or with Sumari poetry, or in finally approving his own psychic writings. The disapproval was still present, however; yet now and then through the years would come a period of release, of sudden ease and sudden physical improvement—each time when he suspended self-disapproval, and when for your reasons you began to suspend your own.

The situation and the faith that you managed to build up in Framework 2 have come to your aid. The ommm exercises and the rune exercises are showing results because some of the material has come through again to you from the sessions, and you are jointly suspending your self-disapproval. In religious terms, you would realize you were saved, or a child of God. You have stopped to a degree <u>identifying yourselves</u> with any limitations.

When this happens you actually symbolically say "Let thy will be done," meaning "Let my greater nature, my spontaneous nature, flow through me without impediment, and without quibbling." Then the benefits from Framework 2 can begin to flow without impediment. The body can right itself, and the methods that you use <u>work</u>.

Do you want to rest your hand?

("No, I'm okay.")

Ruburt's eyes are definitely improving these last few days, as the strain is being relieved from the rest of the body—the neck area particularly, the jaws and muscles of the brow. <u>Nearly</u> all eye difficulties <u>are</u> related to other stresses in the body.

(I should have asked Seth what he meant by nearly.)

Ruburt is quite correct: his vision has fluctuated through the years, and in periods of mental ease, understanding, and physical improvements, his vision also improves.

You both became extremely depressed, thinking in time terms and concentrating upon past failures, <u>with which</u> you identified. The notes Ruburt wrote yesterday are extremely important, with their emphasis upon my old "the spontaneous self <u>is</u> the guardian," and added to that "from which your very life springs." You <u>can will</u> your spontaneity to express itself, even as you can will it not to. Tell Ruburt that if he continues in this manner, and if the two of you can manage to maintain your peace of mind long enough—over a two or three day period, for example, then you can expect rewards in all areas. The inner keys have been turned once again.

(Seth's material here on the use of the will came about, I think, as a result of some older material I gave Jane to read this afternoon. It concerned the amazing powers of her will, and is from Session 713, Volume 2, of "Unknown" Reality. This happens to be the session in that book that I'm working on now. I recommend that it be kept in mind and referred to every so often, for it certainly contains many clues to individual capacities.)

(10:45.) <u>Now</u> I bid you a fond and encouraging good evening.

("Can I ask a question?")

You may.

("This is off the subject, but your material about Christ reminded me of a letter we received from a young woman not long ago. She wanted to know what really happened to Christ, if he wasn't crucified.")

Give us a moment.... That question in the larger context is very difficult to answer.

(Eyes closed:) There were several men who together performed the exploits reported in the Christ story—exploits occurring only roughly in the 33-year period given *(for Christ's life).*

A man was crucified, but he was not one who made up the Christ entity. You understand from stories that have come to you the elaborations and half-truths that people can be convinced are true. None of the men who made up that entity were crucified. They each died—one I believe in India. People do not understand that their dreams become reality, and that the greater dramas of history and myth often bear little resemblance to the actual occurrences, but are greater than the physical events.

End of session. *(With loud good humor:)* You will get bits and tidbits on that now and then.

("Okay. Thank you, Seth."

(10:53 PM. See Chapter 21 of Seth Speaks *for more on the Christ entity. According to history, Christ was crucified, and the other two members of Seth's Christ entity, John the Baptist and St. Paul, were beheaded. Seth hasn't mentioned India before in connection with any of the three, so that information would be new. It would be interesting to get more data on the whole Christ question. As I told Jane after the session, Seth's Christ material tonight reminded me of the idea of the Christ book, which Seth mentioned in* Personal Reality.*)*

DELETED SESSION
JANUARY 14, 1978 9:40 PM SATURDAY

(After supper tonight Jane became aware of a noticeable straightening of her right leg—the shortest one—so that it appeared to equal her left leg. I measured the angle of change, of opening up, as we talked and saw a good increase. Over the last two days she's stood taller walking, so this change had been in the works... Her right side generally has been improving from head to toe also. She has walked faster at times, and there has been improvement in the musculature definition of her knees.

(Earlier today I'd asked Jane if Seth would comment on my chest symptoms, re causes that I'd arrived at through using the pendulum. It appears that my own hassles are related to my fears that Jane's improvements may not continue. More is involved, however, and we've obtained considerable insights in recent sessions. Today the pendulum linked my reactions to certain foods to the chest symptoms, but these I question.)

Good evening.

("Good evening, Seth.")

We will begin with some rather general statements.

Because of the nature of your society, a large number of people cultivate what I will call an outside-attuned consciousness. Naturally, sensation and knowledge must of course come through enjoyment and use of the physical body, and through the data received from the physical environment, with which the body must necessarily react.

The outside-attuned consciousness, however, is <u>almost</u> dependent upon exterior stimuli for its sense of life and enjoyment. I do not want to oversimplify, yet such a type of consciousness is far more interested in exploring the nature of itself <u>as it relates</u> to exterior conditions or circumstances. It becomes, relatively now, opaque to subjective personal conditions, since it has no secure exterior framework against which the inner condition can be judged.

Primarily, such a consciousness knows itself, or tries to know itself, <u>only</u> in relationship to others or exterior conditions. It avoids introspection. No consciousness is purely tuned into outside conditions only, of course. This type, however, is a cultivated specialization of consciousness in which its nature is known through the impact of exterior rather than interior conditions. Generally speaking, and only generally, it represents the consciousness familiar to many in your society—most likely, the majority.

I do not want to set up polarities. I do want to give you some background, however, for some of your attitudes. From childhood in your society, you were as children told in one way or another that it was healthy to enjoy sports and outside activity, to join in games, to be outgoing with playmates, and all of that is of course quite true. Children are also taught, however, that reading for anything but short periods was somehow unhealthy, that daydreaming or staying alone for anything but a brief period meant that the child was withdrawn, and that his activities—or hers—were somehow unnatural.

Children were urged in one way or another to be aggressive, competitive, and generally to fit the conventional idea of the extrovert. It often seemed that there was no in-between point, and if you did not fit one mold, you must therefore take your stand and be the other.

Many men and women in the same fashion, who do not fit the conventional sexual frameworks, take stands in the same way. A man may decide he wants to be a homosexual because he cannot fit into the usual pattern. There is obviously, however, no contradiction between habits of subjective thought and creativity and the physical enjoyment of the body and its abilities.

If you believe, however, that you must have one at the expense of the other, then you will always face a dilemma between exterior and subjective activity. Your friends the Gallaghers inhibit their subjective natures strongly, both of them *(as I was speculating about the other day)*. They are indeed afraid of aging, and so press onward in more and more exterior activity, because they fear that age will show itself there first. They forget the nature of "youthful thoughts." They believe there is a polarity, and they have chosen the other side.

When you were both children, to some degree each of you felt that you were different because of your intense subjective activity—and <u>to some extent</u>, and different for both of you—you felt that you had to "fight for" the freedom to pursue subjective reality.

Since you are obviously able to enjoy physical activity at times, you chose to remain alone rather than "play with the others." As you matured you each to some degree carried beliefs that physical activity and subjective activity were somehow, and to varying degrees, opposed to the other—one being accepted by society, and the other frowned upon.

(10:05.) I do not want to duplicate material. At one time, however, you briefly curtailed physical activity for what you considered the sake of your subjective freedom. You quickly dismissed that idea after a taste of it. Ruburt accepted that idea, believing he must make a choice. All of this, you see, must be considered in the light of our last session, for it involves varying degrees of self-disapproval and polarities of thought, so that the contradictions occurred in your experience—though there were more, of course, in basic terms.

You believed that you should be outgoing, vigorous, somewhat competitive, and you believed you should be socially oriented, while at the same time you believed that those things conflicted in a basic way with other drives. You felt you should be introverted, have periods of isolation, time to sit and think, to write and paint, to look inward rather than outward. In periods of intense inner activity that were enjoyable and productive, you disapproved of yourselves because you were not at the same time socially oriented, vigorously involved in exercises, or physically oriented pursuits, and so you disapproved of yourselves.

When you were both working outside with jobs, out in the community, going to bars and dancing, seeing neighbors often and having parties, you disapproved of yourselves because you were not sufficiently subjective, isolated, et cetera.

You felt you could not merge the separate groups of attributes because they were diametrically opposed in your minds. Instead, of course, there are gradations of behavior, and patterns or rhythms in your lives that would naturally flow one into the other, released from the artificial polarities. The polarities <u>are</u> artificial, but there is no doubt that in your society and times the exterior-tuned consciousness is the most paramount. It, of course, by its nature, is not given to introspection, so it does not question its stance as deeply. So some of this disapproval has to do with your own attitudes about the attitudes of others as they view your lives.

You find yourselves landowners somewhat. You see others shoveling their walks themselves. You disapprove of yourself for not doing so. You feel you <u>could not</u> do so—that you are not physically that vigorous *(as I told Jane today)*. This is symbolic of course of your attitudes. For you feel that the life-styles are completely different, and polarized.

Physically, for example, you are in much better physical condition than Joe Bumbalo, but he is a prime example, to you, of the exteriorized consciousness—and while on the one hand you envy his shoveling the walk, you are <u>to</u>

some degree underneath all that, somewhat contemptuous—somewhat, now; I do not want to speak too strongly, but simply help you become aware of some feelings you might have submerged because you think they are not nice.

This does not mean that you should begin shoveling walks tomorrow, with your attitude. There are classic, distorted stories of the weakly scholar as opposed to the hearty sportsman. To some extent the same applies to Ruburt. You are surrounded by propaganda saying that the body will not perform in a healthy, vigorous manner, if you indulge primarily in subjective activity—if you sit at your desk, for example.

Much of the propaganda is nearly invisible. It appears everywhere. The body and mind are one. Bates's book, or rather philosophy, suggesting that the eyes were not made for reading, is an example of a different kind, implying that there were no books when the eye was created—and so therefore it is not natural for the eye to see letters—while it is natural for the eye to see, say, trees. The body adjusts its rhythms in a quite healthy manner to your activities, and without polarized habits of thought, periods of deep creativity will automatically be followed by periods of walking, natural exercise of one kind or another, in which subjective thought and body motion are synchronized.

That is background. Now give us a break, and we will continue.

(10:28. "Well, once again we find ourselves at odds with society," I said to Jane as we talked. "This time it's over exercise and related ideas. I don't know whether to get mad at our friends, or ourselves, or both." Actually I felt pretty resentful about the whole situation. I guess; it seemed that Jane and I were incredibly dense about understanding what had been going on for the past decade. I remarked about the opinions of others when they read our deleted material after our deaths, for instance, whereupon Jane said that more than once she'd had the idea of destroying all our personal material when we were older.

(By way of contrast, I want to add here that this week Jane has been notified by Prentice-Hall of their most enthusiastic reception of her children's book, Emir. *Not only that, it appears that Prentice-Hall may have found at the same time the ideal illustrator for the work; black-and-white copies of sample illustrations have been sent to Jane, done by the female artist, with Tam's assurances that the color is brilliant.*

(In addition, there is the interesting news from Alan Neuman, regarding his giving Seven *to a well-known movie director, as well as showing it to another agent, etc. Jane has records of this activity, but I wanted to mention it here.*

(In addition. Prentice-Hall will send us additional copies of Seven, *if they have any left. Larry Davidson called from San Francisco, during which he agreed to ship us some copies from the bookstore where he works. This the day or so after I'd had the idea of calling him to ask him to do this.*

(All of these events are clear-cut examples of the operation of Framework 2, I told Jane—including her obvious physical improvements. Perhaps we are learning—slowly. Resume at 10:35.)

You chose to be leaders rather than followers, and you would not have it otherwise.

By nature, leaders are not so much at odds with their world as they are ahead of it. The Bumbalos, for example, envy you, as do the Gallaghers, but they are afraid of subjective reality. They have taught their consciousnesses to conform.

These ideas, with the last session, have to do with Ruburt's partitioning of his spontaneity, for he also felt that you had to choose one way or the other, and that to protect your subjective freedom you had to inhibit the externally oriented spontaneity that was sanctioned by most of the society, because you could not do both. This is, again—and to some extent—on both your parts, black-and-white thinking.

Here, as opposed to the apartment, where the life-styles were seemingly in a more transitory situation, you have both again dramatized yourselves to some degree as outsiders in a negative fashion, disapprovingly seeing yourselves in relationship to your neighbors, but not constructively. You could instead have stressed your positive and constructive differences, for your move to the neighborhood, again, to some extent—excuse the constant qualifying—your move has helped the neighbors see themselves in a different light.

Conventionally, they enjoy having what they think of as highly creative people in the neighborhood. Your lives make them think of their own hidden aspirations. You bring up questions for them. In a strange way, they feel comforted by your presences. They know there are differences, but they are far more willing to see the creative aspects of your lives than you give them credit for.

You have fallen for the same conventionalized beliefs that they have, only you chose the subjective side. They were so afraid of subjective thought that they ran willy-nilly in the other direction, and they envy your choice—again, to some degree. In summer, you think you should do the lawn. You feel that conflicts with your subjective interests, and that the two are not compatible. You see Joe frantically mow his lawn. You are contemptuous—somewhat—and envious at the same time. The same applies to the snow, so you disapprove of yourself whether you have the grass or the snow taken care of—or whether you try to do it yourself.

(10:49.) Give us a moment.... Ruburt has had excellent results with *Emir*, and you should rejoice. You do, yet you think at what expense did *Emir* come—what restrictions of physical activity—and had you been somewhat different,

would it all have been necessary?

At the same time you think that Ruburt is at least spontaneous in his art, while it seems to you that you are not spontaneous enough in that area.

Give us a moment.... Some of your inner feelings are difficult for me to express, because they are in so many layers that I am not sure of their relative importance. To some extent, again then, the sale of a book, a new sale, is somehow connected in your mind with disapproval of yourself, Joseph, in that Ruburt seems able to express what I think you interpret as competitiveness, that you feel you are not expressing—and you add that to your arsenal of disapproval. *(Very good.)*

All of this is connected with the chest difficulties. The food is not basically related, except as it reflects other issues *(as I told Jane this afternoon)*. Those are relatively shallow, but do operate—that certain foods are good for the body and others are not—that heart disease is connected with cholesterol and dairy products, while skim milk is innocent. The chest difficulty reminds you of heart trouble, and you react negatively then to whole milk.

Now, I want to stress that you must not emphasize your feelings that you are at odds with the world. To some extent or another each person feels at odds with the cultural environment, or worse, with their most intimate companions. You cannot expect to be involved in creative activity of an important sort, and at the same time see through the eyes of others.

The 1973 session book Ruburt is reading has helped him, simply because it rearouses the feelings of psychic, creative and physical improvement he did achieve, and because it contains in capsule form all—most all—of the important material I have given, though some of it no longer applies.

At certain stages your experience relatively coincides—relatively—with events in the past, so that some material attains double strength. Generally, however, your hopes and faith in Ruburt's recovery became somewhat eroded. Your feelings of hopelessness were the result, as given in the last session, but nowhere did you thoroughly work out in the past the problems of self-disapproval; or if one managed to attain a foothold, the other did not, so you could not properly reinforce each other creatively, and became quickly discouraged.

This summer, you compared your way of life with those polarized ideas, with the way of life of the construction men, for example. The disapproval causes you to exaggerate the differences, rather than glorify them as you should — though glorify may be too strong a word. Ruburt's physical condition becomes a materialization of those concepts, exaggerated, so that he is not able to go forth in the world, believing the polarity so great, with him and subjective activity having the disadvantage.

(11:09.) You believed to some degree—varying degrees, but jointly—that subjective activity and creative activity must be achieved at the expense of some physical expression. You obviously did not fall for that to the extent Ruburt did —and all of this must be considered also in the light of the religious and scientific views, with Ruburt particularly, in which the spontaneous self was considered the psychological villain of the society and the individual. The spontaneous self <u>is</u> the guardian—that is what Ruburt is learning.

The Gallaghers trust spontaneity only when it is expressed through physical motion. <u>To some extent</u>, again, Ruburt trusted it only when it was expressed through subjective motion. I suggested that you take walks, Joseph, some time ago, simply to rearouse your natural love of that activity.

Give us a moment.... You can see how Ruburt's body responds when he suspends self-disapproval, and when he allies himself with his nature, and when you both suspend your sense of hopelessness in that area. If you continue as you are, you can indeed expect quite startling improvements—but you are not to compare, either of you, Ruburt's condition with the Gallaghers' skiing, anymore than they could compare their attempts at subjective journeying with Ruburt's inner soaring. Avoid absolutes.

All Ruburt wants is normal motion. You saw the response in his leg this evening. The important neck and jaw areas are definitely releasing, and the eyes will swiftly begin to resume their normal activity—if you continue as you are. Your own physical vigor is there, and can express itself, comparatively speaking —comparatively speaking—with far greater ease once you rid yourself of those polarized concepts and the disapproval that goes with them.

Ruburt stands taller—observably. He is using muscles in new ways. Gaining strength and vitality. Your body is already in excellent shape, in general terms—we are not speaking of athletes. It would need, naturally, some period of training if you were thinking of climbing mountains, or expected to ski down a good slope tomorrow—but it is well prepared for normal activity. Only your beliefs impede it—so work with those beliefs before you shovel the drive. It is the dilemma behind the whole thing that is important, the implied conflicts between subjective and objective activity. And the <u>responsibilities</u> you <u>feel</u> this entails.

You have both moved through many periods of understanding, where others might have stopped, and the going-ahead always involves new challenges. Your friend Bill Gallagher's operation represented a triumph on his part, for he regained his health in one important area—an achievement of worth. But it also represented a failure of a kind, a stopping-point at a certain level of development.

This does not mean that medical help is always detrimental at all, for the intents of the individual always apply. The tension between the two couples, and yet the latent sympathies, are what unites you—that is, are what unites you and the Gallaghers. For Bill does have significant psychic abilities that he inhibits for fear they will operate against his survival in the world of business.

Give us a moment.... I do not want anything to impede this not new important work of progress. Now, walking would not be particularly constructive for you. The ommm exercises, or simply some quiet yoga breathing exercises, would however, and either would relieve the feelings in the chest considerably on the physical level.

Ruburt's vitality, reemerging, shows itself in his desire for physical intimacy, and will hopefully, as you continue this path, be reflected in all other areas of life.

Do you have questions?

(Of course I did, yet I seemed to be peculiarly numb mentally: I couldn't think of any. "No, I guess not. Probably—but I can't think of them.")

The 1973 book would be a help for you also, if you find the time to look it over. I bid you then a hearty good evening.

("Thank you, Seth. Good night.")

(11:34 PM. Jane had "just slightly that sicky feeling" in her stomach, as she sometimes does when the material is particularly good. She immediately turned on television to get her mind off the feeling. I thought the session was excellent.)

DELETED SESSION
JANUARY 16, 1978 9:38 PM MONDAY

(Today I read the deleted session for June 24, 1973—one of those in the 1973 deleted book that Seth suggested I read, in the last session. I was dismayed to realize that some four and a half years had passed since that session had been held, and that we were still struggling with the same problems—indeed, that Jane had lost much ground physically in the interim. I read the material and it plagued me through the day. I explained my feelings to Jane as we sat for the session, and as I talked felt myself sink into a deep depression. Once again, I wondered what we'd been doing while all that time passed.)

Now: I have a little to say, for that notebook contains important insights.

Ruburt read it, and is reading it, looking for those feelings that allowed vast improvements to occur at the time—and for once he did not look into the past with his usual self-disapproval. To some extent he began to recapture some of those feelings. With what he has learned, and with that emotional touchstone, he has indeed made good strides, which are quite obvious for both of you to see. . .

I have given you endless material on the importance of significances, and how you build upon them according to your focus. In that one area of Ruburt's condition, you focus upon the improvements that occur. You do not compare the present situation with a past one in a detrimental manner. You live in the present. All of the recent material I have given you has enabled you to see some considerable results because for a time you have managed to give yourselves <u>some</u> peace of mind—at least enough to move ahead.

Ruburt recaptured that sense of acceleration, at least momentarily. In *Personal Reality* I stressed many of these points for our readers, but you yourselves forget to apply them in that one important area of your lives. The last sessions managed to rearouse your faith, but you yourselves must tend it, as indeed, Joseph, you tend your plants. Do not identify with what you think of as past failures. The point of power is in the present, and when you believe changes can occur, they do indeed happen.

Framework 2 begins to open doors in all areas, and only you and Ruburt can possibly stand in the way of excellent developments that have begun now in all avenues, including Ruburt's condition. They are activated. Old patterns of thought can at times rearouse feelings of hopelessness and failure. A little extra effort on both of your parts can help you not only to recognize the feelings, which you do, but to decide to suspend them for now. Agree to give yourselves a breathing spell from them. Try to counter them.

If Ruburt is showing improvements, then let these rise to your attention. The material in the last two sessions explains why it is so easy to feel disapproval. To some extent the same attitude applies to whatever you do physically, for you compare it to what you think you should be doing that is perhaps more vigorous. You can break those habits of thought. Ruburt certainly has made some strides of late, and so have you.

Those thoughts bring you precisely what you say neither of you want. I suggest you read the late sessions again, and I imagine that by our next session you will both be in a better frame of mind, unless you allow your discouraging feelings to predominate, which would be a vast mistake.

<u>To some extent</u> the perspective one, two, three material is related to Frameworks 1 and 2, for the symbols of your mind grow in their own fashion, changing shape and form, but following the emotional content rather faithfully. If you truly understood what I am saying, you would realize the importance of encouraging optimistic, jestful feelings of faith, of cultivating them—for it is

far more important to collect them than money. They represent far greater security, defense, and strength. They are far more practical than any negative considerations, regardless of how realistic those might appear at any given time.

End of session. I want you, however, to take this to heart, for simple as it sounds the session is of significance. My heartiest wishes to you, and a fond good evening.

("Good night, Seth.")

(9:59 PM.)

DELETED SESSION
JANUARY 21, 1978 9:16 PM SATURDAY

(Before the session Jane said that in the last week she: 1. Is reading much better—"damn well" on Seth's book. Psyche, and on Emir. This applies to her copying work on the typewriter also. 2. Her newspaper and other small-print reading has been better overall, although it's not even in quality. But still there have been definite improvements. Her intermediate vision needs the most work. 3. "My legs have changed quite a bit during the week. I'm definitely taller. I can stand taller most of the time." These changes were accompanied by perhaps three days or so of muscular soreness, which has now largely disappeared. All of these things Jane considered to be her "two-week report," as discussed in the deleted session for January 7, 1978.

(My own chest difficulties are much improved, although at the same time I'm not doing any additional hard physical labor. I'm simply mentioning ordinary activities—chopping a little wood, etc. I still haven't shoveled any snow, in spite of the series of massive snowstorms we've experienced within the last week—the worst in over a decade. I have been rereading the latest sessions on self-disapproval, and these seem to have made the difference. Jane has also been working on her feelings of self approval and disapproval, and credits her efforts with her improvements.)

Good evening

("Good evening, Seth.")

Now let us look at the roots of self-disapproval from another vantage point.

When man identified with nature, as given in *Psyche*, he did not imagine that the gods disapproved of him when storms lashed across the landscape. He did not at that time, as is supposed, do sacrifice then to win the gods' approval. Instead, identifying with nature, man identified also with all of its manifestations.

This of course gave you at that time a different orientation of consciousness. Man did not see himself pitted against the elements, but allied with them, whatever their mood or behavior. I have explained that kind of consciousness fairly well in portions of *Psyche* that Ruburt is reading. Man could exult in nature's energy, power, and splendor, even in the midst of the most fierce storm —in which, indeed, his life might be in danger.

He felt himself to be a <u>portion</u> of the storm, however, and felt the storm as a vast magnification of his own emotional reality—even as he felt the body of the earth itself to be, beside itself, the magnification of his own emotional reality and that of others.

In your terms, with time, historically, he began to lose this identification, so that an emotional separation began to occur between man and the elements, between man and the other manifestations of nature. He still sensed nature's grandeur—*(louder:)* but that grandeur was no longer his own, and he felt less and less a part of it. Nature became an exterior power, more of an adversary, even though man has a love for the earth, the fields, and the grain that they yielded.

With that loss of identification storms for the first time became truly threatening, capricious, for man's mind could not intellectually understand the intimate and yet vast connections that the intuitions and emotions had once comprehended. It was then, and in the terms of this discussion, that men felt a division between themselves and "the gods," for it was then that man began to personify the elements of nature.

Once this was done, nature it seemed could be dealt with, could be cajoled, tricked, or reasoned with as circumstances warranted. If a large area was besieged by stormy weather of any kind, then obviously a god must have somehow disapproved of human action. It was vital that the person so disapproved of be cast out. If any doubt was present then another person would be cast out or sacrificed. Acts were scrutinized so that those offending to the gods could be clearly categorized so that men would not unknowingly offend. Tribal life became a series of ritualized activities. If certain patterns of behavior were followed and the weather was pleasant, then those patterns of behavior must be ones that were safe. If the weather turned disastrous, the people were in a quandary, reexamining the patterns of behavior, finding perhaps minute differences, suspicious variations, that seemed to occur just before the storm—so these became the new sins.

Self-disapproval <u>in that context</u> became a virtue, for indeed survival depended, it seemed, upon constant self and tribal evaluation. None of this has anything to do with natural guilt, as described in *Personal Reality*. Now man does feel a certain amount of natural guilt when he loses his identification with nature, for that identification leads to intuitive connections with nature's greater source.

(*Long pause at 9:41.*) Your religions have been largely patterned from such self-disapproving bases. The thrust of your civilizations has been concerned with manipulating nature. Your latest snowstorm is an excellent example. Not only of nature's power and its effects upon civilization, but it also provides you with a very small hint of the other side of the picture, for man despite himself has not lost entirely that identification with the elements. People still feel a part of nature's power. Storms often, oddly enough it seems, bring out a feeling of adventuresomeness and neighborliness, because people are united—not against nature, as they may think, but <u>by</u> it. The good skier feels a part of the snowy hill, yet most skiers feel that the hill must be conquered. When you take a walk, you usually think of walking through nature, not realizing that you are a part of the scene through which you walk. The loss of a real, sensed, appreciated identification with nature has been largely responsible, however, for man's attitude that self-disapproval is somehow a virtue.

Again, the animal approves of himself, <u>whether</u> he is sick or well, slow or swift. The sick animal wants to get well. It does not disapprove of <u>itself</u>, however, or even think of itself as "a sick animal." In those terms it might think of itself as an animal who was sick—a big difference—and even then no self-disapproval would be indicated.

You are different than animals, but in this case the same issues are involved. You must have a basic approval of yourself. This is information not only for you two, of course, but for others—but <u>you must trust your basic being</u>, with its characteristics and abilities. You have them for a reason in all of their unique combinations. You should also avoid labels, for these can stereotype your perception of yourself.

I will give you some (*stereotypes*): Ruburt is stubborn. He never forgets a slight. Ruburt is fiercely loyal. Joseph deals in details. His mind is logical rather than intuitive. Ruburt is spontaneous. Joseph is not. All of these are labels, and quite relative. Ruburt is loyal to <u>you</u>. He was not loyal, <u>in those terms</u>, to Walter Zeh, or he would still be with him. Ruburt is spontaneous—but if he were all that spontaneous he would be walking better. You, Joseph, <u>are</u> spontaneous. <u>You</u> do not have to think before you cross the floor—where there Ruburt is aware of the slightest detail—the arrangement of his body or the furniture, the lay of the floor.

Do not label yourselves, for then you often try to live up to those labels, and they can be highly limiting. I do my own part in these sessions, and if I may say so (*highly amused:*) very well indeed—and yet there is certainly something in Ruburt's mind and abilities that allows him to speak, regardless, over the years, an immense amount of material, some of it highly detailed and orderly. So how can Ruburt say that he cannot deal with the details, and thus disapprove of himself?

You have disapproved of yourself, thinking yourself not spontaneous, and so your belief has often hampered your <u>natural</u> spontaneity, so that you struggled for notes because you thought you must; that was the kind of person you thought you were.

Disapproval of that kind prevents you from perceiving your own abilities, and limits of course your appreciation of yourself. To some extent your acts become ritualized, as those of our tribesmen mentioned earlier.

Since disapproval will never bring abundance or pleasure, it gradually cuts down on your options, until there is little about yourself you approve of. Again, I am speaking generally as well as specifically.

Take your break.

(10:03—10:15.)

To an important degree, each of you have believed that self-disapproval <u>was</u> indeed constructive or virtuous. You were not on the lookout against it, therefore.

When you look for "what is wrong," you are feeding self-disapproval. When you are looking for the reasons behind a condition, that is different. The two attitudes, while they may seem similar, are really quite opposite in their intent and effect. Ruburt recognized self-disapproval today *(after her nap)*. He saw that the feeling itself was the culprit. He disapproved of himself because of his condition, or so he thought, and he has felt that way often. The self-disapproval causes the condition, however, and not the other way around. This got through to him.

Your own ease in *"Unknown"* now is the result of your suspension of self-disapproval, and would be the same if you were doing appendixes. You do need to support each other in that regard, helping each other to approve of yourselves.

Ruburt's entire body has stretched noticeably in the last week and a half, the legs in particular. He has implemented that stretching so that he is indeed taller walking. The lower back is becoming more elastic, and <u>that</u> allows for a greater loosening of the knees. Those back muscles are strong and vigorous, but they were tightened in order to hold this lowered pose *(with gestures)*.

His eye muscles <u>are</u> basically elastic, not weakened. The fact that they are responding in closeup reading is a case in point. Many eye difficulties have to do with body posture. <u>I suggested hot towels for the knees</u>—and said that this would help the eyes. I repeat that recommendation. The position of the knees is tied into the positioning of the head and neck areas. The heat, applied to the knees when the body is sitting and relaxed, releases the neck tension, and that helps bring the eyes into better balance.

The yawning is excellent, and also helps the entire head-neck area. Ruburt does not like to take his new teeth out. Taking them out at night, however, would give the jaws greater leeway for relaxation.

You spoke of the pendulum *(at last break)*. Again, labels are somewhat implicated, for you each thought you worked well with the pendulum, but that Ruburt did not. It can be used most effectively and in the past at times Ruburt used it well, particularly with your help—largely because he believed it necessary. Make sure you do not look for what is wrong, however, but for reasons behind behavior.

The pendulum will not work, of course, if your self-disapproval is paramount, for then you cannot trust your own answers. Ruburt <u>should</u> concentrate upon his ideas and creativity. I have said this so often, and yet I repeat: concentration upon a problem magnifies it.

You, Joseph, are making gains as you know—again, because you minimize self-disapproval, and therefore bring into the range of your attention abilities of your own that before you quite inhibited

This is quite enough for this evening, since I expect you to take an almost equal amount of time not only to read this session together, but to explore at the same time the ways in which your own self-labels may have added to your own self- disapproval. <u>That</u> exercise is a part of this session.

And now I bid you a fond and a hearty good evening.

("Thank you, Seth. Good night."

(10:38 PM. Jane had feelings of emptiness, that "sicky feeling" in her stomach after the session—the feelings she often gets when the material really hits home.)

DELETED SESSION
JANUARY 23, 1978 9:34 PM MONDAY

Good evening.

("Good evening, Seth.")

Now: on your television screen this evening you saw a little girl *(in a European country)*. She said that she had asked in a prayer for proof of God's existence. After a short time an earthquake occurred *(in Romania)*, and the child was afraid that she had caused it. She was convinced that God had answered her prayer thusly.

Because of the beliefs of religion, the child expected God to show his power through some disastrous act by which sinners would be punished. child's life already carries the marks of her beliefs about religion, God, pow and mainly in the belief that nature is a tool in the God's hands—to be used against man at any time.

When consciousness becomes <u>overly</u> exteriorized and no longer identifies strongly with nature, then it no longer properly identifies itself with the inner nature of its own actions. One's own actions therefore seem to be as exteriorized, or apart from consciousness, as trees or rocks seem to be. The exteriorized consciousness will always see such an event as an earthquake by viewing only its immediate, sometimes tragic, results. Those results will seem meaningless, chaotic. Men caught in such an event will question "Why should this happen to me?"

The conventionally religious will be certain that the earthquake is a punishment for sin. The scientist will see the affair as relatively neutral —an event, however, in which man is certainly a pawn, caught by chance in a catastrophe that he would otherwise most certainly avoid. The earthquake is a mass natural catastrophe, seeming then to be perpetrated upon man and his cities by an earth that certainly does not take man or his civilization into consideration.

Private events of tragedy seem in a smaller context to happen without man's knowledge or without his consent. The overly exteriorized consciousness has cut itself off so that it no longer perceives the inner order of events. The world with its wars or disasters, its illnesses or poverty, its mass or private tragedies, seems to be thrust upon man or to happen—again without his consent.

The emotional identification with nature meant that man had a far greater and richer personal emotional reality. That love of nature, and appreciation, quickened and utilized inner biological capacities, also possessed by plants and animals, so that man was more consciously aware of his part in nature. He identified with natural events. It is almost impossible in your time to describe man's reality when he was consciously aware that he would die and yet not die, and when he was everywhere surrounded by those inner data of his psyche.

Those data were equal in his experience to those physical data of the world, so that the two kinds of experience constantly enriched each other. Man then understood that he did form his own reality in all of its aspects, both privately and en masse, and in terms of natural earth events, as well as for example the events of his society. You cannot of course limit your world to the world of facts at any given time, though you may try to do so. That little girl's experience with the earthquake, and her beliefs about it, have little to do with the bare facts involved. She is dealing instead with an inner world of myths.

more powerful than any facts, and they carry with them the [...]'s own emotional force as it is interpreted through man's [...] rtainly seem to be provable in your world. Myths are generally considered to be distorted facts, interpreted by primitive minds, or the result of creative acts of the imagination. That power is little understood, much less its reasons.

When man identified with the grandeur and energy of nature, <u>then</u> he knew nature's reasons, for they were his own as well. He knew his death, his personal death, was only a transition, for his identification allowed him to feel the mobility of his consciousness, and allowed him to feel a sense of communion with the passing seasons, and with the ever-constant renewal of plants and fields. He did not need to look for a reason for nature's destructive aspects, for he knew through experience the great sweep of its vitality. He knew no Gods were sending down vengeance.

(10:06.) That inner knowledge is behind all of his myths. It is said that there must be something, surely, to the story of Christ, since civilization was so altered. And for one-thousand, nine-hundred and seventy-eight years Christianity has flourished in one way or another. For a time it fueled both the arts and political life. It peopled the world of man with saints, sinners, priests, and it peopled space with a God, a legion of angels, and a devil and his cohorts—so surely Christianity must be based upon fact.

When people say this of course they mean that fact is true and myth is false. If I say there was very little factual basis for Christianity's beginning, then people will interpret this to mean that Christ's reality had no basis in truth. That is not what I am saying. There were other religions in other times that held a sway over civilizations for far longer periods. There were changes, but in general the religions of the Egyptians and the ancient Greeks are cases in point. The longevity of <u>those</u> religions and their effects upon those ancient civilizations are certainly not taken by "modern men" as proof that those religions had any basis in fact. Instead, they are considered as myths, pagan stories. Those peoples considered their Gods to be quite real, to have a basis in historical fact. Those religions had as great an effect upon their cultures as Christianity has had upon your own.

The first Gods began the process of man's exterior consciousness, so that the portions of nature with which he no longer identified were gradually deified, and put outside of himself. I have told you that your physical habits of perception are learned, and that the world can indeed be physically put together in different fashions. Events such as hallucinations give you hints of this.

At first, then, men perceived the Gods physically. These perceptions were different however than what you think of as ordinary ones. They appeared and disappeared as man perceived, and then did not perceive, these inner realities. These inner realities <u>were</u> "real." These were what you might call vital, responding personages, born of emotions of creativity. Perhaps you could compare them to the natural psychic or emotional <u>equivalent</u>, the psychological equivalent, of nature's clouds, sun, storms, or seasons.

They are quite as real in the emotional landscape of man's psyche, as the elements of the skyscape are above his planet. Myths always weave in and out of historical context, even as dreams are related to daily life. Myths usually include, then, some "provable facts," either of people historically known to have lived, or in terms of places or physical events of a natural kind. These are often taken then as proof that the myth is fact.

The interweaving of "dream reality" with the world of facts, however, is precisely what causes a myth to begin with, and is the source of its tremendous power, for it combines the two realities into a construct powerful enough to charge civilizations with new vitality, and literally to reshape man's course. Fact alone could never do that.

Both before and after "the time of Christ," as historically given, there were men who claimed to be the messiah. The messiah was a myth waiting for factual clothes. Many men tried on the fit. <u>In a manner of speaking</u>, now, it would make little difference which man was finally given the kingly robes—for the greater reality of the dream was so encompassing that it would come to be, whether one or 10 or 20 men's lives were historically joined together to form the Christ.

(10:37.) Christ tried to return man to nature. In a manner of speaking, again, there was no one Christ, historically speaking, but the personage of Christ, or the entity, was the reality from which the entire dramatic story emerged.

Are you tired?

("No, I'm okay.")

Get our friend a drink then, and come back.

Christ of course was a common name. Crucifixions were normal punishments. Conflicts between the priests and righteous members of the congregation were frequent. Many men dreamed of being the messiah, yet the dream went even beyond the confines of Jewish identity, and was far more international than any would-be messiah realized. Some of the stories have absolutely no basis in fact, as you think of fact. Others are distorted versions of factual events.

One of Christ's purposes, meaning the entity, was to teach man to see beyond the so-called facts of existence; not to deny death's physical event, but to show the greater dimensions of that event, and man's emergence into a new reality.

(*Long pause at 10:47.*) The greater creative drama involved occurred for centuries. Christ tried to tell men that he was everywhere, but they could not understand. He did not want a church, but an inner brotherhood. He was not born of a virgin, nor was his physical history any more factual than that once given for Zeus, or Apollo, or the Egyptian gods. His reality however did change the consciousness of man.

Historically speaking, the ancients understood man's psychology, his psyche, far better than you do now, for they were far more aware of its context. Their identification with nature gave them a sense of man's emotional power. They understood that dreams represented a reality as valid as the physical one, and they did not see the two worlds as separate. The early gods carried remnants of that grandeur.

Give us a moment.... As a people you are geared, say, to the exploration of the physical world. You climb mountains. It seldom occurs to you as a people that inner landscapes are as real, or that there are, say, psychological structures, usually unperceived, that are quite as real as any physical one. You are unable to see your own events as they interrelate with others. You do not understand that an idea can indeed change the world, unless you see firmly that the idea has a factual basis.

The inner landscape is no less real because you do not generally perceive it. In Framework 2 that inner landscape <u>is</u> the reality, and it is from that world that your physical events emerge.

(*11:02.*) You may want to separate the session at this point.

If in your private subjective reality you label yourself, unthinkingly now, in too-limited a fashion, then you can see yourself for example as the isolated artist at the brunt of society, the misunderstood poet that must be protected from the world's ways—mythic material that falls short. Such ideas can have strength only if you forget to identify yourself with the great inner order of nature, and with the physical <u>natural</u> world.

When you identify with nature you automatically fulfill your own world. Your dreams instantly come to life, and appear in your experience as aids and guides. You need not pit yourselves then against what you think of as a society that does not understand you, for that society falls into place as simply being one present aspect of a vaster natural world in which you are indeed firmly rooted. You can therefore naturally draw from Framework 2 all that you require.

Again, have Ruburt remember his love of nature. I will say nothing about the "fact" that you have not together studied the last session, or that Ruburt has not used the hot towels, for I do not need to. I do want you to approve of yourselves as natural creatures, for that approval automatically brings you in contact with nature's greater source, and your own.

End of session—
("Okay.")
—and a hearty, <u>natural</u> good evening.
("Thank you, Seth. Good night."
(11:14 P.M.)

DELETED SESSION
JANUARY 28, 1978 9:25 PM SATURDAY

Good evening.
("Good evening, Seth.")

I would like to give you an explanation for last evening's events, presuming you are both interested. I would also later like to make some comments about *"Unknown" Reality.*

Last night's events cannot be discussed without a brief preview of the time since our last session. Yesterday in particular, however, provides an excellent example of the way approval and self-disapproval work, and of the ways in which the habit of disapproval can cause you to misinterpret events, and then of course act accordingly.

Since our last session, you both made considerable efforts, so that you momentarily managed to suspend self-disapproval for some periods of time. As far as Ruburt's physical condition is concerned this was the pattern, as once or twice I believe he mentioned, by the way. I want it understood that I am not exaggerating. However, the pattern was thusly: in rhythmic patterns of activity, the entire body, part by part, stretched itself from head to toe. This was done in the body's own order. It <u>was</u> obvious to both of you, I believe, that at times Ruburt would stand a good deal taller. On some of those occasions all of the areas from the hips upward were stretching, while the legs would more or less be bent in the usual fashion. On other occasions the areas from the hips downward would stretch considerably, with <u>much</u> new activity in the knee joints and the ankles.

On many of those occasions Ruburt's back would bend over in the usual fashion as the knees continued their activity, because that was necessary as the adjustments at that time were made. The body could not, standing, stretch that fully all together and maintain balance, because part of the newly stretched muscles are not as yet that strong, where other portions that he has used are.

In between, there were periodic periods of new stability, where the newly activated portions moved and held. This period would last several days, when the process would begin again. That pattern began strongly enough for you to notice changes in Ruburt's height several weeks ago. Last week, however, keeping approval in mind, the process was activated further. Ruburt managed to stop worrying for a while, except for a few lapses, and you yourself made strides also there, and met your own challenges. The rune exercises and yawning in particular also helped.

By yesterday several new and significant changes appeared. Two or three times Ruburt found himself getting up, not only easier but easily to a considerably higher position. Finally he felt the impulse to walk without the table, used the plunger as an aid, and did not need to put his weight upon it. That meant that at that point newly activated portions of muscles and joints were working more or less in unison. He had to bend over, but the elasticized back was simply holding itself in abeyance. The muscles in the high portions of the legs, in the back, are the ones that need to be strengthened to unite the body in the flexibility that various portions of it are achieving.

The important head and neck areas are definitely healing themselves, and Ruburt is aware of those sensations. That improvement is also apparent in his rune exercises.

Until evening everything went well. Your pendulum exercises were most beneficial. They open up dialogues between various portions of the self, and of course bring these to the surface, amplified for your conscious attention. Ruburt was aware of rousing energy, then, as conflicts were aired. The pendulum also serves of course as a dialogue between the two of you at various levels, conscious and unconscious. You were both pleased when Ruburt walked from the bathroom to the table with his plunger. So what went wrong? It is important that you understand.

Ruburt felt like seeing company—a good sign. You encouraged him in that respect, but not too actively. You went along, however. When Ruburt could not reach O'Neill's, and pleased by his reactions during the day, you acted on impulse—a good sign, and suggested you both go for a ride. Up to here, all is well.

Ruburt in the meantime had felt his body relaxing. He wanted to go out in order to show that his attitude had changed. And to please you. You said "Don't go out because you think you should." He felt like crying all of a sudden, and he mentioned that. He went to the bathroom, and as he did he knew at once that his bodily situation had changed. At that point he immediately took it for granted, with a rush of self-disapproval, that this was a sign that he had learned nothing, and that his body was objecting to the whole idea of going out, and therefore challenging him—in other words, that his negative beliefs had risen to challenge new healthier attitudes.

It was obvious in the bathroom that his legs, which had been stable for several days, and showing improvements, were now trembling and insecure, but he interpreted that bodily message with self-disapproval, at the end of the hallway he had to sit down. You interpreted his situation precisely as he did, and for the same reasons, so of course there was no answer for this manufactured crisis, except that he ignore these bodily messages and act in spite of them.

He made a half-hearted attempt to get out of it. You then made a remark, voicing his own fears as well as your own, saying that you would not let him get away with it, meaning you would not let him get away with not going out as a pattern. So you were both in the middle of a crisis. What happened physically was this. Ruburt's body had extended itself on several occasions that day, stretching and using new postures, giving him the impulses toward further activity, exercising itself through that small-enough but important walk. It then relaxed.

The back and neck areas began a new expansion. The knees in the meantime, and the lower portion of the body, would ordinarily have rested. The body was sending messages simply that the time was not right. You both took it for granted, however, that despite what it seemed Ruburt might have learned lately, negative beliefs were rising in rebellion, and forcing a crisis that you then had to meet.

(10:02.) Ruburt went out to his room. The phone rang. Ruburt was given what he wanted—the psychological stimulation of a friend, who was all ready to visit you because Ruburt's message <u>had</u> gotten through. The psychological activity would have allowed the body to continue its process. The impulse had been a good one, to have company. Even then Ruburt was tempted to have Wade come, but his own disapproval, and yours, made it obvious that to do so would certainly be a copout. His body was not ready.

Because of your fears, going out has become an issue. Not walking properly is the issue—otherwise there would be no problem. You were pleased when Ruburt walked across the floor with his plunger, without the table, yet both of you expected him to walk down steps, small as they are, and walk around the car in the garage without his table, or there is something wrong. You expect different kinds of behavior in the house and in the garage.

Ruburt does the steps, something he does not do inside—a change for the body, and a good one—but in his position an <u>exercise</u> in itself. Both of you even refuse to think of using the table in the garage, so Ruburt forces his body into the most unnatural of positions so that he can lean upon the car. Those positions would aggravate anyone. He made it to the car, knowing that on the other occasions that his body had so protested he had had difficulty. He used his resources to try to change the situation. He used suggestion. He tried to concentrate upon the ride.

On your return, considering the situation, he gallantly tried to gather his resources, and made it halfway around the car before the protesting muscles had their say. The newly activated areas of the day repeated that they were being overworked, and they pulled other muscles with them. You, of course, took it for granted as he did that this was an excellent example of the negative or still ignorant portions of the personality coming to the front, and this is what was responsible for your own somewhat ungallant behavior.

You helped Ruburt physically, but you heaped upon him a barrage of disapproval. That disapproval was in a way quite natural, considering your interpretation of the event. It made the situation worse, of course. You both managed at the end to not fall into the kind of situation that in the past you might have, considering the conditions.

Ruburt's body earlier signaled its desire to move, its readiness. He obeyed the impulse, which was excellent. The other bodily messages were as valid, and there was no need to take it for granted, as both of you did, that some element in Ruburt's personality was rebelliously and purposefully sabotaging you at that time.

You may take your break.

(10:18—10:25.)

Such self-disapproval can color your interpretation of events, then, forcing you to act accordingly.

You both did very well up until that point last evening, and afterward Ruburt in particular did well, though both of you managed to avoid pitfalls that might otherwise have occurred. When you left yourselves alone, as you did generally speaking, during the week, you not only attained some peace of mind, but definite improvements in those areas that concerned you both. Ruburt's eyes have been improving, as his typing *Emir* shows. Not only did he see better, but his hand and eye coordination considerably increased, as did the flexibility of his fingers. During your ride, he noticed that his vision then was a good deal better.

Now a few remarks about *"Unknown."*

I repeat: you made no errors, as far as putting that book out in two volumes is concerned. With your attitudes, you would have been no more pleased, either of you, had you put it out in one. In fact, it's possible you would have been less pleased.

I am dealing with probabilities—but I do not believe it would have been out at all yet, and your own attitudes would have made that an even more regrettable situation. There was nothing held back in that regard. Ruburt's attitudes, now, were known to you, as were your own. Let yourselves be for a while. Ruburt will feel like going out. There is nothing about outside, in those terms, that frightens him—that is from the house into the garage, symbolically speaking. There were times in the poor weather, when physically he felt like going out. When you make an issue, however, you manufacture a crisis.

Not only then do you have a manufactured crisis of one minor variety or another, but Ruburt is expected or expects his body to execute the steps, walk without the table or any other aid, and behave entirely differently, and of course better, than he does inside the house. Neither of you would even think of a chair in the garage; any aid would be a copout. There are some days when his body can perform in that regard, and some days when it cannot at this point.

His shoulders and arms are beginning to release considerably. He could consciously move his shoulder blades in the back for the first time this evening, and the arms are very important in bodily balance. He was beginning to try to walk without the table for small periods—commendable in the house, but expected, no matter what, in the garage.

Basically, it is this self-disapproval that forms artificial crises, that then impede your progress, cause you to misinterpret events, and act accordingly. This of course applies in the area of *"Unknown,"* as well as in situations in which either of you compare yourselves unfavorably with, say, your neighbors' physical activity. It is unhealthy not to want to go out. You interpret that statement, however, in social and moral terms. Of course the healthy body wants to go out in nature. It is not morally wrong at any given time to want the opposite, or overall to prefer mental to physical activity—nor, overall, is that preference unhealthy.

When Ruburt does not go out, however, it is never a simple issue of the body's condition at any given time, but a moral dilemma in which, basically you see, you are misinterpreting events. Ruburt felt like having company. Your own improved mental habits of the week, your pendulum work and his own improvements, released energy that under those conditions sought release—and his impulse showed him in what direction.

On another occasion, he might have wanted to go out, to take a drive; and the impulse will also be the result of the body's knowledge that the time is right. He was relieved during your bad weather because the artificial crisis was lessened. You have made gains, and important ones. Ruburt's body messages should be heeded. He heeds them if they follow your ideas of improvements. If not, you both take it for granted that the body is not in the middle of a process, but that some immediate challenge exists.

The disapproval forces you to make a pattern in which the improvements become <u>insignificant</u> rather than significant. You could not understand the body's performance last evening because you <u>took it for granted, and without question</u>, that some portion of Ruburt was challenging other portions.

(*10:52.*) *Emir* is a delight. Your own painting is showing definite advances. If you want challenges, learn to challenge your self-disapproval, and to question those beliefs that you take for granted as truth. No part of Ruburt rose in rebellion last evening, to defy either of you.

Self-disapproval always takes resistance for granted, and sees it at every turn, therefore of course leading to battles of one kind-or another. I do not blame you for wishing that Ruburt's table were not necessary, but he is showing signs that he will be able to dispense with it. I do not blame you for wishing he did not need a stool at the sink, but that area has no conflict now, and Thursday he had an impulse to do the dishes without it. Yet, aids in the garage also were considered copouts.

His bathroom behavior is not only good, but even with the various rhythms mentioned, has shown improvement. His grip is stronger. Last night's experience could, and in the past would, have severely set you back, because then your self-disapproval simply would have been deepened. You are therefore to understand what I am saying, and not to further disapprove of yourselves or your reactions, but to be pleased with your additional knowledge—for that will enable you to look at events with clearer eyes.

Now I bid you a very fond good evening.

(*"Thank you, Seth. Good night."*)

(*11:01 PM.*)

SESSION 822 (DELETED PORTION)
FEBRUARY 22, 1978 9:27 PM WEDNESDAY

(*The following material is from the 822nd session.*)

(*11:13.*) I have two comments. One is for our friend Frank. Give us a moment.

These are helpful hints for him to consider. He is used to feedback from others. He enjoys ideas, but in that regard he does not trust himself. When he is alone and writing, the distrust of the self becomes apparent. He does not trust the expression without the feedback.

Sometimes a particular desire, as when he does estimates, will allow him to work unimpeded, because in that area experience has shown him that his estimates are usually more or less correct. There he has anticipated future feedback that he relies upon.

The direct expression through writing confuses him, for he is faced with a different kind of construction, say, than one might feel in a kindergarten, where blocks of wood carry the alphabet, and physical blocks might be moved around to form words. At the same time he is afraid of feedback, and he has learned to minimize his hearing to protect himself from criticism. The writing represents strong portions of Frank's personality that are intently concerned with the expression of subjective feelings—feelings that appear nebulous at times because they cannot be expressed—so it seems to him—in a direct fashion.

The writing became a <u>symbol</u> for the expression of thoughts that could not be verbalized in childhood. This carried over into the writing, and comes to the forefront now because of his father's condition. He wanted to express love for his father as a child far more openly than he felt his father would allow. He felt that his father would consider such demonstrations not masculine.

When he learned to write, he thought of <u>writing</u> to express such thoughts, and was always tempted to use writing as an expression of those subjective feelings he felt were forbidden—not just directed toward his father, but feelings of which he felt his father would disapprove. Writing therefore became a charged activity in any area.

(11:30.) The condition becomes more worrisome because it now bears the brunt of an unspoken or unexpressed love that is hidden behind his conscious attitude and behavior toward his father. Frank's father himself was afraid of showing unseeming love, in his terms, toward his family. Frank avoided that kind of behavior with his children, but did not fully surmount the pattern as far as his own father was concerned.

It seems that such expressions of love would now come too late. Expressing such love now, however, would show immediate benefits.

One other small comment. Ruburt simply identified with too-small a portion of himself, not realizing that left alone his abilities would draw from Framework 2 <u>all</u> that was required for their fulfillment—all of the impulses, desires, and circumstances. He thought, as you did, that artistic abilities were like alien flowers in an unfriendly land, that had to be force-fed and protected at all costs.

Have him read over my sessions again, to remind himself that his abilities spring from Framework 2, and do not need such overprotection. It does not help, and it definitely hinders his creativity, that he so misguidedly tries to protect. Overall, you cannot be simultaneous in one area while you hold down simultaneity in many others. He must allow himself the freedom of his being, and from that freedom his work will further develop. Creativity is above all high play.

If you trust yourselves, and approve of yourselves, all of your problems literally dissolve, and playful creativity bursts into its full flower.

End of session, and a fond good evening.

("Thank you, Seth. Good night.")

(11:42 PM.)

SESSION 824 (DELETED PORTION)
MARCH 1, 1978 9:40 PM WEDNESDAY

(The following information is from the 824th session.
(11:26.) A note for Ruburt, and to some extent for you.

Forgive the terminology, but you each believed in "magic," or the sessions never would have started. You believed that reality had more to it than the senses showed. You believed that together you <u>could achieve</u> what had not been achieved earlier—that you could somehow or other offer meaningful and real solutions to the world's problems.

Of late, I hear more and more from you both in your private discussions, in which you voice opinions to the effect that overall man can hope to learn little—that the individual can only do so much, that you can at best glimpse the most minute portion of knowledge. With attitudes like that, the sessions would never have begun. With Ruburt's condition you forget your own abilities almost completely, relatively speaking.

Let Ruburt remember the playfulness of games. And above all remember that pretending is not a lie *(re Cinderella)*. He can pretend to be well and flexible if he remembers that, without feeling any contradictions at all.

The symbolism in the birth dream *(of Jane's)* is obvious. That is all I will say for now—but apply the book dictation tonight to your own lives. End of session.

("Thank you, Seth.")

A fond and most affectionate good evening.

("Thank you. The same to you.")

(11:34 PM.)

SESSION 828 (DELETED PORTION)
MARCH 15, 1978 9:53 PM WEDNESDAY

(The following material is from the 828th session. A note: This is the third anniversary of our moving into the hill house.)

(10:51.) Ruburt hit upon some pertinent points this evening, that will be clarified for him. For now, let me say that in his writing and psychic activity he has learned to largely forget the levels of consciousness that are limited to cause-and-effect and time continuity.

In the physical situation, this is hardly the case. I want him to continue helping with *"Unknown"*—but also to follow the suggestions I gave a while ago, and devote some time each day to free, creative, playful thought. During that time he automatically refreshes his body, by placing himself in a state of consciousness that is at least <u>capable</u> of opening up all kinds of help, inspiration, and undreamed-of considerations.

This is only a hint for now, that will automatically lead him in certain directions. Those states also automatically help bring about necessary physical relaxation, for the relaxation of course first exists at that other stage.

End of session, unless you have questions.

("No, I guess not.")

Then I wish you both a fond good evening—and both of your dream activities should continue to be quite vital.

("Thank you, Seth.")

(10:58 PM.)

DELETED SESSION
MARCH 20, 1978 9:41 PM MONDAY

(We sat for the session at 9:10. As we waited Jane said several times that she felt "a sense of reassurance" from Seth, that he was organizing some kind of material or program for her because of her physical situation. She didn't think there would be a regular session this evening. Finally, as I began to write these few notes, Seth came through:)

Good evening.

("Good evening, Seth.")

Now: I am preparing some special material for Ruburt. Some will be given in session time, though not this evening, and other material will be given at various levels of consciousness. There will be no regular session this evening, except for these comments that are meant to reassure Ruburt. He worries otherwise.

There are rhythms that exist, as I have mentioned before, and over a period of time, had you the time to check your records you would see that overall we have about the same number of sessions over a yearly period. There are many cycles that are involved—some connected with the two of you, with myself, or with other conditions quite apart.

Some of those conditions could be called the result of psychological atmospheres that surround the earth, say. I do not travel physically in a UFO *(with amusement)*, and yet my mental or psychic journeys must occur in a medium of some kind. There are rhythmic activities in that atmosphere that I count upon and use. As for example a sea captain might use the rhythm of the waves for his journeys. Those inner atmospheric "waves" have a certain regularity. They are more intense at certain times than others.

Tell Ruburt to be looking for some of the mentioned information, and some I will deliver.

End of session, and a fond good evening.

("Thank you, Seth."

(9:49 PM.)

SESSION 830 (DELETED PORTION)
MARCH 27, 1978 9:18 PM MONDAY

(The following material is from the 830th session. Break came at 10:25, after Seth had delivered material for his book on the mass psyche. The notes that follow were written during that break, and would usually be presented with the regular session; however, since they're more personal than usual, they're given below instead. Jane's quotations in them do apply, however, to material Seth had given as dictation for Psyche.*)*

(10:25. Jane was rather unhappy when she came out of trance. She said she was "mad"—an adjective I'd heard her use several times earlier today as she talked about her own physical state, beliefs, control, etc. I asked her now to dictate to me exactly what she wanted me to record: "Now *he's telling us that to take conscious control of your beliefs and life and everything* does *involve a new manipulation of consciousness, where I'd been knocking my guts out thinking it should be something you can do real easy. So how come I'm so dumb, I've been thinking. After all these books*

he tells us that. All of this is my interpretation," she said, *"based on what I remember I said in trance."* She was more than a little upset. *"Like now he's saying 'Well, there are a few difficulties involved,' where before it all seemed so easy. A little bit tricky—"*

(Resume at 10:53. Seth did go into the two questions I'd asked at the start of the session.)

That was the end of dictation.

I may have slipped up, but I do not think so: I do not believe I gave the information about you and George in book dictation *(for "Unknown" Reality)*, in order to keep the material simple enough for the reader. But you and George are and are not counterparts. You do share psychic memories, and hold in common the memories of other selves who did live in the time of the Roman-soldier incident.

Those memories exist as patterns. In this life, you come together and part, come together and part again, forming a counterpart relationship when it suits your purposes, as streams of consciousness might mix and merge, and then separate.

These counterparts are psychic relationships, formations that in the deepest terms flow into historic time and out of it. Some, in your terms, last a lifetime. Others represent psychic encounters that happen between two individuals at several points, say, but are not continuous. They may be no less intense, however.

Your experience concerning Jack Wall *(on March 23, 1978)* was quite legitimate, although it happened some time ago, in your terms *(a point I'd wondered about)*. It was triggered by your associations immediately previous. In a way, Jack found it inconceivable that he should die. He wondered at first why Elizabeth did not perceive him, and he remained unconscious of his own funeral. He did perceive such a light *(as I sensed)*—the light of understanding.

Now give us a moment.... You should both read tonight's session, book dictation, with Ruburt's situation in mind. You have tried to maintain stability while you work, and have schooled yourselves so that it is not disrupted. You are still both afraid—Ruburt primarily, of course—of really trying for fear you will be disappointed, and worried at the disruptions that might occur—again, Ruburt primarily. Most of all, however, he has identified of late with what he thinks of as his failure.

He became afraid of trying again to disrupt the old patterns. You of course do give tacit consent, and give up whatever role of leadership you possess in that area, which is far more considerable than you allow yourself to admit. Ruburt is often afraid he has little control over the situation. This prevents him of course from breaking the patterns.

<u>You</u> tell yourself you have little control over his actions, or that your feelings make little difference in the face of his actions, but that is the other side of the same coin. He begins with the pendulum and drops it, but neither do you encourage him to persist.

The winter doldrums always affect him, but are of course reinforced. Today's visitor *(Josette)* came in response to Ruburt's need, bringing him appreciation and a new encounter—but tonight's session dictation can be of considerable benefit to you both. Ruburt simply drops the issue for a while—and then he feels panicky—at times a quite normal reaction to a sense of powerlessness. Neither of you have persisted with the Framework 2 methods.

(11:00.) The lack of persistence simply shows that in large measure your way of life suits you both, regardless of its consequences. You are obviously dissatisfied, however. Again, in the session there are strong clues, but you—or rather, Ruburt primarily must take advantage of them. The pendulum is excellent, particularly when you do it together. It can be used to advantage, particularly together, in the mornings for suggestions. Only a brief time is required. The intent is the important thing—and then for another <u>short</u> period to search for current reasons behind behavior. There should not be a concentration upon the problem—<u>as a problem</u>.

You are in the middle of a learning process. Do not think one portion of the personality is sabotaging another portion. Instead, one personality is working with a system of beliefs, and trying to attain an overall synthesis. That is all for tonight's session. My heartiest good wishes and a fond good evening.

("Thank you, Seth." 11:06 PM.)

DELETED SESSION
APRIL 3, 1978 9:33 PM MONDAY

(The story of what we've been up to the last few days can be found in Jane's records of her pendulum sessions since March 28. Of course, she has been trying to find out causes for her physical symptoms. I've helped her somewhat, but plan to do much more. Several times lately she's remarked that she's "desperate," so when she did so again in bed recently I told her that from the next day on we would put her needs first, regardless of all else. This means working with the pendulum, suggestion, self-hypnosis, whatever's needed, to get at the root of her troubles. We'll do this first thing each morning, for however long it takes each day, until we see signs that results are what we want them to be.

(*It appears that we've already made a small beginning; through the pendulum we've arrived at several categories of belief to explore. For the first time in many months I feel that we might be onto something, and so does Jane.*

(*No session was held last Wednesday while Jane worked on the* James *galleys. I mailed them to Prentice-Hall this morning.*

(*We wanted a session tonight on Jane's problem, although we'd settle for something from Seth each time, along with his other book dictation, or whatever. As a result of our work with the pendulum this morning, Jane was so relaxed by session time that she didn't know whether she could manage a session. I suggested she try, so that her mind would be at ease. Tonight's session was excellent, and should of course be studied in connection with the material we've already accumulated through pendulum work.*)

Good evening.

(*"Good evening, Seth."*)

A private session. Some of this material has been given before, but it is important here.

First of all, it is important to realize that Ruburt's unconscious, so called, is not working against him on purpose, sabotaging his projects. The subconscious does reason, but it also reasons according to the information that you give it.

I want to begin by reminding you that these divisions to the self are rather arbitrary, for the sake of discussion. The ego, again, looks into the physical world. The source self, or inner ego, has its prime reality in Framework 2. Between the ego and the inner ego, you have what you think of as the unconscious. It gets its energy of course from the source self, and its primary directives to insure the fulfillment and the survival of the person. To some extent then it must depend upon conscious deductions and reasoning. With that as background let me continue.

You have a good point of organization with your pendulum work today. Fear of the kind mentioned (*scorn and ridicule*) is behind the symptoms. Whenever our sessions, your own efforts, or other events, have convinced Ruburt either of the personal safe universe or of the basic safety of the self, that reassurance helped quiet the unconscious fears, and allowed him then to direct his will toward physical improvements.

The fears were never granted validity, however, though sometimes given vague intellectual recognition. They were considered cowardly, unadult, unreasonable, degrading, and both of you considered them in that light. "How abject can you get?" you would both think.

Now let us for a moment look at the situation from the point of view of the unconscious. With the information it has received, and in the light of what it considers Ruburt's lack of understanding, lack of gratitude, and determined refusal to understand its position.

We must start with the fact that Ruburt did not feel secure as a child, but was made somewhat to feel responsible for his mother's illness and breakup of her marriage. He was then sent to a home. He was a high-spirited child, and was taught there that he must toe the mark and do what the others did, or he would be punished.

Later, when he returned home, he learned that he must toe the mark again, or Welfare would put him in another home. <u>He must not make waves</u>. It was not safe to stand out. His food, clothing, and survival depended on toeing the mark. The church provided a family of sorts, but that family also was dependent upon religious obedience. Ruburt's high spirits and abilities fought against such circumstances. He finally broke away from the church—running to college—a college considered by the church at the time as communistically inclined, antireligious, and so forth.

His survival in college, since he had a scholarship, was dependent upon toeing the mark, and even then he refused to do so; and was quite unceremoniously kicked out on his independent ass.

He refused several marriage proposals, having determined he would not toe the mark at all in a conventional marriage. He tried a relationship with Walt, but his high spirits and abilities would not stand for <u>that</u> kind of repression. When he met you, he turned to love <u>and</u> science, for by then he had set upon science and the intellect as a safe means of containing his abilities and expressing them.

Your own joint sexual love was too hot for either of you to handle, and you both tempered it with intellectualism and caution; but for all of that it has endured. Ruburt's abilities and energy kept seeking fulfillment. Through those years he considered himself an outcast from society, and he did not know where his abilities were leading. He tried to toe the mark while doing his own thing. He did not identify with the world or its people. He identified mentally, however, with science, with the avant-garde, and so was sustained. At the gallery, for example, when your psychic work began, he did not speak out, and you encouraged him not to, and you both considered this as a scientific kind of breakthrough. When Ruburt discovered that his energy and abilities had led him to a point where he was at odds with religion <u>and</u> science, and had no place to roost, thematically, he became very worried.

(10:00.) If you did not toe the mark, you were punished severely, or abandoned; or your sustenance was cut off. His unconscious had learned to tread a

careful line, to let Ruburt use his abilities while seeing that he was protected at the same time. Its ideas were largely gained in childhood, and there was a give-and-take between Ruburt's fears and hopes. Gradually, however, the give-and-take gave. He held back the fears, thinking them beneath adult behavior. He stopped giving his unconscious feedback in that regard.

A point also from the past—if he did not toe the mark with Walt, Walt also threatened to abandon him—once, in the middle of the desert.

He found himself with you and his work. He would do what he would do anyway, protecting himself as he thought fit. When the feedback stopped, the subconscious became panicky. Since so much of Ruburt's life was involved with yours, it felt that Ruburt must now toe the mark with you also—at least topside—so that he must not express any contrary opinions, or that you would abandon him also, in which case he would be utterly alone.

Give us a moment.... Ruburt did not approve of fear. He felt it was, again, cowardly. It was given no validity, nor acknowledged as valid. As the books continued to sell, several conflicts arose. They served expression and creativity, and they insured financial security—but at the same time they made Ruburt's unofficial "dangerous" thoughts publicly available. They told the <u>world</u> he did not toe the line, and he feared retribution, ostracism, scorn.

He fears the books will not sell, because he is afraid, as in childhood, that if you do not toe the line your sustenance will be taken away. Remind him that <u>financially at least that not toeing the line has paid off very well indeed</u>, and in your pendulum work inform the subconscious of that.

Tell the subconscious that you understand its purposes, and thank it for its concern. Apologize for cutting off the important give-and-take of feelings, and admit that under the circumstances it was given, its own fears were justified. You did not give it all the facts. "You" here is Ruburt. You did not grant its feelings any validity. Remind the subconscious that its origin is with the source self; which will indeed provide it automatically with the necessary conditions for safety and survival.

At the time the subconscious developed these fears, it believed that its survival was dependent upon other people, for Ruburt was young and frightened. If you did not do what other people said, you were in trouble—and deeply. In the face of that belief Ruburt still determined to do his own thing, only with the safeguards.

As his abilities blossomed, the safeguards turned into fortifications. He could not <u>counter</u> the fears because he would not acknowledge them. The unconscious therefore felt forced to take stronger measures.

(10:20.) Give us a moment.... At times, again, inroads would be made. I

have probably mentioned before that in college Ruburt would cross the street often rather than meet a group of students. The pattern simply intensified. The Gallery of Silence affair was simply another episode, in which fears were pooh-poohed, but he was afraid that those people would come here, and he felt threatened.

His new room gave him the view that he wanted, but no protection—and not only that, but then he was the one who met guests head-on.

All of this goes back, forgive me, to fears that the spontaneous self will in one way or another get him in trouble.

Give us a moment again.... Obviously the unconscious is spontaneous, but his early experience taught him, as given earlier this evening, to use that spontaneity with care. The subconscious feels that it is doing its job, because Ruburt has not allowed feedback; not approving of fear, not allowing the feelings release, and therefore also cutting down on experience that could <u>counter</u> the feelings and show the subconscious that the fears were exaggerated.

(A note: We should ask Seth what sort of countering experience he has in mind.)

Ruburt does not think that you are afraid, for you seldom voice any fears. He feels, therefore, that he is a coward, that fears make him seem abject, that they are unacceptable. On various occasions, when the suggestions in his papers worked—you follow me—they worked because at the same time Ruburt was writing down his feelings: his aggressions and his fears.

(This may explain why the 1973 suggestions, which Jane still refers to often, worked. It's worth checking.)

He felt that aggressive action was also threatening, for the same reasons as just given. You do not bite the hand that feeds you. The feelings of panic are the result of fears usually buried, when they simply reach a point of intensity that seeks acknowledgement.

I believe that is it for the evening.

("Okay. Very good.")

Thank you. I hope it helps.

("It will. Thank you. Good night," I said. I knew, of course, that the session had many good things in it. Less than half a minute passed, as Jane and I talked, when Seth returned at 10:35.)

A note: I had not intended to say this again. Because it seems to do no good. I would like to mention, however, that neither of you make any <u>serious effort</u> to change your beliefs about the world of men.

What I have said on that issue has made little inroad there. You are self-righteous, both of you, and intolerant of your fellows. You look for evidence of their poor intent, and chicanery, and you seek out evidence of their flaws. In your terms, I do not share your humanity, in a fashion. I am not directly concerned with the exuberance, vitality, creativity, joys, sorrows, or tragedies of life.

My standards of spiritual behavior, I would say, are as pertinent as your own, as "high," yet I can honestly say that your self-righteousness blinds you both to the good intent, however misguided, in say even political actions. Look how Ruburt's unconscious tries to protect him, with symptoms that you certainly find most disagreeable, because Ruburt has not given his unconscious, say, all of the facts.

In a different way, countries try to protect themselves, or people will believe that they must perform certain acts that are deplorable. Yet you both collect data confirming man's nefarious nature.

I will ride my good fortune tonight by telling you that such actions do not help either of you at all, and that they are not realistic or objective attitudes, though you may believe that they are. I will carry my sacrilegious remarks further to tell you personally, Joseph, that the Rockefellers are not driven by any evil intent. And with that remark I leave you, daring not to trespass any further upon your cherished beliefs. A fond good evening.

("Thank you very much, Seth."

(10:45 PM. Seth's remark about the Rockefellers came about evidently because I'd read an article recently claiming that the Rockefellers were making loads of money out of the country's inflation troubles, re the Arab oil crisis, etc. I'd forgotten it. At this time, however, I'd have trouble believing the Rockefellers weren't making out like bandits.

(I mentioned to Jane a question I'd thought of during the session but hadn't interrupted to ask: If the subconscious can reason, as Seth tells us, why doesn't it understand that at times it can go too far sometimes?—that obviously the idea of self-protection can be very damaging if carried to extremes. Why wouldn't it back off somewhat in such a case? Its own domain could literally be threatened or obliterated if it didn't act within bounds. Jane listened, but didn't get anything from Seth in answer, so it's for next time. She did say that Seth indicated that class helped her to some degree, in that she got approval from it, as in a family situation.)

DELETED SESSION
APRIL 5, 1978 9:37 PM WEDESDAY

(We've learned a good deal about Jane's symptoms, working with the pendulum since Monday's session. We're keeping a list of all questions, with the daily

answers, and are now seeing some notable shifts in answers, indicating improved communication between her conscious and unconscious selves.

(We had several questions for Seth, including the one noted at the end of the last session: Why didn't the unconscious realize it was going too far in its protective role? Why didn't it back off? Jane wrote the question up on a separate list, so that we'll make sure the inquiries that develop are taken care of by Seth. Two corollary questions I came up with yesterday are these: Does the unconscious know there is a physical body? If it does, what is its conception of that body?

(This afternoon Jane had a very revealing dream about the whole question of protection, the male aspects of her personality, etc.; a copy is attached to the session.

(I also wanted Seth to comment upon my very discouraged reactions to the mail today; the letters were certainly not the kind we wanted in response to our efforts, I thought.

(As we sat for tonight's session we made two important connections; 1. When the refrigerator turned itself off I expressed relief at the sudden quiet. But Jane said the silence bothered her—the kind of remark I've always heard her make. Then she said that as a young child she was always uneasy at home when it was too quiet—that those were the times when she worried about what her mother was up to. When Marie had been making noise, involved in noisy activities, Jane had felt much better, safer. 2. This insight led Jane to an obvious one neither of us had ever made before: that when she gets a letter in which the writer threatens suicide if Jane doesn't help him or her, this is like Marie threatening the young Jane that she will commit suicide.)

Now: a private session.

The points Ruburt brought up immediately previous to my speaking involve connections made because the subconscious was responding, and trying to give you further information.

I want to begin, however, by making some rather neutral but important points. You age of communications has significantly altered public and private life, so that for example by mail Ruburt might receive as many petitions as the king of a country in times past. People of no other age, historically speaking, have had to contend with the dimensions of public exposure that are now possible.

The public man, the man of letters, et cetera in other centuries, and the public man say of Rome, or of the Middle Ages, or of the 19th Century, involved personal interactions with the public, but in very limited, controlled situations. The private image of the person was largely unknown. A king could travel through his own lands and not be recognized if he wanted it that way, for no television screen flashed his image into the homes of his people. The line between the public and the private was much more clearly drawn. There is much more that could be said, but I simply here want to mention that such issues demand far more of a gifted personality.

Give us a moment.... Art always serves as some self-disclosure, in which the art stands for the person, and the art is sent abroad, for example. The art stands for more than the person. In a way it reaches higher than the person, in that it expresses dimensions of imagination or inspiration that are heroic, and often by nature it speaks of capacities that cannot be fully expressed except through art.

The person, therefore, often "cannot live up to his art." Ruburt wants to <u>embody</u> his art. He expects himself to possess all of the qualities that his art tries to entice from human nature. If man can be a natural healer, and he says so, then he personally should heal others and himself. That is his reasoning. If he is gifted with words in writing, and gifted in speech, then he feels that he should go out bravely into the public arena, and speak out his message to the world.

I am not making value judgments of my own here in the following remarks. His subconscious, however, knowing its own beliefs which were given it by the conscious self, after all, feels highly threatened, for it knows not more about Ruburt than he does, but more than Ruburt will <u>admit</u> he knows. He expects himself to do such things, and the minute he gets better, he says, he will go thusly out into the world.

This is the same person who on the other hand used to put up barriers of bookcases at one end of the living room to protect himself from any neighbors or miscellaneous callers; who objected when Mr. Gottlieb dared to cross into his private working area and glance at a paper. In the face of those fears, Ruburt did progress from someone who was afraid to read poetry to friends, to someone who ran an excellent class of nearly 50 people—all of the time denying that any fears existed. Not faced, the fears grew.

Now, to some extent, in pragmatic terms, you must look at your backgrounds. Your father greatly distrusted the public and public events. When his battery shop closed and the public turned to the new inventions, that made his livelihood passe. He disliked the public from that moment on, and felt resentful toward those whose pictures he took, that his livelihood would be at the expense of their favor.

You felt that commercial art would work financially, because it belonged to the times, yet even then the comic book market, you felt, was falling beneath you as the public's ideas changed, and *(Mickey)* Spillane's comic strip fell beneath censure. You simply would not, later, curry the world's favor with your paintings—even if, through hard work, financial success might follow. You did not trust people to know good work when you produced it.

(10:05.) In one way or another, both of Ruburt's parents had little use for the world, and did not trust it. None of your parents, in other words, had an easy give-and-take with their fellows in that regard.

Ruburt decided to brazen it through—to do his thing and be paid for it. At the same time Ruburt carried the fears mentioned. He hoped for the world's approval, for he knew his work was good. On the other hand he carried the beliefs of this afternoon's dream—that originality made a person instantly suspect, and that in the ordinary world, if you put yourself in the world's eye its people would hunt you down. In opposition, he carried the belief that he <u>should</u> go on television, make tours, and so forth, and expose himself in direct opposition to those fears.

(Along in here I had an insight as I wrote, no doubt triggered by Seth's material. It was that although Jane's eye condition might be caused by my delays with getting "Unknown" Reality to the public, another reason was also involved: namely, that she saw the revealing notes I did for "Unknown" as a threat also.)

Because the fears were hidden, they could not be countered through, say, fresh experience that might show them to be at least exaggerated. They could not be reasoned with, and the unconscious was left holding the bag, so to speak.

The <u>exaggerated</u> fears carried threats not simply of scorn, but as you so clearly put it the other evening "Those people would burn us at the stake if they had the chance." To save Ruburt from such possible assassination, the symptoms were not considered too strong a measure. But in the face of that <u>kind</u> of exaggerated threat they were considered very strict, but reasonable enough under the conditions. The subconscious was not too pleased with them.

Take your break.

(10:15. I told Jane about my insight, involving her eyes and "Unknown" Reality. She agreed. We'd finished with Volume 1 in early 1977—February, say, and she recalled that by March she'd started having eye trouble. But what's the connection between eyes and the threat of exposure? I told her she didn't have to answer the question now. It should be listed, though.

(Jane was getting that "slightly sicky feeling in my stomach" as we talked about fears. I got her a glass of milk. "I'll do what I can about the session," she said. She was yawning again and again. I reminded her of my two questions from Monday's session, plus the one about my reaction to the mail today. Seth didn't go into the first two, but the following material did have to do with reactions to those who wrote us. Resume at 10:27.)

Now: Ruburt has had nearly enough for this evening, considering today's activities, but I will get to all of your questions in the very near future.

You have those <u>down</u>, but I want to mention some matters you are not aware of.

Ruburt became frightened, for example, of out-of-body travel when he began to get it in his head that "all the nuts" were doing it too, and that out-of-body activity involved him in an <u>inner public environment</u>, in which he might meet "all those fools" who were then not bound by physical restraints. He did not fear death, for example, at the hands of others, then, but too close emotional contact. He felt people "could get at him" that way.

In a strange fashion because of his fears, now—and these particular fears can be countered with communications with the unconscious, and with understanding—he was afraid simply that so many people knew of his existence. To some extent that would have been involved no matter what field of endeavor he chose, if he became well-known.

The secrecy of childhood is connected because of Welfare, and your own statements to him often, years ago, <u>not to tell people anything</u>. Those statements reinforced earlier beliefs.

Now you <u>are</u> exceptional people, and exceptional people in your work are quite simply exceptions. You deal with relatively rare, different kinds of achievements and challenges. Many of your correspondents are quite average, though to you they seem deplorable. They are not used to dealing with imaginative concepts, or conceptual thought, or of applying the intelligence to the realm of the imagination. Often they cannot discriminate between good work or poor work, artistically. They are drawn to what emotionally arouses them or offers them hope, even though they may only be able to put a small portion to practical use. They deal with emotional realities that are rather apart from your own concerns.

Your interests place you in a position in which you question the theories of your times, and the people who uphold those theories are not about to seek you out. You do not realize the exhilarating nature, again, of your own endeavors in comparison to those of, say, the majority.

The Framework 2 material provided Ruburt momentarily with enough faith to show some physical improvement. Faith will indeed dissolve fears.

Give us a moment.... Fears turn into severe anxiety, however, formless, when they are not identified and understood. The Silent Gallery people epitomized Ruburt's fears in a fashion, and though I have given material in several ways pertaining to the fears, Ruburt never <u>consciously acknowledged them</u>, but shoved them under. The subconscious should be reminded of the help that is available from the source self, for its fears began before it had that information, and the fears themselves caused blocks that prevented assimilation of the knowledge later.

The subconscious can be told to take advantage of that additional knowledge and help, and it will gladly do so. Remind me of other questions at our next session.

A fond good evening.

("Thank you, Seth.")

(10:45 PM.)

JANE'S NOTES
FRIDAY, APRIL 7, 1978

(*I feel more hopeful today; and almost as if there might be something from the libvary on the principles of conservatism and originality as in the* Cézanne *book. In the meantime though, I want to paraphrase material that came from Seth off and on last night—in the john and bedroom. It came in that circular fashion, like a concentrated minisession but it's hard to write out for that reason too, so I only have a few highpoints.*

(*The idea seemed to be that creativity, mine and anyone's, is initially playful, curious, seeks expression—and is one of the highest kinds of psychic play—the artist playing with concepts no matter what the art; and actually inserts his or her reality onto the world, superimposed upon it. But the creative basic part of the personality enjoys* that; *the doing, primarily—the art will always be an individual interpretation and recreation of the world—that exists for itself and* is *its own meaning.*

(*Its very difficult for the practical world—for people who aren't primarily "artists or creators" to deal with that sort of thing; they don't know where to place it and ideas* alone *make them uncomfortable—they aren't real or unreal according to their way of looking at reality.*

(*My personal problems developed in force when I began to be overly concerned with my creative "work" as work, as it applied to the world, as it would be received and interpreted; when I tried to compare its reception to other officially accepted activities—that people understood—when I tried to look at my "work" through their eyes, and when I began to expect the kind of honor and approbation given to others—who conformed.*

(*I am right—meaning in accord with my own nature—when I "forget" each book as it is done...* Basically *the creative play exploration, writing, is the main core of my creativity—and I do that for the love of doing it.* I am *"lucky" that the books sell, and that does mean that the world does accept "my work" to a certain important degree. But basically creativity is not a career in usual terms. It cannot be treated like a lawyer's career or a scientist's or whatever. When I started doing this, I aroused* *the protective elements—the conservative elements—of my personality... which immediately wanted approval for my books—not that I shouldn't want approval per se but that I began to <u>demand</u> that my art provide <u>all</u> my needs; to financially support me, to give me honor among my fellows, a sense of belonging, etc. Now this can be expected to some degree for a noncreative career; but it can damage creative activity; the need for creativity naturally is... the <u>creation</u> of something new that disrupts the conservative principles; and that freedom <u>is paramount</u>. If you confuse the issues you try to temper your creativity (to gain approval, etc.) which can dilute the work; <u>or</u> you set up protective measures to protect yourself against the worlds disapproval or scorn.*

(Late Friday afternoon—I begin to read Seth sessions for last summer and a line reminds me of what else I was getting from Seth last night and today.

(It was: distinguish between the natural and cultural or social world and assure myself I am safe in the natural world.

(Then to read a session he gave about... asking yourself how many actual people I've met who scorned me... or hated me or tried to physically attack me... and to remind myself and the subconscious about responding to <u>actual experience</u>... remind it also that its experiences with scorn or whatever, as written down—were not all of its experience by a long shot. There were people like Blanche Price or even Father Trainor. It's important that I find and read those sessions.

(To remind the subconscious of its love for the natural world and walking alone or with Rob; being out in the elements. Ask it to revive those loves and desires.

(Remind subconscious to be responsible to all of its life—)

DELETED SESSION
APRIL 11, 1978 9:44 PM TUESDAY

(The session was not held last night because of Tam Mossman's visit.... I told Jane before the session that all day I'd been thinking that there was still a cause or causes for the symptoms that we didn't know, or hadn't uncovered yet. Perhaps a relationship between the intent to publish the sessions, and the idea of exposure or threat for not "toeing the mark." [Tam is Jane's editor at Prentice-Hall.]

(I also asked Jane why she hadn't done much about her eye condition since it began a year ago, other than an occasional pendulum question, or the sessions Seth had mentioned it in. A little later she said that she was "upset" by the question, that it threatened her. She added that it touched something within, leading to feelings of hopelessness—and that now she had to get out of <u>them</u> before she could have the session. I mentioned that the question had probably touched upon hidden defenses, fears

that the "protection" furnished by the eye condition would be taken away, and she agreed.

(The next day, before I began typing this session, Jane outlined material she'd picked up about her eye condition this morning, evidently in response to the question of the night before. I don't know it well enough to quote it here, but suggest that she write it up and add it to this session, for it sounded very good.)

Now a private session, not for publication.

Ruburt's early environment was far from perfect. He chose it, because it did indeed provide a framework that would make questioning prominent. He began in his own way to form his own theory concerning the nature of God and reality at a young age. He expressed these theories and feelings through poetry, which was itself an unconventional activity.

The poetry provided a direct expression of his ideas, and a protective coating as well. He lived by those ideas, however. As stated, this brought conflict with the church—a painful-enough period for Ruburt, but he was sure in his convictions. At the same time, poetry was and is creative play, and it sprang from the depths of his being. You do not have to try and make poetry practical.

Our sessions began, really, as an extension, a natural enough development, the results of a personal search. Give us a moment.... I have given more material than I can say on the subject of Ruburt's attitude toward creativity and what happens when he <u>emphasizes</u> the idea of work as work, or as a career, <u>above</u> his spontaneous creativity. I got my message through to some degree on several occasions for example, when his arms were suddenly free. It is the <u>overemphasis</u> upon work and career—overemphasis, now, that brings about or triggers the fears behind the difficulties.

When he is emphasizing his own creativity, encouraging it, encouraging its spontaneity, then that flow has its own impetus and direction. It is freeing spiritually and physically. That flow releases or incites solutions, and is overall, say, of itself fear-banishing.

It keeps him in touch with the powerful portions of his personality that search for truth, out of joy in the activity for the quest itself. The <u>doing</u> is important. When he considers <u>work as paramount</u>, however, or thinks in terms of "the work of my life," that emphasis inclines *(with amusement)* him to think primarily of results rather than of doing. It <u>inclines</u> him to see his ideas as existing in direct conflict to those of your contemporary times. That focus <u>inclines</u> him to a quite literal insistence that his creative material should in its way act like some supernatural doctor's prescription that can be at once taken like a pill to solve each and every problem of each and every correspondent, and of course to solve his own problems as well.

Then he feels that he is in at best an ambiguous position, for the world continues doing as it will, and his correspondents, solving one problem, immediately write with another. This kind of situation of course then triggers old fears of doubt or threat. Those fears are then not admitted, for he thinks that they must indeed be beneath a person <u>whose entire life work</u> is devoted to a search for the nature of reality, and therefore a person who must possess, or try to possess, the answers to all of the questions.

In such a situation, Ruburt thinks of work as work, and finds himself wanting—for a doctor after all heals patients, a lawyer solves cases or whatever, so it seems to Ruburt that his work <u>must</u>—underlined three times—make truth practical, and of course beneficially so. That emphasis alone, with the material I mentioned, and the triggering fears, further opens the door to other worries.

The truth, as he interprets it, is no longer the joyful, curious, creative, free search for truth, let it lead where it will; but the idea of a life's work makes him think "Who's following me? My truth must be the real truth, for I do not want to lead others astray."

Television becomes a threat because he feels he is being asked to prove the unprovable, and yet since this is his life's work he feels responsible to do so.

He did not want me to tell you this—but your seriousness, much as it is well-intended in *"Unknown"* 2 and its notes, bothered him. They inclined him further to think in terms of his life's work as a highly serious, no-nonsense endeavor, a body of work to be set against the world's other great works.

(10:15.) Of course the personal material did threaten him, with his beliefs, for how could the person responsible for such a weighty lifework have any weaknesses? Certainly the weaknesses said that the material was not true – because when he <u>emphasizes</u> work over creativity he becomes overly conscientious, overly concerned with responsibility, and puts himself in a situation where old fears are indeed triggered.

In those circumstances, free creativity itself almost becomes suspect, for supposing his creativity turns up an element that is contradictory? Or again, that will be misinterpreted, that will be used "wrongly" by others? In that kind of a climate, both inner and outer worlds to some extent must be protected against. I have given material saying that most clearly on innumerable occasions.

(10:20.) Give us a moment.... That entire climate arouses feelings of disapproval, for the individual can never live up to impossible aspirations. That is what happened for a while to Seven. You both have your own characteristics, and if you understood that, or if Ruburt did, he would be better off.

The sessions I gave on spontaneity and work should be most helpful now, as long as the fears are now being admitted. There is nothing wrong with fears.

Unidentified fears are something else.

I want to comment on your pendulum sessions, however. First of all, the fact that you do them together is highly significant and beneficial, more significant than you realize. Ruburt's experience with you in the bedroom was an excellent example of your enduring loving relationship, and represented your single and joint decisions to utilize your love and devotion to solve the difficulty.

Ten pages is too much to do in one session with the pendulum. Look at your questions as if you were asking them of a person, so that in one session do not act as if an answer given before has not been given. Do you follow me?

("Not really.")

If the pendulum says it does not regard.... Give us a moment.... I want to think of some clear examples. *(Long pause.)* If on page 2, say, the pendulum says that it feels the symptoms are no longer necessary, then in following questions for that day take that answer as given, and do not ask questions that would undermine the given answer, as if you do not trust it. That becomes a cross-examination.

It was important that Ruburt state his position, for example, by saying clearly that the symptoms threatened him, and that they threatened him more than any scorn, and important also that he state that the symptoms inhibited his writing. Once the pendulum shows you that the subconscious does understand, however, it is all right to check now and then, but those statements can act as negative suggestions otherwise. Each session should be thought of with its questions in consecutive terms, so that later questions follow the reasoning pattern already given.

Questions like "Are you lonesome?" certainly need not be not asked each day. I am simply asking that you not give the subconscious too many issues to deal with at once, and the last part of each session should always reinforce any positive steps you have made and end with a few, very brief, clear positive suggestions.

(10:40.) Rest your fingers.... The most important thing, of course, is that you have set up communication, so that Ruburt's fears are no longer being inhibited. But those fears must be considered in the light of the material given this evening. Remember, I am speaking of an <u>overemphasis</u> upon the idea of work, not about a normal concern about book publications, or career concerns, those are certainly reasonable. The overemphasis brings up the public image idea, so that Ruburt compares himself personally against some composite image that he imagines other people have of him. First of all, truly creative "work" is timeless. It must appear in time, but its nourishment is not like that of a baker's

loaf, and its "practicality" cannot be reduced to such terms. Ruburt's lifework so far has been produced—again, so far—because despite such erroneous beliefs he has still allowed himself a creative spontaneity. But in the recent past that spontaneity has had to emerge against those resistances.

You asked the question about the subconscious this evening, before the session, and Ruburt immediately interpreted it in the light of the following: the weight of the responsibility it carried for all those psychologists, and all of their patients, and his <u>responsibility</u> to obtain, in capitals, <u>the answer</u>, not only for himself but for all those other people. The idea behind the question does of course spring partially from your private, practical concerns right now, and yet it also springs from Ruburt's and your great natural curiosity.

I will answer it, and at our next session, when you remind Ruburt of the great creative climate in which it can be "answered."

The <u>overemphasis</u>, again, upon the <u>work</u> alone triggers the old fears about poverty, and toeing the mark and so forth, for it arouses worries about "making the work pay." Remember, when Ruburt wrote short stories he slanted them for the market. The woman could not win out in tales for *Playboy*, so when Ruburt thinks in that fashion about work, he thinks he is not only <u>not slanting his material</u> for the market, but often telling people precisely what they may not want to hear at all—hence this would arouse worries about the sale of the books.

That is enough for this evening, but the session, again, can be most beneficial if it is taken to heart. You have been highly active with Ruburt, though you do not remember it, both of you in Framework 2 clearing up old issues, forming closer communications with each other, and dropping old beliefs.

The question about the subconscious's view of the body will be answered along with the other one, and at our next session. Your own support of late in particular is highly valuable. End of session, and a fond good evening to you both.

("Thank you. Same to you."

(11:00 PM. I was pretty depressed by session's end, since it seemed we had so far to go. The first question Seth referred to was the one about why the subconscious didn't realize it was going to far, when it imposed or brought about symptoms, as in Jane's case, that were proving to be too damaging to the body, compared to what they were supposed to protect the body against.

(To do: read sessions in Chapter 15, Personal Reality. *Check pendulum for good things done in past. Check pendulum for <u>good things done in past</u> we're pleased with now.)*

JANE'S NOTES
TUESDAY, APRIL 18, 1978

(Eddie Albert calls again today telling me he just finished Speaks, *asking about world problems, starvation, good and evil, etc. After I mess around with a few plots for* switch; *then do some on* Oversoul. *Nap. When I awaken:*

(I think my symptoms are all the worse because of what I do in contrast. Eddie seeing me might think understandably: how can she offer any hope for mankind, etc., when she cant even walk across the room? Like ... I'm not getting this clear but the feeling was like you're supposed to demonstrate truth through your life and my symptoms sort of were the opposite, or indicated the opposite; not only didn't I heal others but not even myself. I forget just how those feelings went, but that approximates them, being ashamed of my condition as if for Christ's sake, they blemished my art, or ashamed because they blemished my work. All this quite apart from the normal feelings about health. I mean that in my mind the symptoms were associated with my work as if they cast aspersions on it—quite apart from worrying about what they did to me. *Following these came feelings of disapproval because I fussed happily around with* switch *plots when... what Eddie wanted were answers to those weighty problems, and I come up with* switch *plots, that any other writer could do... I didnt spontaneously come up with impressions for example about switch programing...*

(I told Rob these feelings. He said... if I have this right... that I was afraid of my own energy... maybe afraid that I was *supposed to change the world or try to... afraid ...of what? Not sure here, but that I hadn't outgrown old religious beliefs and training or come to terms with my own energy or abilities.)*

DELETED SESSION
APRIL 19, 1978 9:35 PM WEDNESDAY

(This afternoon I reminded Jane that she should read the 657th session in Chapter 15 of Personal Reality. *It contains Seth's material on the present point of power; I came across it while checking out a reference for Volume 2 of* "Unknown" Reality. *Looking it over, I saw at once that it contained the key to Jane's solving her challenges with the symptoms. At the same time, it depressed me deeply as I thought of the opportunities we'd missed through the years. My depression grew through the afternoon, the session, while I slept, and woke again. At the same time, I do think we've made some progress through our own work with the pendulum.)*

Now: *(Long pause.)* Personal fears never exist as a result of personal experience alone. They are always connected with larger belief systems that belong to some extent to the person, and to the person's age as well.

Personal Reality, a book Ruburt may have heard of, does indeed deal precisely with such issues. No particular episodes alone, though they may seem to do so, ever cause a particular condition, say, of illness, though such episodes may be used as catalysts. Instead, the framework of belief in which the episodes occur has prime importance. Fears should not he inhibited, but encountered, and yet behind all of them, in your time at least, lies the feeling that the individual is powerless against the conditions of his body or the events of the world.

Intuitively Ruburt blazed through such beliefs—<u>intuitively</u>—and his books and mine are evidence of that. Intuitional knowledge and conscious assimilation are some poles apart, at least in your society. Both of you found it quite necessary to take a strong conscious, critical look at the material from the beginning, for your trainings told you, in the terms that you understood them, that the "subconscious" could be very misleading, though creative, and that therefore you must critically examine any intuitive productions that profess themselves to stand as truths rather than as creative fictions in your world.

Because Ruburt was the person most involved, he became in a way the most critical. Therefore to some extent he has not been able to use the ideas on his own behalf nearly as effectively as he might.

The material in *Personal Reality*, however, contains psychological and psychic truths. Those truths have indeed, and as of now, helped millions of people. Those people were not involved in such a psychic initiation, however, in your time, so they can in your terms afford to use such helpful information, and do not feel any need at all to hold themselves apart from it as Ruburt has.

If the material does not work, they can always blame Ruburt, you see.

Now: your friend Tam quite happily gives readings with Ruburt's experience behind him, and he says "I simply say, I take no responsibility for what James says." Ruburt, however, takes the responsibility for what I say.

In that regard he becomes overly conscientious. We have never told anyone to do anything, except to face up to the abilities of consciousness. Because of that attitude, however, and because of the critical—or, rather, overly critical stance—he has held himself more aloof than necessary from using the material itself. The ideas, for example, in *Personal Reality* are exactly those that will resolve his doubts and remove his fears, and the techniques given do work.

There are other reasons, however, that have added up to a feeling of powerlessness on Ruburt's part in regard to his physical condition. Both of you have a tendency to concentrate upon the ills of the world—and so that applies also to the mail, for you remember the letters of those who are in difficulty far more than other letters—and Ruburt thinks that he is simply one more person with a problem that seemingly cannot be solved.

He is himself a person who brought about a vital breakthrough in his own knowledge, an acceleration of creativity quite extraordinary, that led to these sessions, and these sessions have literally expanded the realities of many, many people. His abilities and powers of concentration are not ordinary. He has however thus far not nearly utilized the information that he has, and in the meantime he became frightened that his will had little power to change the course of events.

Your pendulum sessions have been of benefit, and one reason is because they represent a united, joint and determined effort on both of your parts, and Ruburt feels your support. He therefore feels less lonely in his efforts. The subconscious is of course a hypothetical terms that stands for the portions of the self at which normal consciousness and the source self meet. There are really no hidden beliefs. The pendulum method is simply a technique that is effective because of your beliefs, and brings to light your own quite conscious ideas—those that you might not approve of, and so conveniently appear to forget.

(10:05.) In those terms, the so-called subconscious has your own concept of the body. There is however a body consciousness that carries on more or less automatically, seeking health, expression, and the full vitality. Its power comes from the source that gives it its life.

You must understand that <u>basically</u>—basically—both body and mind are mental. You are dealing with translations of impulses, beliefs and feelings into flesh, which in itself is composed of consciousnesses also. It is difficult to verbalize, but your question "Why doesn't the subconscious know when to stop, if its defenses actually become too dangerous?" is asked in too limited a framework, though I understand your concern and what you mean. The self knows it has many lives to live. It knows no limitations last. The body and mind are one, and in that unity, regardless of appearances, one is the materialization of the other.

However, the source self always attempts to send new information, inspiration, or whatever help is required. The personality—each one—with its own challenges, will seek to solve its problems in its own way. The source self, sending out all assistance that it can, will still not attempt to <u>override</u> the conscious personality, for such actions would ultimately deny the conscious personality its powers of decision and control.

Your immediate situation and all past ones, regardless of personal fears, which should not be discounted, result from Ruburt's until-now determined decision to stand critically apart from his intuitional knowledge. That knowledge, in other words, consciously assimilated and used, <u>can</u> solve any of the personal problems.

Before I continue I would suggest that if others "use *Personal Reality* like a bible," Ruburt could at least take it seriously. He does not like people to speak of the book in that way because it arouses, of course, thoughts of those who <u>followed</u> any dogmas without using common sense—dogmas that blindly led people into further feelings of powerlessness. Both of you are critical enough. I would most heartily suggest then that Ruburt use that book.

(*A <u>true</u> use of* Personal Reality *would be to use it like a bible – although not slavishly – but such use would <u>unite</u> the critical and intuitional faculties. The critical approach <u>would be to use</u> the book.*)

Now in the past I have not emphasized it. I want his beliefs written out. I want all the exercises done that he tells others to do, and I want both of you to consider your beliefs about the world <u>as</u> beliefs. Do not accept them uncritically, as there you do. I want you both to discuss together the ideas in the book, and to literally begin a program in which your purpose is to put those ideas to use where you need them.

Ruburt's mood of powerlessness must be broken, and you can help him there. Such a program will have effects in your life also, Joseph. Ruburt's fears, again, should not be buried, nor should they be emphasized, but the book will tell you how to handle this. I mean both of you. (*By having <u>faith</u> that in the future things can be better—thus, <u>no</u> conflict.*)

Ruburt is back to writing, which means that he has made inroads again. He has been emphasizing the problem, which adds to the feeling of hopelessness. There has been however on both of your parts a new determination to do what is necessary, an impetus not to let matters ride, and a new quickening at other levels of your own relationship with each other, so that your love for each other in Framework 2 is coming to your aid now.

Ruburt's new inclination for house cleaning is an excellent sign of intent and impulse, and your own support marks your own determination. You saw the bodybuilding program *(Pumping Iron)*. Ruburt's body is making a valiant effort to readjust and to strengthen itself. When bodybuilders work together they have guidelines to follow. Their muscles hurt. They are aware of each group of muscles. As Ruburt's muscles exert themselves they often also hurt, but there is no one for him to compare his situation to—and because he has not trusted the body he becomes alarmed.

I want the suggestion given again, then: "I can trust the physician within, and the ancient wisdom of my body." You each have achievements, but you let these fade in your concentration upon the problem.

This session can indeed be a turning point, if you accept it as such. The point of power is in the present. Understand that, for this session can indeed be a turning point, and you can both determine that this be so. There is nothing else to prevent it.

End of session.

("Okay.")

And a fond good evening.

(10:41 PM.)

DELETED SESSION
APRIL 24, 1978 9:38 PM MONDAY

(We're still working with the pendulum six days a week. Our questions change continually in a slow rhythm, we've noticed, constantly evolving into what we hope are more penetrating ones as we continue to learn. We've learned much, and Jane's body seems to be initiating good responses.

(At the same time, her responses are at times very uncomfortable as the body begins readjusting various portions of itself, like long-unused mechanisms that need prompting and lubrication to start working more smoothly. Today, for example, her left side, leg and knee were all moving in unaccustomed, more flexible ways, she reported, thus affecting her walking. At times such changes make it very difficult for her to get around, yet they are obviously signs of change for the better.

(In addition, she's done more around the house in recent days than she has for many a month—all signs for the good. She's exclaimed about the additional feelings of freedom these new activities have given her again and again. Some of them involve her pushing herself about in her chair.

(We've also talked over Seth's answer in the last session about why the subconscious doesn't back off when it's obvious that it's gone too far in a protective role, say. I said that I understood his answer to my question all right, but yet that I felt there were still things there to be discussed; that in individual cases, for instance, the subconscious could go too far when there was no need to, and that in such cases it seemed to ignore the wishes and desires of the conscious personality involved. I felt, then, that there should be a more intimate give-and-take between all portions of a personality. Since in numerous cases throughout the species' history, I added, this hadn't happened, I thought there could be important insights there that we might learn from Seth. But primarily, my original question had to do with Jane's own case, and at this time that was the one we were still interested in gaining insight into.)

A private session.

I would like you both to try a slightly different emphasis—but a highly important one, in the way in which you look at Ruburt's situation.

Think of him as being simply "out of condition," for that is indeed true. Your bodybuilders start of course from a better position, and yet many of them are quite puny. Because of their relative inadequacies they decide to overcompensate, seeking for an ideal that in certain terms can only be held for so long.

Ruburt is beginning from his own position, and he is seeking the normal, free motion of his body. All of the equipment is there, and there are no disease elements. The body has not been used, however, in a normal manner. As mentioned, when bodybuilders build up certain muscles, they do indeed experience great distress <u>at times</u>. They understand the reason for the discomfort, for they are building muscle—but in their cases they often overdo it. Nevertheless there are others with whom they can share their discomfort.

The reasons behind the condition, causing the condition, brought about the secondary group of mental habits. The bodybuilders look forward to their workouts, for they have a purpose in mind. Ruburt instead developed habits that discouraged him from using his body, except in certain ways. As much as possible, I would like Ruburt to remember these comparisons, for he is just becoming aware of certain habitual thoughts that accompany motion—walking, say, or getting up or down. With your help, he has tried to temper some of these.

A bodybuilder begins with certain weights that he can handle. He does not berate himself because he cannot yet achieve greater weights. As much as possible, then, think in terms of Ruburt not so much as having certain symptoms, but as being simply out of condition and trying to reestablish certain physical skills. Do not concentrate upon the lacks. This alteration of perspective can be of great help.

Now: you are working very well together, and your suggestion about the use of the chair *(to get around the house)* was the result of Framework 2 creativity. It took Ruburt a day or so to accept it. He was afraid of wheelchair connotations, but he triumphed over that negative idea. Your suggestion was important for several reasons. It was practical, and could be done at once. Its most important benefit, however, was that it freed Ruburt from mentally seeing himself in only one corner of one room, and immediately aroused his normal leanings toward love of whatever home you share.

It rearoused his desires to clean—desires that had been inhibited. Immediately he began to think in terms of physical activities he <u>wanted</u> to perform. Physically used in such a manner, the chair does exercise his knees and feet, while his weight is not upon them entirely, and his thoughts are not on exercise.

Moving the chair backward some is also excellent, for it moves different ligaments than he normally uses. Using the lightweight carpet sweeper will also help, and aid in coordination.

Try not to use the word "symptoms" in your pendulum work from now on. There are other ways, but the word has served its purpose. "Is my body out of condition because," for example. There are endless other ways, but the change of focus as I have suggested will automatically bring a change in your questions. <u>Always</u> end your pendulum sessions with the new beliefs you want to instill, reinforcing whatever you have learned from that particular session. The idea of those pendulum sessions should not be to find out <u>what is wrong</u>, but to discover Ruburt's feelings and beliefs, and to ascertain how they can be changed to bring about more favorable conditions.

(*10:05.*) Give us a moment.... You cannot say that any of Ruburt's attitudes were "wrong," nor can you say <u>in larger terms</u> that his method was "wrong." You cannot say, and should not, place moral connotations in such situations. Each personality is different, and affects the body in a different way. You think of health as physical only. If you think in terms of an unhealthy relationship, for example, then you may at least begin to glimpse the ways in which individuals will seek prerogatives, so each case must be seen separately.

In normal terms in life, while the conditions for life are given, the nature of physical time means that practically speaking life will be full of surprises, for in usual terms you do not know what will happen tomorrow. In that context people take "risks." They set up prerogatives. They do not usually concentrate with the same intensity in all areas of their lives, so there is seldom what you might think of as any ideal balance. If your health is bad enough, of course, you will die. If you are poor enough, of course, you will starve, or freeze to death in the wintertime. If you are lonely enough you may go mad, as people do in isolation cells.

In between excellent health and death through disease, in between wealth and perhaps gluttony, and poverty and starvation, in between a glittering social existence, the comfort of a family, and the utter loneliness of isolation, there are literally infinite variations and gradations of behavior, according to individual differences and prerogatives. Most of this refers to your question, and is by way of giving you a fuller explanation.

In those terms, the subconscious can consider the health of a relationship quite as important as the health of the body, or even more so. It will go along with enforced starvation, deprivation, or whatever, if the individual in mind is in pursuit of something else that it feels it must have to insure its existence.

In those terms, when the subconscious considers health, it must also take into consideration the individual's strong intents, in which case it is insuring the mental and emotional health in a somewhat different fashion.

(10:22.) I simply want to stress that health in those terms does involve more. The "subconscious" will try to save an individual from great disappointment. This may mean the incidence of a disease, but the disease may save a person's sanity. So the issues are not nearly as clear as it would at first seem.

Rest your fingers.... Ruburt's particular case is rather clear and exaggerated in that respect. It is not murky at all. I have given this material in the past. He thought of his father—he <u>thought</u> of his father—as spontaneous, free, and undisciplined, as somewhat stupid and somewhat dangerous. He thought of his mother as possessing a strong will. His mother was authoritative to a degree. His father was lax. He feared his mother far more, however, and he tried to temper his own behavior, to ally the intuitions and the intellect or will.

He wanted to use his intuitive abilities fully, but felt that great caution must be used. He thought mainly of the health of your relationship together, and the health of his work. He became divided, seeing these as <u>opposing</u> tendencies in his personality, rather than as complementary ones that quite naturally met <u>in</u> his personality, so one was set against the other. Much of this appears in your pendulum work of late, but you both then project those ideas upon the world, so that you think of your readers as overly credulous, or of critics who are overly critical. This leads of course to people who are for you, but dumb; or against you but intellectual.

It leads to Ruburt feeling physically that relaxation means letting go into laxness; as I told him in the past, however, letting go means motion and the ability to respond. It also means the natural aggression of motion.

Take your break.

(10:36—10:55.)

Choices are a vital ingredient in life.

If this were not so, the subconscious would not only see to it that the body was in ordinary good health under any conditions, but it would automatically refuse to allow any individual to put its health in jeopardy.

High risk sports would not be allowed—excursions across the seas undertaken with "inadequate" provisions, or with rafts. It is not easy, you see, to draw the line, and the species obviously puts itself in risk situations often; and often attains certain triumphs as a result.

Now there are some people who consider overall balance a prerogative, and you will usually find them in decent health, with average concerns, and you will not find them taking risks. <u>The</u> subconscious does not exist, of course. "It" is a highly personalized portion of the self, uniquely tuned. Some people enjoy risks. The body may be in excellent health, and die that way in an accident. But the subconscious knows that the quality of life for that individual involves such exhilaration, and such a person literally chooses that rather than, for example, what someone else might consider a well-balanced long life.

That "well-balanced life" might well be considered a slow death to our risk seeker, and no moral judgment can be placed on such behavior.

One flower may die before another. One may be blemished and the other not, but none are the less flowers for that. Ruburt was convinced he needed certain protections. His judgments, and yours to a lesser extent, <u>can</u> be regarded as the flower's blemishes, though I am aware it is not easy for you to see this in that light.

It is imperative, however, that you make an effort not to think in terms of "the symptoms" any longer, but instead to think of ways that Ruburt can condition his body, realizing that he need not be at the mercy of old fears.

Your dream showed you the opening of another probability that has emerged as a result of your joint efforts. The dream took place at 458 because it is an offshoot of an unrealized probability that opened there on two occasions *(in 1973 at our apartment at 458 West Water Street, Elmira, New York)*.

One was at a time when Ruburt began *Rich Bed* and the first draft of *Adventures*. He was examining beliefs, expressing aggressions naturally, and freeing his spontaneity. This led to the birth of new creative material as well. His beliefs and hopes arose again later when I gave the sessions on spontaneity and work that I want him to reread. But those probabilities did not materialize.

Your dream shows that Ruburt's determination—with your own determined involvement—have strongly attracted you to that probability again—and this time in the dream you saw it actualized. The suggestions I have given this evening are to lead you toward that actualization.

Your other dream involves Miss Bowman's desire for death—her knowledge that although her mother died at an old age she is young and active at another level of reality—and it was Miss Bowman's image of her mother as a younger woman that you saw. Your parents were simply symbols to you. They were not active in the message. *(Miss Bowman was my high school art teacher.)*

Ruburt is doing well with the point of power exercise, and I suggest he take the same amount of time to open himself up to intuitive material from the library, or otherwise. It is natural-enough that when he is beginning to use his body more that at times he becomes more aware of it, and of the time involved, and so forth. He must also remember Sumari time, for the creative imagination works no matter what you are doing.

End of session. My heartiest regards and a fond good evening.

("Thank you, Seth."

(11:23. As we talked, Jane said that Seth wanted to return for a moment. Resume at 11:25.)

One point: I wanted to stress that when muscles are reactivated, to Ruburt they "feel sore." The muscles' experience is quite different. They experience sensation to a heightened degree, where before their sense of life was not that active.

The sensations activate other ligaments, muscles, and so forth. They signal activity. After disuse the sensations are exaggerated. Most people are not aware of them, for example. In the past, and with beliefs not understood, Ruburt would become depressed, or you would, so it is important that that activation be understood.

That understanding will prevent anxiety from cutting short progress. Since various groups of muscles and ligaments come into motion in their own order, the soreness will come and go, or appear in one place and then another. If he recognizes this, he will get to know when slight activity of the parts will help, or when resting them will.

And that is all.

("Thank you.")

(11:32 PM. Seth's last point above was well taken. It's the next day as I type this session from my notes. At its beginning I wrote about the soreness Jane was experiencing throughout the left side of her body. Today, that soreness has let up, or nearly so. Instead, she's aware of soreness in other parts of her body on the right side.

(The two dreams Seth referred to took place on April 24, 1978. See my dream notebook for their accounts. A copy of Seth's interpretations from this session is attached.)

DELETED SESSION
APRIL 26, 1978 9:57 PM WEDNESDAY

Now: a private session.

The circulation has increased considerably in Ruburt's legs, knees, and feet as a direct result of the increased activity. Today the knees were activated almost constantly, relatively speaking, because he did follow his impulses. Since he is moving more, just about every portion of the body takes new positions. It is natural enough when he begins such activity if ambiguous feelings emerge. They should be accepted, for they often show conflicting beliefs that are then out in the open and more easily contended with, because a specific incident will usually be involved.

Each such incident is like, now, a small morality play, with a lesson to be learned, and therefore each such incident is a step ahead in terms of progress and understanding. Almost immediately after your chair suggestion, and with the work you are both doing, Ruburt's mind and body began to respond. Mentally he began to think of doing things that previously he had simply put aside. The <u>definite</u> improvements are therefore the result of Ruburt's determination, and your support, but also of the body's resiliency when it is allowed to follow its natural impulses.

Ruburt's lapses have become quite noticeable to him, in contrast with the renewed air of freedom that he has indeed felt lately. He has also, however, begun to project, in small ways, in a quite positive manner, and felt impulses that before he denied.

He at least wished he could go into the yard this afternoon, once he imagined that he could make that step out. He wanted to pick his daffodils. He could not give in to that impulse yet, but before he would not have allowed it, because his position would then seem so hopeless in contrast. There are then several other such instances that he has forgotten, that are at least as important as the lapses that seem to loom so large. Such activity increases his sense of power, minimizes his physical hesitancy, and mobilizes physical activity.

The arms have been exercised in new ways. He has <u>felt</u> like performing some physical activities—getting the meal today. *(Jane's first in many many months.)* The impulse automatically led him to perform physical acts that before he simply would not have done, so desire and impulse mobilize the body.

The exercises—or rather, the exercising—automatically stimulates all portions of the body, and will lead to periods of relaxation.

I have mentioned this before, but your environment is a symbol of your inner life and beliefs; one appears physical to you while the inner life does not. The physical body responds to stimulus from outside and from within. Ruburt's newer activity enlarges the physical stimulation possible—the different view of your house and grounds, for example; or preparing one meal automatically reminds him of others <u>that he will want to prepare</u>.

He takes new interest in what food is in your cupboard or refrigerator. The interest propels him to look. Today through such activities he found himself, if in a simple fashion, taking a few steps without his table to get where he wanted to go. I am going into this material because it shows how desire works in any area. His thoughts were on what he wanted to do, though he very definitely had to consider the means, the getting about.

(10:15.) To him, it seems like the kitchen is suddenly a room, because he has opened a room up in his mind. You cannot exactly say that each object is a

symbol of a belief that specifically, and yet any alterations that you willfully make in your behavior with the objects of your intimate environment represent alterations of beliefs. There is a constant give-and-take between the two. In mundane terms each piece of furniture is a symbol—you have conscious feelings about it. When you change a room around you are altering beliefs in an observable way.

(Long pause at 10:20.) Now give us a moment.... Ruburt is doing the point of power exercise well. I do suggest the pillow pounding, for it encourages the expression of normally aggressive feelings through bodily release, rather than repression through bodily tension.

The body likes to exert force, however, beside that. It enjoys using its strength, so the pillow beating need not be necessarily tied in with the release of aggression alone, but can serve now simply as a way for the body to express its sensations. You are getting ahead of the game because daily you are not letting things slide, and therefore cutting down on the buildup of tension.

Now many beliefs that are unfortunate, in your terms, are worked out through creativity at other levels, so that dreams, intuitions, and mental processes work together with bodily expression toward a resolution. Some of Ruburt's exaggerated fears, for example, become minimized automatically as he realizes that he can do some activities that he had given up.

Following his natural impulses automatically brings issues out into the open, so that today he worried about not writing, and so was <u>consciously</u> aware of the conflict and of its reasons. He therefore reminded himself that he could and must trust his own individuality and rhythms.

The fears are not hidden in the past, but are obvious in each day, remaining buried only when you choose not to challenge them. Your work with the pendulum brought them to notice. The feedback allowed the subconscious to question the data it had been given in the past. The species is much more plastic in its nature than you imagine. Its "instincts" are not as set as with the animals. Children have to be taught, because the abilities of consciousness in human terms cannot be held to such dictates.

You must realize that the inner portions of the self are aware of the greater framework in which individuality takes place. Men will die for an ideal. A man will die to protect his children. If pure personal survival were all that mattered to the so-called subconscious, such acts would be impossible—and in fact, they would be inconceivable on man's part. And the selfish gene has nothing to do with any of it *(emphatically).*

Excellent health is to be sought, it would certainly seem. Men have committed crimes in misguided searches for an ideal. Great acts of heroism have also resulted, however, and men, it seems, have spent themselves in following an ideal that they hoped to actualize for the rest of mankind. Why does the body not protest if men have nearly starved, or become the scorn of their fellows, or whatever? The answer is that as beneficial, as desirable, as good health is, and the performance of an excellent body, man's pursuit of other kinds of accomplishment, his equally strong desire for knowledge, and his insatiable curiosity, his pursuit of the ideal, often lead him into pathways that result in the body's difficulties.

Yet in certain individuals, life, fully healthy or otherwise, would be meaningless otherwise. You both decided to do what you wanted to do regardless of any "psychic field" of endeavor. The term is meaningless. The fact is that you decided to use your minds in certain ways that you felt were not approved of in your society—and that pattern goes way back for both of you; when you, for example, decided to bow out of a <u>career</u> in commercial art.

Take a short break, and get our friend some beer.

(10:45—10:47.)

You could have "amended your ways," but you both insisted upon what you wanted, and persevered in your highly individualistic ways of looking at your world—and in pursuing questions and accomplishments that you knew from the beginning were not those of the official world.

You had a period of acceptance under your belt, in comics, that you left. Ruburt did not. *(An important point to remember.)* He was determined to go his own way. His being demanded expression through the use of its abilities, and despite his need to be accepted by others he began to exaggerate the threat of their disapproval into scorn. When he began to sell his work, he felt to some degree, now, dependent upon the acceptance of the others in the world—for if they did not accept him at all they would not buy his books. Your own feelings about the world did not help in that regard.

He took excessive means, as he said today, to avoid going to excess.

(Jane made this revealing remark this afternoon as we talked. It's worth keeping visible for reference.)

The two of you <u>exaggerated</u> your position. You saw yourselves in opposition to the world. Ruburt was afraid his need for the world's acceptance might lead him out into it again, where he would necessarily meet scorn, for he thought in absolutes.

It is important that he used to promise himself that he <u>would</u> go on tours or television if he became well. This was actually a threat he held over his own head. You must both realize <u>that he can indeed recover completely</u>—and you must both want him to. Do not forget Framework 2. Ruburt need not go abroad in the world to promote our ideas, nor have I ever suggested it. The ideas are best promoted through these sessions, and books—and not by hasty encounters on television, where answers must be simplified and ideas diluted, but in the reasoned writings that build in their own way, tell Ruburt, resting upon the great framework of the intuitions' knowledge. And remind him that spontaneity knows it own order.

He is afraid, of course, that if he "gives into" impulses other than writing for a day or so that he is lax, yet the exercise and relaxation of the body refreshes the soul and allows the intuitions their clear vision. <u>If</u> he can stand it, I would like him to take until Monday to follow his impulses, whether or not writing is involved. Then, as of Monday, he can begin to correlate the new physical activity with his writing, gently, by settling upon three hours a day of the basic "time put in"—but with the stress upon creativity, ideas, and free creative play that may or may not include *Seven* on any given day.

(11:07.) His creative abilities will see to it that *Seven* is finished. He enjoys doing it, for that matter. Thoughts of work, however, do not work. You are not to compare yourselves with people who have jobs, or to say "They put in so many hours"—for you set up comparisons <u>that do not apply</u>, and that hamper your creativity.

You might feel like applying yourself to *"Unknown" Reality*, and you might feel like writing steadily for many hours. Well and good. I am aware of your difficulties with time, practically, and yet freeing yourself of the ideas of work as you have begun to do lately with *"Unknown"* frees your creativity, and you concentrate better and more clearly. This applies in double fashion to Ruburt.

Ruburt's way of forgetting past books is a natural and good one <u>for him</u>. It conflicts with <u>your</u> natural way. The two ways can complement each other if you understand this, as you are beginning to. In your society, with your ideas, you have paved a way for yourselves. The books sustain you financially. People do accept you, and in a way that is quite important to their pocketbooks, and in times that are not financially good. Forget the taxes. If they seem unfair to you, they are unfair to many—you are not being singled out in that regard.

The increased activity and the release of impulses with these sessions, and your pendulum work, are once again arousing Ruburt's body and mind, and your own, so that you have an excellent chance now for Ruburt to recover. Do not let issues go underground. There are improvements, and considerable ones. You want more. Remember what I said about muscular activity, so that when Ruburt does have a sore day, say, you do not become discouraged.

Give us a moment.... Alterations of schedule or of activity are excellent, now, because they serve to break up associations. They act like gentle "shock treatments."

Unless you have questions, end of session, and my congratulations thus far.

(11:21. "Do you want to say something about his dream of this afternoon?" Jane's copy of her dream is attached.)

The eyeglass dream portion: the old black frames of the glasses represented old beliefs. They were dropped into the water, the realm of Ruburt's fears, by a young man who represented an earlier self who thought success was a male prerogative. The glasses came up cleansed, but together again, and the frames were updated—so that Ruburt's fears, encountered as he is doing of late, actually allow him to see better and clear his vision. For they dissolve, and vision is restored.

He was afraid that they were lost. Then he thought only one lens was saved. This shows that he was worried for his vision, and thought that only the one right eye would operate properly. He discovers the glasses intact, however, better than before, and no longer curved outward and thick.

This portion of the dream represents his realization that his eyes are clearing. The fears are being washed away. Before, he was afraid to go down into the fears, represented by the water. The fears dissolving, however, turn into cleansing agents. The part of the self responsible for the fears was the part that thought success a male prerogative, so that the woman had to exert extra discipline. That was also one of the reasons behind Ruburt's fear of the world's scorn.

That is enough for this evening. One small point: as you realize, the adolescent children did represent emotional conflicts in the dream that Ruburt managed to force his way through.

My heartiest regards, and a fond good evening.

("Thank you, Seth. Good night."

(11:34 PM.)

DELETED SESSION
MAY 1, 1978 9:43 PM MONDAY

(Both of us wanted Seth to discuss the sudden relaxation of her upper body that Jane experienced last Friday afternoon when we made love. She's written her own account of this. But the event provided us with an obvious clue—any body that can undergo so spontaneous a change can hardly be one that's permanently fixed in a stiffened condition.... We've already obtained some interesting pendulum answers, this

morning, about the event, concerning emotional factors that lead to physical restraint. We also wanted Seth to comment on Jane's eye condition, which lately has taken a variety of states, some of them momentarily excellent.

("I do feel a lot of material there, on all of this," Jane said as we waited for the session to begin.)

Good evening.

("Good evening, Seth.")

Let us begin slowly.

First of all, what have you done recently that was of benefit in your situation? Which of your efforts paid off, so to speak? The things that paid off, the things that were indeed quite effective, were these: again, your chair suggestion —remind me to return to that, for I have not mentioned some other reasons why I would like it stressed—it being the chair; the table in the kitchen, with all of the implications of additional cooking and involvement; your remark *(last week)* that Ruburt's face looked much better than it did in those old photographs; your bringing in the flowers; your lovemaking, which I will discuss; and Ruburt's point-of-power exercises. The pendulum work was important because of the togetherness it entailed, the joint determination it symbolizes, and Ruburt's decision to uncover any or all fears rather than hiding them.

The points I have mentioned were highly effective, and they were the most easily and naturally accomplished. I will return to them in a short time. They led Ruburt into periods of time in which he enjoyed simple pursuits—the making of a meal, for example. The impetus further led him around the kitchen, usually in the chair, but often to take steps in a different way from one point to another. He was reacting to new stimuli, as is natural for the body. He stretched just about every muscle in a new way, and made new demands upon the body, that the body quite agreeably tried to meet.

He tried out new motions, getting up and down from the stool, for example, without his table, and Saturday he reaped certain benefits, getting up surprisingly easy often, and gaining <u>some</u> new confidence.

In between, there were periods of body soreness in one area or another, which he and you handled well, remembering what I said. Your lovemaking, as you found to your surprise, led to a sudden, though momentary enough, excellent release of Ruburt's trunk. There are sessions hidden away *(with wry amusement)* that should have explained that episode. However, I will discuss those reasons now.

They have to do with communication, and with your individual and joint ideas of how feelings are to be communicated, and above all about your beliefs as to <u>which</u> feelings are to be communicated.

First of all, again, the situation, the living situation you have chosen means that you both place a good many demands upon the other, that in a family situation, for example, might be dispersed. Each of you then must meet many needs of the other. You are to be mate, lover, friend, companion, working colleague, each to the other. You are with each other constantly. With that as background, what do you think about communication?

Basically, Ruburt is verbal. Basically, he is highly affectionate. He believes in communicating through words, and he believes particularly in communicating "in a positive manner." He does not believe in communicating disapproval or aggression. The reasons, as given many times, lie in his background, where it was not safe to express disapproval or aggression. He equates silence with disapproval. He does believe in communicating love verbally and through touch, whether or not sexual feelings specifically are involved.

(10:07.) Now, my fine feathered friend: you never really trusted the verbal expression of feelings, while you trusted the verbal expression of ideas. You were particularly distrustful of the verbal expression of love, tenderness, or devotion. You felt it imperative to verbally express dissatisfaction or disapproval, generally, now—that is how words were used by your parents.

You felt that love and devotion should be understood, and that they did not need to be stated. In a way, both of you meant different things by communication, and used it to express only part of the spectrum of your feelings. It is Ruburt's nature to yell at the cat, but he feels the noise upsets you—a small point, but important.

In the past you felt that the touches of affection were ambiguous. You did not know what to do with them, or whether or not they should lead to a sexual encounter. Ruburt enjoys your combing his hair, because then you are touching him. The latest bedroom encounter took Ruburt by surprise. He was unhappy with some attempts he had made in the kitchen, and after some due consideration decided in this new mood of openness to discuss his feelings. He expected some understanding mixed perhaps with mild exasperation.

Suddenly, however, the wells of love within you opened, uncritically. He felt that, and was moved, as always. But for all your talk about "wanting to help him too," you seldom take the initiative in that regard. This time you began to caress him. The response was immediate, spontaneous, and as complete as the moment and his physical condition allowed. Many people spend hours, now and then, caressing each other's bodies, massaging each other, or simply relaxing in such a way, whether or not a sexual encounter occurs or is expected.

You need, each person needs, that kind of touch. Love expressed through touch, in whatever way, has a reviving effect upon the body and the mind. It restores the spirits. In Ruburt's particular case, it speaks volumes.

It was easy to see how the body could respond, and only provides a hint of what such future episodes could bring. Healing through touch of hands—why is it ever effective? It happens spontaneously when no healers, per se, are involved, millions of times, anytime a body is touched with love, compassion, and understanding. The organism instantly responds.

Now let us look at yesterday *(Sunday)* morning, and for background remember the bodybuilders, who purposefully shut out all annoying distractions. You began your day, first of all, by verbally expressing your dissatisfaction about the late delivery of the paper, by projecting into the future the late delivery of it for a year, and then by discussing critically and in disapproving tones the educational system, and so forth.

It is legitimate enough, but whatever other feelings you might have had of a more positive nature you did not express, and so your day began on that note. Other people would read the same paper, yet all of them reacted in their own ways. <u>If</u> peace of mind is a goal, <u>if</u> it is, the late delivery of the paper is ludicrous. It is not allowed to color your day in such a way. The bodybuilder would dismiss it without a thought.

Now the bodybuilders and sports teams have coaches, who remind them constantly of the goal in mind, and arouse their enthusiasm. They say "There <u>are</u> odds, but we will beat them." You need to be your own coaches in that respect.

Take your break.

(10:33—10:45.)

Now: there is nothing particularly wrong about you expressing your disapproval of the world, or whatever.

You inhibit the expression of feelings of love, approval, devotion, and this means that your verbal communications are <u>largely</u>, now, of a disapproving nature.

Ruburt needs approval. He needs the verbal expression of love and affection, not only in regard to his work, which he appreciates immensely, but in terms of his person. He used to try to trick you into such remarks. Sometimes he pleaded, and finally he decided they were simply against your nature, and so he must forget it.

You would go out of your way <u>not</u> to give such approval, by making a joke or whatever, because you did not believe that verbal communication should be used for such purposes. It made you feel inadequate, fearful of falling into cliches—or worse, trite expressions. It is good that naturally at least Ruburt <u>is</u> given to such expression, though that is not followed through as spontaneously as it could be. Ruburt, however, feels that it is not safe to express disapproval—the opposite of your habit—and so he feels threatened to some extent because your verbal expressions are so often of that nature, even if they are not directed to him, and he inhibits his own expression of any disapproval he feels, or frustrations. Lately he has made an effort to speak out.

Now: use of the chair is important because it <u>does</u> increase his mobility in this stage; but also because it exercises the knees while the rest of the body is in a comparatively normal position, with the back, shoulders, and head fairly upright. It also provides exercise to the feet without the weight imbalance that presently operates when he walks.

Activity in the important neck and shoulder areas has increased, so that the eyes have been highly variable in their behavior. Part of this becomes more noticeable as he looks upward more, say, in the cupboard, and as he changes the positions of his neck far more often.

I told you that the knees and the eyes were connected, and again, the hot towels will help. If you fully trusted what I am telling you, you would understand that that activity changes even as the muscles in the legs might be different from one day to another.

(Jane detected good evidence of the relationship involving her eyes, knees, toes, and other portions of her body the next day. Her description was very similar to the material Seth has just given.)

Give us a moment.... The eye condition is not separate, and now the more active muscles are arousing greater activity on the part of the ligaments, which will begin to loosen the joints considerably. The neck ligaments are involved here. They are moving constantly, releasing the muscles leading to the eyes, and making adjustments. When Ruburt relaxes he does not stare so, and the relaxation periods are of great benefit to the eyes.

After Saturday both of you became frightened again, and your joint beliefs and habits of pessimism to some extent at least meant that you began to doubt the gains that had been made. This morning's pendulum session, while helpful, for the general reasons given earlier, was also however more of an exercise in what is wrong, again, and was not followed by any constructive suggestion at all.

I would like both of you to read the chapter on affirmation *(in Personal Reality)*, and to keep it in mind daily. You, incidentally, are afraid of expressing verbal states, et cetera, for fear of being made to feel a fool because your background with your father was so loaded with such connotations.

The pendulum should be used to uncover feelings, to allow feedback between portions of the self, but mostly as a way of implanting new knowledge and constructive suggestions and feelings of safety to the "subconscious."

Your encounter with Leonard *(tonight)* was beneficial, because it allowed for expressions of friendliness on all of your parts, and the suspension of disapproving attitudes.

(*Jane and Leonard worked out a price for the purchase of Leonard's dining room set; we gave him an electric coffee pot also.*)

I want you to follow the advice in the chapter mentioned, and unless you have questions that is it for the evening.

(*"I guess not."*)

I wanted you to know what you did right, and use that knowledge to structure your current behavior. Framework 2 operates beautifully when you let it, as per your suggestion about the chair, and the kitchen table. Those are examples, and there will be many more if you keep this in mind.

A fond good evening.

(*"Thank you, Seth."*

(*11:14. For a while, listening to Seth, I found myself wondering if I'd done anything right since Jane's troubles began a decade ago. I didn't voice my thoughts, which were kind of low; then Seth returned almost at once:*)

One additional point: Ruburt can indeed recover. Not only that, but his recovery <u>can</u> be fairly easy, but your joint habits of pessimism color your attitudes. It is as if the team coach shouted "Try as hard as you can—but we will probably lose because that is the way it is."

Now: you have begun to change that attitude. Simply keep in mind those significances. Notice how you are focusing. The bodybuilder does not think he is inhibiting his expression if he chooses to focus on his bodybuilding to the exclusion of distractions that may be quite real but detrimental to his purpose. Feelings of pessimism regarding Ruburt's condition are detrimental. You both did very well on many occasions recently, so try to duplicate versions of the behavior I told you was helpful—and focus in those directions.

The old coach bows out for the evening.

(*11:20 PM.*)

DELETED SESSIONS
MAY 3, 1978 9:45 PM WEDNESDAY

(*Jane asked that Seth comment on her fear about time, a question we'd uncovered recently with the pendulum. Her bodily changes continue, and these are detailed in her own notes mainly. Actually she wanted Seth to comment on her overall condition, what was happening, etc.*)

Good evening.

("Good evening, Seth.")
A personal session.

More or less, your nature sustains you. The nature of the earth sustains its creatures, and overall, while there may be floods or earthquakes, you can rely upon the sustenance of the earth.

The sun will shine upon you whether or not you think you had a good day or a bad day, and it will shine upon "the sinner" and the religious man; it will shine upon you without judgment. As I have said, animals have an inbuilt sense of their own worth in that regard. They trust their nature, and the greater nature from which their existence springs.

Without going into background information again, and regardless of the reasons, people in your time have been taught to regard their natures with suspicion. Since Ruburt's nature was rather—<u>rather</u>—extravagantly different from what he considered the norm to be, and since he possessed abilities that were not common generally and specifically to his sex, he became even more unduly suspicious of his own nature. He believed then that he needed safeguards.

Each person's nature, however, innately possesses all of the qualities and characteristics necessary to bring about its own fulfillment. It will automatically find frameworks that are suited to <u>it</u>, though perhaps to no others. When that nature is trusted, there are no interior impediments or conflicts, even though the individual may feel himself to be in conflict with certain elements in the world at large.

None of Ruburt's characteristics are "negative," bad, or dangerous. All of them, recognized as a part of his nature, would basically work together in the most auspicious, satisfying, and fulfilling of fashions. When he fears his own nature, however, then the qualities are not put together as smoothly, so that one can appear contradictory to the other. Thusly, Ruburt felt that there were contradictions between spontaneity and discipline, the intuitions and the intellect. Therefore he tried to be either spontaneous or disciplined, or intellectual or intuitive, but with the implied supposition that these were somehow opposing conditions, or opposing elements of behavior.

The physical body runs itself spontaneously, and yet with an inner automatic discipline and order that is indeed almost impossible for you to understand.

The vast majority of intellectual deductions are based upon unconscious, intuitive realizations, and the edifices built by the intuitions have a dazzling framework of high intellectual content and reason, so brilliant that the mind itself often cannot follow.

When you two make love in any manner, you are involved with a spontaneity and discipline, again, that literally cannot be consciously ascertained. In Ruburt's situation, such encounters are particularly of the highest import, for spontaneous motion is elicited. Impulses are aroused. The nervous system is regenerated. Nerve impulses quicken, as does circulation. More than this, the body automatically, spontaneously responds to emotion, and yet in that spontaneous activity what inner discipline reigns.

The inner order of the body is hidden within its great spontaneous abilities. Now Ruburt once felt that he had to discipline his impulses, lest they spontaneously lead him where he felt his purposes, or safety, might be threatened. If he understands now that his own nature provides for his sustenance, and automatically leads him into fulfillment, and couches his existence in perfect safety *(leaning forward)*, then certain things will become clear.

(10:10.) Give us a moment.... He has been painting lately, quite happily anticipating the next painting period, yet at the same time worried that he is not writing instead; or when he does write on *Seven*, he does so because he thinks he should. So he experiences a conflict. He did give in to the impulse to paint, however. The painting is providing a mental rest, aiding in the coordination of hand and eye, and allowing him to work at certain inner challenges in a different way. His nature knows he needs the variety—the creative variety.

The visual activity itself stimulates different portions of the psyche, and allows mental concepts to be rearranged while he is thus occupied. New intuitional insights grow while he is not thinking in those terms, and if he trusted his nature more fully he could enjoy the painting more while also realizing that other levels of the self had their own reasons. The impulse to paint, therefore, fits in with the same kind of spontaneous "discipline" that is so magnificent in the activity of the body.

Because of your age difference, Ruburt felt he had to catch up, and he became more conscious of clock time. I want those sessions read again that I gave about his attitudes toward "work." They were designed specifically for him and his nature, for when he <u>forgets</u> about work, with its connotations for him, then he is at his most intuitively creative, and inspiration springs naturally and quickly at his beckoning.

You have both done well since our last session. Ruburt on his own began to give the old suggestion "My legs and knees <u>can</u> bear my weight," for he suddenly realized that that was indeed true. His fears, unexpressed, now being given expression, led him to certain beliefs about the body. I am giving this material again for your easy current reference. He can indeed walk easier and better now —another suggestion that he can begin to use. There will be variations, however, as you must understand from material I have given you recently.

Since our last session, very significant activity has accelerated in the entire head area. Basically, it results from the chair activity, and activation of the knees, while the upper body is not in a state of stress. Those areas are being released, and the process, continued, will release the eyes.

He should resume yawning again, whenever he thinks of it through the day, for that will help quicken the process. So will hot towels *(with gentle amusement. We have yet to resume using them).*

It will help if the two of you together discuss your feelings about time and work. Ruburt's nature will see to it that he has time to do all the important things he wants to do in any given day. Becoming more aware of his desires will activate the body so that it performs more quickly in order to meet his goals. In the past he cut the desires down, to make sure that the most important prerogatives would be met, but his picture of reality was too small. The body and mind both need stimuli, variety, and richness, and his nature automatically seeks expression, not repression.

That is the end of the session unless you have questions.

("How about my dream with John Wayne?")

John Wayne represented old lines of conventionalized beliefs about the male. Wayne represented feelings about the male that you received in your background from your father, and through boyhood movies, in which the male could afford affectionate behavior or conversation—only with his horse *(with amusement).* In other words, the uncommunicative male, who was afraid of open sentiment. The dream was in response to our last session, in part, and of your own musings as a result. You saw yourself as separate from Wayne, and able to manipulate much more quickly. And your feelings in the dream toward him were your feelings toward those old beliefs.

("How about the young couple trapped in the burning car, in the dream?")

The couple represented old fears; again, interpretations of your father's beliefs, that young couples become trapped by the fires of desire, and could not escape; that the man could not hold himself apart, but would be devoured by the sentiments of love that would consume him. Those fears of your father's were given a less frightening, more conventionalized and safer image in John Wayne, who escapes such situations by refusing intimate entanglements, and is "free to roam the range."

(10:42.) You are the "victor" of the dream, in that you are apart from those images.

Do you have other questions?

("Have Jane's dreams changed in character since we began our latest efforts to help her?")

Ruburt has not remembered, and yet in the dream state he has been working through such issues. Physically, rooms in the house have opened to him, as with the kitchen, and the table *(just delivered by Leonard)* in the new room. Those represent the opening of inner rooms, of course, and will further trigger the opening of still new intuitive areas.

End of session, and a fond good evening.

("Thank you."

(10:45 PM. Jane was surprised at the quick end to the session, and I was willing to continue longer. A copy of Seth's analysis of my John Wayne dream is attached to the dream in my notebook.

(I might add that today, Thursday, Jane experienced a dramatic further release in her neck and other areas of her body, so we are getting results with our program. Her new release began this morning as we worked with the pendulum, and she can attach her report to this session if she wants to. We voiced the idea that three key words seemed to symbolize her physical hassles—fears of scorn, criticism, and flamboyance. As the morning passed and we continued to exchange ideas, we saw of course that all these reflected Jane's fear or distrust <u>of her own nature</u>—a situation that simply must be remedied. I made a brief note about the three words on a sheet of our pendulum questions.

(Our exploration of "flamboyance" came about through Seth's use of "extravagant" in this session, as I scanned the original notes this morning while coming up with some new questions. I guess the realization that the basic mistrust of one's own nature could have such dire results was what triggered our conscious realization that we could <u>do something</u> about the whole business of symptoms, etc. Jane began to show results as we discussed the subject; after lunch, she was so loose, including her knees, that she wondered whether she could get to the john—which she did, by the way. But she reported "new things" releasing in her head area, and the back of the neck, that had been "tight as a fist." Very encouraging, and we plan to continue working with these thoughts.

(After lunch we discussed her own notes on the morning's work, and stressed that she should use the word "flamboyant" as part of her own true nature, attaching only positive meanings to it, being proud of it, realizing that it gave expression to her abilities in a way that few could match. This of course meant, as we said, that she needn't go about any longer pretending to be like the normal housewife next door, or whatever inanity—since nothing could be further from the truth: She is <u>not</u> like the normal housewife next door, should not want to be, should not be in alarm at their criticism, and should thank God for whatever abilities she has of her own that do inevitably make her different, superior, talented, etc., with something unique to offer the world—an opportunity few possess, and that should be used with the greatest joy

and abandon. After all, I said, people come to her for help, she doesn't go to them. To stand in fear of the criticism or scorn of others is now, we see, the worst possible behavior. This must be eliminated, and we intend to work unceasingly at the task until its accomplished. I see no reasons to prevent our succeeding.

(All of this sounds very simple in the telling, of course, but was opaque to us until we'd gone this far with the pendulum work, evidently. Seth has said the same thing many times over the years. The difference now, I told Jane, was that we were paying attention to those ideas.

(I also stressed that our changing attitudes would be sure to change our attitudes toward others—that instead of trying to act "normally" toward strangers when they came here, especially when they were unannounced, we should simply be ourselves, secure in the abilities of our own natures; if any of these actions could be taken as "flamboyant" in a negative way, then so be it. That would be their hassle, not ours, I added. Our goal now is to simply speak our minds, if in a nice way, usually, to others, and let the chips fall where they may. I added that it would be ironic and hilarious indeed that if this new behavior brought to us everything we'd always wanted for our life's work.

(They don't have the talent, Jane—you do! Always ask yourself: "Do I want to be the one who's trying to do something, or the one who criticizes the efforts of others?")

DELETED SESSION
MAY 8, 1978 9:43 PM MONDAY

(Today is Jane's birthday.

(I explained to her, as we waited for the session to begin, my dilemma about Note 6 for Appendix 22—my feeling of time wasted after I'd spent a couple of days writing it very carefully—only to have it fall apart at the last moment because I'd forgotten to deal with one crucial point. I found my evident lack of skill at planning quite depressing. See Volume 2 of "Unknown" Reality.

(Today Jane has had a steady barrage of bodily sensations of incipient release and change—her most active and encouraging one so far, since we began our program on April 3, 1978. Today was also one of her most uncomfortable, however, due to the muscular soreness involved as little-used muscles in her trunk began to act. At the same time, her knees are much looser. However, we've learned by now to have the confidence that by tomorrow, say, the soreness in her shoulders and arms will have lessened, and that another part of the body will begin loosening itself.

(I hadn't had time to buy Jane's birthday presents, although we both know

what she wants—hot plate for the kitchen, and a summer bed spread. We've had a succession of visitors, all but one of them unannounced, and have lost work time as a result. Saturday, for example, I wasn't able to get out of the house to go food shopping.)

Now: tell Ruburt I said "Happy birthday."

("Thank you.")

Bodily motion is obviously of itself healing in nature. Ruburt's new and more ambitious movement about the house, using the chair, has activated the body's motion, of course, so that massaging-like effects occur. In his particular case, as mentioned, the knees and legs are allowed far greater exercise than before, while the body is in a more or less normal position.

That activation has indeed begun now the highly important release of the upper portions of the body. Areas are being reawakened, and circulation greatly increased in certain areas. It is not necessary to trace nerve pathways, and yet the stretching of both legs and muscles reawakens and quickens nerve impulses. <u>All</u> portions of the body are now being stretched.

Before, relatively speaking, each portion of the body reinforced the position of each other portion in such a manner that little leeway was possible. Ruburt now is at the stage where each portion of the body takes a more positive, active position, and gently nudges each other part to greater freedom. In other words, the new changes do not meet with such <u>resistance</u>, but now the definite improvements can begin an overall acceleration.

The greater release of the knees allows for a greater freedom of the trunk which in its turn further frees the knees, and so forth.

(Today, even though she was so uncomfortable, Jane was still standing taller than she has done for a long time.)

Ruburt has done very well in understanding these body changes, and has been aided by your support there. I am pleased to see that he moves about in the chair more and more. That intent to move further activates the body, and sends impulses through it, for it knows it is meant to move about on two feet. Those impulses quicken the physical changes, so that the two go together; as in the kitchen he now feels like standing, or wants to walk from the sink to the table.

(9:56.) Give us a moment.... I want to point out that the Seth groups throughout the country are far more significant than you might realize, for they are not formed as a result of any kind of promotion. They arise spontaneously, and despite the fact that you do not actively encourage them, or even pat them on the back.

In that respect they are grassroot, coming from the people themselves.

Those people interpret our books from their own levels. They regard the books as their discoveries. They buy the books for friends and relatives. They try to pass on the ideas to parents or children, and to interpret them through home life, and through areas of work and community. They invest time and enthusiasm—and that kind of grassroot development is in the long run more apt to change the beliefs of a society than any authoritative dictums from the specialists, whatever their field. You are reaching tomorrow's "authorities."

To reach today's authorities you must make too many concessions, and that is true of anyone who hopes to produce great work in any area. Men in the sciences have years and years invested in a particular system, upon which their reputations, self-respect, and livelihood depend. They have inbuilt leanings, then, quite understandably if regrettably, that mitigate against their looking with clear eyes upon work that shows the gaps in their own understanding or systems.

Your work, in any case, is the interpretation of reality through your own experience, providing a new and creative view of man and the universe. You want that view for yourselves. It has always been your individual and joint search —a private determination to glimpse what you could of the nature of man, that was not glimpsed before.

Your original purpose was the purpose of the creative artist or of the mystic, and that kind of purpose automatically brings you in rebellion against official authority. Your original purpose did not involve gaining the respect of those authorities, and it is, if you will forgive me, overall shortsighted to worry about the approval of such people in your time. It can make you bitter for no reason, for this kind of creative work exists outside of its time, and will still be read when the old authorities no longer exist, in your terms.

You must do what you want because you want to do it, and if the authorities listen, well and good, and if not it is their loss.

The ideas will grow in any case. Whenever possible then outside of normal considerations, both of you should concentrate upon the creative, intuitive elements of what you are involved in. Forget such things as impressing the authorities so that they somehow will change the world. Do not expect the books to sell like novels, as I have told you. Free yourselves from such considerations, with their implications.

Those implications are the kind of things that trigger in Ruburt worries about meeting scorn or criticism, worries that then set up their own chains of reactions. Don't be bothered that parapsychologists are not knocking at your doors. Ruburt's abilities lie outside of their realm, and they know it. They are doing the best that they can in their framework, but you do not fit into their framework.

This may sound simple, and yet all such considerations serve to weigh you both down, and they color your attitudes far more than you realize.

I know you both fairly well. For now, I suggest that you not contact your famous agent *(Scott Meredith)*. You are not being treated like merchandise at Prentice, whatever Prentice's faults might be, and you would be treated like merchandise by the high-powered agent, who would consider you a fine property, and expect you to act accordingly.

(This rather humorous material from Seth was in reference to a talk Jane and I had, at my instigation, several days ago, when I idly speculated about asking Scott Meredith to personally represent us. I think I got off on that tack because I was concerned about getting money that Prentice had withheld against returns. [That dilemma has since been resolved.] In the meantime, both Jane and I had forgotten all about the Meredith question.)

You are making a good living. There is nothing at all wrong with wanting, say, to become a millionaire, but if you simply concentrate upon the creative, personal elements in your lives—your writing in the notes, your painting, Ruburt's writing and psychic freedom, then everything else will fall into place. You will each have more frequent and fulfilling psychic experiences as a result. The other ideas I mentioned, to some extent now cast an unclear light, so that the attitudes they evoke are in conflict with your original, most persuasive goals.

(10:28.) In Ruburt's case such considerations make him feel set against the world, where actually that social world <u>has</u> rather agreeably enough allowed you room and a certain platform on its stage, through your readership. You have a considerable number of people, considerable, in all walks of life who wish you well. There is no need for Ruburt to anticipate scorn. There is no need either, however, for him to imagine that he has any responsibility to go out <u>into</u> that mixed social arena to do tours or appear on television.

He anticipates scorn if he did so. He would indeed meet a large range of reactions. Scorn would be the least of them. He would meet honor, belief, respect, disbelief, anger, love—and some scorn. Such a career addition would be bound to change, of course, the foundations of your lives. I do not believe you are willing to meet people on that basis.

("Would <u>you</u> mind doing that?")

Do you want me to go on the Johnny Carson show?

("I don't know.")

Under certain conditions, I would certainly appear on television, for I have done so. But I also have your natures to think of—quite lovingly, by the way.

Your pendulum work continues to be a help, because it keeps such issues before your eyes. Ruburt should read our last session particularly, once or twice a week, for it will reinforce your pendulum work.

Ruburt's body is geared for full recovery now, so keep that joint determination in mind. Trust your nature, and then you will see that what you consider mistakes are simply insights that come out of place, so to speak, and that has to do with your remarks before the session.

I am closing the session early. And *(whispering)* in the time left over, I would like Ruburt to soak his knees.

As you read this session, however, try to see how those attitudes that I mentioned do clutter up your minds to some extent. You set yourselves, if you will forgive me, eternal goals. Along the way your livelihood has been provided for, and you have a framework in which to work. Many people hold you in respect and regard. In larger terms, however, your goals are not temporal, so do not become overly concerned—overly—with temporal considerations. They impede your private psychic experiences, for they add stresses you do not need.

(10:45.) End of session.

("Will you say something about my dream of last Saturday morning?")

As you noted, the dream provided a distorted glimpse of your visitors.

The older man was the one you saw. The apples did provide the painting connection with the girl, and the dream was very simple—a distorted view into tomorrow's mirror. I am more concerned that you each to some degree have inhibited your subjective freedoms, and not allowed yourselves the opportunity for an even richer diet of dreams and psychic experience. I hope this session would rectify the situation, and it should.

("How about those people selling those tapes? Should we forget about that?")

(Recently Jane was told that a complete set of class tapes, with transcripts was being offered by someone on the West Coast for around $255.00 for 55 of them—$5.00 or thereabouts a tape. During a call to Tam this morning, he advised Jane to "put a stop" to the affair before it went too far—to at least write the people involved a letter. Jane has asked Sheri Perl for the names and addresses to do this, and plans to write a letter. We think the quality of the tapes must be very poor. There's also copyright infringement, since some of the class sessions have been published. Jane is against the whole thing on esthetic and invasion-of-privacy grounds, not monetary ones so much, and I guess my feelings about it all are too ambiguous. At the same time, it all sounds familiar, as if we heard about someone doing the same thing last year, say.)

(With a smile:) I had hoped you would not ask, for my situation is not yours.

At the most a letter from Ruburt. My framework is different from yours. I do not see how such people can hurt you in any way. If you wanted to make money from the tapes, you could have. If they make money from the tapes, you do not make less.

I am quite aware, however, that such affairs can appear quite complicated, but your situation cannot be threatened by such people unless you allow it to be. Good ideas are going out into the world. The tapes are not artistically produced. They are not tapes of quality in that regard. They <u>are</u> tapes of quality in another regard, and they cannot be reproduced forever.

End of session, and a <u>fond</u> good evening.

("Okay. Thank you.")

My comments this evening are simply made in response to my knowledge of your original goals, and Ruburt's. Only in <u>their</u> light are those other attitudes detrimental.

(10:56 PM.

(A copy of Seth's comments about my dream, which did contain some precognitive elements, is attached to the dream in my own notebook.)

DELETED SESSION
MAY 10, 1978 9:30 PM WEDNESDAY

(Jane wanted material from Seth tonight on her "blues"—the mixed emotions and conflicts she feels at times when waking from her afternoon naps. She'd felt that way today "as if I'll never get inspired again—I mean in a big way, like I did for Politics....")

Now: another personal session.

What of your letters and visitors lately? For one thing, the number of excellent, well-meaning letters, and the birthday cards *(and telegrams)* were meant to show Ruburt that he was regarded with affection and honor and not held up in scorn.

They were also meant to show appreciation for your work, jointly, when it seemed you needed it, and therefore to revive both of your spirits. The same applies to your guests, and particularly to the two young boys from the Sunday school, hopefully showing Ruburt that all <u>conventional</u> churchgoers were not closed-minded, but were also seeking out new knowledge.

The young man *(from Maryland)* with his gift, represented his generation, in a way, and so in bringing his gift he brought it symbolically for others. The longer visit, with the cheesecake woman, was meant to give you a closer look at the kind of person who gives lectures about us, and so forth—so she was symbolic of others. The young girl was helped by her visit here, and symbolizes many others who are helped by the books alone.

(*I also found a bouquet of carnations laying on the front step Monday afternoon, after a heavy rain had evidently knocked them over. No card was enclosed, however. No big deal, but from last Saturday noon until after supper Monday evening, we had eight callers, all but the first two, Rusty and Hal, being unannounced.*)

These were interruptions, and because of your attitudes you thought of them as troublesome interruptions: surely you would have sailed through your work otherwise, or performed chores that you wanted to accomplish; and so because you still do not really understand the effectiveness of Framework 2, those visits added to your sense of concern and hassles with time. Framework 2 knows of all of your purposes, as I have mentioned. The visitors took Ruburt's mind off of his condition, provided new stimulus, provided reassurance, and allowed his body to continue its improvements.

Neither of you really, however, took full advantage of the reassurances those visits were intended to give <u>each</u> of you. You have a right to refuse guests, of course, and yet if you learn to work with Framework 2 with greater faith you will find that other issues are usually involved than those immediately apparent.

I may return to the subject of time later.

(9:44.) It is obvious that Ruburt's body is responding, and it is responding eagerly to the approaches you are now using, because it is dealing with the entire picture. The area at the right side of the back of the head, in Ruburt's case, physically speaking, is a trigger point for motion. The blockage there, in those terms, has been <u>largely</u> responsible for the difficulties in locomotion, and for the eye difficulties as well. That area is finally in the process of releasing itself. The ligaments in the legs are responding beautifully, and as I said earlier, there is a give-and-take between the trunk and leg areas.

The neck area mentioned is also <u>largely</u> responsible for the arm angles and all of that is now beginning vital release. This is an overall body process, then, and you are both handling it now very well. It is quite natural that Ruburt becomes irritable at times. He should not pretend otherwise, for such irritability is short-lived, if expressed, and usually directly related to a particular difficulty in manipulation, or whatever.

Try to respond more clearly, each of you, to the moment, for you have a tendency otherwise not to see given events as clearly as you might otherwise. It should be obvious that comparatively speaking Ruburt feels quite well sometimes. He will be chatting, or yelling at his painting, or whatever. He is quite open often, say, to making love, as you know now, but earlier you colored your reaction to him often through the pessimistic cast that both of you had allowed to slip over your perceptions.

He felt quite maligned earlier tonight, when you did not realize that he was not grunting with exertion as he walked to the bathroom several times today. You did not realize that. It was of course apparent to him, but this is an example of the way in which unthinking habits of reaction can inhibit your perception.

The same sort of thing used to apply in a different way, but does no longer, when Ruburt would see you frown, for example, and would then ignore an obvious cheerful mood on your part, still interpreting your behavior in the light of the frown.

I want to get into some other pertinent material, and will let you take a brief break before I begin.

(10:01—10:10.)

Before I discuss our main material, I have a few comments regarding strangers.

You might make a small sign: "Beloved stranger: we are working. Please do not disturb us." You could add to that "Please write a note," and buy yourselves one of those contraptions for your door. *(A mailbox?)* Or you might decide yourselves upon some hour of the day or evening when such a guest would be least bothersome. You could decide never to see a guest during the day, for example, and inform such people to come back at such and such a time.

You could decide to see such people at lunch hour, and no other time, and put that in your note: "Come back at noon." You could, therefore, make several different kinds of decisions that would give you a free mind for large portions of the time. You would not be rejecting guests at the door, per se, but telling them to return at such and such an hour, or to leave a note. You could compose several such signs, so that one might read: "We are not seeing any strangers today at all," but there are many variations that you could settle for.

Now: Ruburt himself hit upon the "heroic impulses"—and what he meant was this: that ideally speaking the individual's impulses were inner directional signals that, followed, would automatically lead to the greatest fulfillment and development.

He thought of that term before our Framework 1 and 2 material, and his idea was that the impulses came from a part of the self that automatically knew the entire picture of the self's environment and potentials. He was quite correct, for those impulses arise from the larger self's immersion in Framework 2, and those impulses led Ruburt to his intuitive inspirations, experiences of psychic events, and to the books. When he becomes overly concerned about writing as work, or with psychic development as something he should do, then he tangles those impulses, and becomes worried that he will not be suitably inspired again.

To some extent he feels abandoned at such times. *Oversoul Seven 2* began from inspiration, and whenever he turns back to the manuscript he is inspired again. He enjoys the book, yet it has become entangled with his ideas of work and publishing schedules.

He wants to be inspired. On the other hand he thinks "What if I am inspired with new material when I still have *Seven* to finish, and when besides I should be helping Rob with *"Unknown"*?

The reasons behind such behavior are given in the sessions on work. He has been inspired, but to paint, because his impulses are quite correct; the painting of flowers leads him to contemplate beauty for beauty's sake, frees his mind, and also allows for certain kinds of muscular motions that are now beneficial.

(10:29.) The idea is for him to play with *Seven*, to let his mind freely play with ideas, and to follow his impulses. He paints as he writes, furiously involved, in bursts. The psychic experiences, intuitional developments, and dream activity—these refresh him and lead precisely to the kind of inspiration he wants. So the library idea that you had is an excellent one, but it should be done playfully.

I gave the three-hour recommendation because at the time he was worried that he could not correlate the new physical impulses with his other activities. He has done very well there, however.

Give us a moment.... You are both apt to have rather absolute ideas at times. These sessions now are helpful. There is no reason, however, why in the future you cannot freely take a month off from sessions in order to quicken your work on *"Unknown"*. That would not mean, for example, that Ruburt was not using his abilities. As far as impulses are concerned, most likely Ruburt could have three or four excellent sessions a week at certain periods in your lives, and there would be periods of vacation also. Often, however, you both have a tendency there to think in black-and-white terms.

You are each making some excellent and vital readjustments, and our last session in particular should help clear your focuses. In Framework 2, *"Unknown"* is completely finished, of course, and whenever you have any difficulty with a note or an appendix, take a moment and tell yourself that the final, completed, quite excellent version of that note will come to you. This can be of excellent practical help.

Your joint determination is already building up bonuses in many areas, and by all means remember to keep up the personal contact you have begun together again. The suggestion "Help and inspiration are appearing at all levels of my experience," can now again be used by Ruburt to good advantage.

It will be of great benefit for you to make some kind of decision involving your guests, as I mentioned. If you decide you simply will not see anyone during the day, then have a note read accordingly; but be very clear in your own minds, and <u>act accordingly</u>.

It <u>is</u> advantageous from many standpoints to alter your hours, and some alterations do have the advantage of automatically providing solitude. You both seem to like regular hours and habits, however, so any such alterations, to be effective in a large manner, would have to be worked out so that you had a definite framework to rely upon.

I merely want to mention various possibilities that can offer advantages. Ruburt's point of power is progressing well. You own attitude could hardly be better, as far as Ruburt is concerned, since we are not looking for saintly behavior *(amused)*. Some definite decisions about guests, however, will relieve your minds, and allow you to work more freely. Remind yourself, again, of *"Unknown's"* completed form, and if you do so its pattern will transpose itself upon your thoughts as you work, so that you will be tuning into its model in that respect.

Everything that I have said should further help Ruburt, so that he feels more at ease. Remember the use of the playful creative abilities, because again they can lead you to further ideas that would trigger unanticipated positive results in Ruburt's condition, as per your chair idea, the table in the kitchen, and so forth.

Use this session to compose some new pendulum questions also. Now I bid you a fond good evening, and I expect hot towels on the knees. The last session should be read again, for it can reawaken both of your psychic abilities to a greater degree. End of session.

("Thank you very much."

(Much louder, and with humor:) You can always write a note that says "Seth said go away."

("Yes. Good night." 10:52 PM.)

DELETED SESSION
MAY 15, 1978 9:10 PM MONDAY

(At suppertime tonight we read a newspaper article about a 27-year-old man from Philadelphia who'd committed suicide in our area by having himself decapitated by a railroad train. Jane said the first thing she thought of when she read the article was that the stranger might have been on his way to see her for help. I thought

this a very meaningful projection, reflecting her exaggerated feelings of responsibility to the world because of her psychic abilities. I asked that Seth comment.

(Upon waking from her nap this afternoon, Jane again felt blue, deserted, and alone except for me in the world. Feelings about writing were also mixed in, and time, she said. Again, I wanted Seth to comment.

(Our daily pendulum work continues, and continues to get good results. Each day brings something new. Jane has been extremely sore in her arms, shoulders, rib cage, and so forth today, yet she was able to stand taller, by leaning against the bathroom door frame, than I'd seen her do in a very long time. It's part of the rhythmic healing process going on in her body, as Seth described it recently, moving through different areas successively, followed each time by new releases. Jane said her knees felt very light and considerably looser.

(Her soreness vanished by early afternoon. Tonight she stood "even taller" briefly, yet through all of these changes the eyes have bothered her considerably. Again, I asked that Seth comment on it all.)

Now: a personal session.

First of all, the advances, the physical advances, and I will come to Ruburt's physical condition, have come about because he is making certain advances psychologically.

<u>Largely</u>, he has stopped projecting negatively into the future. There are a few lapses, but overall he is changing that habit—and the point of power has helped him considerably there. He is discussing his feelings openly with you. That, plus your pendulum work, prevents fears from going underground again. He is quite importantly beginning to change the viewpoint from which he previously viewed his reality. There is a line in the point of power material to that regard.

He has not as yet changed his viewpoint to that of a normally flexible person, but it is vastly improved from the one he had only a short while ago. It is true that he is quite aware of his bodily conditions, and yet overall he is not concentrating upon them, or regarding them negatively. The new viewpoint, with its new attractions—helping with work, helping with house chores—these automatically take his mind elsewhere, and act as further stimuli. And remember, they are the result of loving creative inspirations, again, the table and the chair, you follow me?—

("Yes.")

—so be on the lookout for further such inspirations.

The body itself is responding beautifully. Ruburt went in a very short period of days from doing relatively little physically to giving the legs rather constant stimulation with the chair. The leg ligaments have released and loosened rather considerably even since our last session. The ankles and feet are beginning to respond to the new requirements, and the knee joints themselves, now, are increasing their lubrication, and gently beginning new motion.

That requires considerable change overall. Remember the alternating pattern I told you of. Those vital neck areas are further releasing. This means that the shoulders, arms, and entire trunk follow. Muscles in the stomach and the ribs themselves are involved *(as Jane has noticed)*.

The releasing action causes the odd stomach sensations. The eye muscles change constantly almost, as the huge motor area of the neck alternately releases and relaxes. There are rhythms, so that Ruburt had, for example, two excellent days—Thursday and Friday. The body was resting, its activity more or less at a state of balance. He cleaned portions of the house, and was quite active.

The weekend brought new activity in that neck area, bringing discomfort, but also new releases to the shoulders and the rib portions, loosening the stomach muscles. It was natural enough that he has periods of disorientation walking—but overall he has handled this well. The released ligaments can feel unstable, particularly when they first relax. There are other times when he definitely feels like putting his weight upon his legs, and walking, and he should be very faithful about following that impulse. As the muscles change, there can be some difficulties with depth perception regardless, since the muscles are used to reaching out only so far, and must change their orientation.

The eyes are growing healthier—meaning more active and resilient. It would be a good idea now and then during the day for him to make circles with his eyes, without overdoing it.

Jaw pressure is being released. These are all very active signs.

(9:30.) The gradations will be less apparent before too long, and Ruburt will be able to do more and more without such obvious changes in the body—that is, they will occur, but in this period, very important ligaments have been released, and they are bound to be felt.

Give us a moment.... The library should be continued, and your private periods, for again these are vastly advantageous—and I might say, to you both.

Yesterday Ruburt received some excellent ideas for *Seven*, which shows that he is beginning to change his attitude, and he should continue to read those work sessions.

Give us a moment.... The creative artist can be in somewhat of a quandary, according to his beliefs, for he wants to preserve the precious moment, the fleeting thought, the daffodils, the perceived insights. At the same time he often feels the need to stand apart from life, from the fleeting thoughts, the daffodils or the insight, so that he will not be lost completely in the moment, but able to form almost a second self with a larger viewpoint, who can then more clearly examine and understand the thought, the moment, or the insight.

The creative artist <u>can</u> be afraid of letting himself go completely in his life, for fear that he will become so involved that he will forget to stand apart, to look or to listen. Now to some degree that is Ruburt's quandary, and to a lesser extent, your own.

You want to examine life, to experience it, and yet in some way find in time a safe dimension <u>apart</u> from time. What you want is a <u>second life in life</u>, in which to appreciate and examine life's experience. The ordinary distractions of life immediately then cause conflict. On the one hand, they <u>are</u> living, these distractions. They are life. On the other hand, they rob you in time of that second life you want, in which to examine your experiences.

Now obviously, if you cut down distractions, or all experiences, there would be little left to enjoy or examine. You both tried to find a framework in which you could have two lives at once in that regard—and putting those two together is taking some doing.

Since you set yourselves such a course, then you obviously have a certain responsibility to both lives. They are your creations, after all. Almost all of Ruburt's difficulty with time, and your own, spring from this basic quandary. For most people do not try that hard to preserve the living moment, or to understand it, while they are still involved with time's physical package. Hence, to some extent your difficulties with *"Unknown"*—that is, with the notes—for you are trying to fit one dimension into another. A bold venture, and one that fits in quite will with your intents jointly to understand and preserve fleeting reality, and one that conflicts with your attempts to do this in the context of one physical time that passes.

(9:50.) Most artists, painters now, are lost, so to speak, in the moment or moments of the painting's creation. The painting becomes the creation, and also it is the passing time of reality. Most artist, painters, do not feel the need, then, to "later" examine the moments of creativity themselves, nor to form still another subjective platform from which to examine the creative process.

You do, however. Ruburt does also in his writing, for he then becomes another self who watches the creative self. So both of you form subjective extensions that you must one way or another put together in physical time. *(With gentle humor:)* My books represent vast creativity, and yet you perform your own additional subjective leaps, forming subjective platforms that then deal with the circumstances of the books.

Ruburt, therefore, became somewhat overly concerned with physical time. He must allow himself greater freedom creatively, in a playful manner, forgetting all thoughts "at the time" of time.

I have a few suggestions for both of you. I am not speaking of schedules. You have a responsibility to time and to timelessness. I would like you to make a list of what you want to do in a day—that is, in a 24-hour period, <u>and to think of that period</u>, now, as a gift of time, to be used as you desire.

Do not think of breaking it up into segments, but rather as the rhythmic flow of desired activities. You will want to paint, to prepare *"Unknown."* Now painting is in one regard timeless, though it will flow into time. *"Unknown"* is timeless, yet it will flow into time. Yard work is not timeless. It can be a joyful exercise of the body, the natural life being reinforced, and it can also provide feelings of timelessness, so that in that regard your love of timelessness can be combined with your love of the moment.

I want you each to make a list, then, of what you want to do in a day. You can quite properly decide, if you want, how many hours you want to devote to given activities, but do not think of schedules, but instead of the flow of timeless energy into time. When you have decided, and see where your prerogatives lie, then stick to them.

Ruburt can begin now with his three hours, this to be a free creative time for thinking, or writing. He likes to paint, but he does not regard that in the same way, so let him allow himself an hour a day for painting, or so many hours a week—whatever he wants.

The library takes little time, but he should turn his focus more toward his timeless encounters, and toward the playfulness of his creative and psychic abilities.

You determine the time you want to spend with *"Unknown"*—time you want to spend, say, in the yard. For now the pendulum sessions are involved. You do not need to worry about hurting your friends or neighbors, who will understand quite well. You have only to firmly state your position, and they will follow, <u>expecting</u> this of you.

Think of the entire 24-hour period, however. If the two of you stick together, there will be no problem, and particularly if you view this not as a schedule but as a way in which you want to mix time and timelessness, and merge the "two lives" that each of you try to live in the one life. Distractions may occur, but you can deal with them if your attitudes are clear, and if you see that overall you are doing what you want. Then any distractions will not be that important.

(10:13.) Give me a moment, since I have your list also in mind *(humorously).*

Truth is not like a specific prescription. It is an aura that pervades all reality. Ruburt is upset on two levels. He loves the pursuit of truth for its own sake, and the pursuit of truth is basically a playful creative endeavor, in which children indulge all the time.

On the other hand, he becomes upset if people cannot make truth work in literal terms. He is very touchy on that point, and yet he becomes very angry if people try to make truth too practical. Why can't truth make people want to live? Why can't truth be used as a prescription? The suicide story bothered him simply because it reminded him of Will *(Ives)*, who had attended classes, and of a friend of Venice's, who committed suicide many years ago, although a session was held for her.

The story in the paper rearoused those old conflicts. But truth involves insights of a most peculiar kind, for they cannot indeed be truly specified, and the more specific you try to make them the more you distort them, or the more you dilute their original power. You make your own reality. You cannot force an individual to live, nor can you force him to die, through the use of the truth. One and one is two—that is a fact in your world, and you can use that fact in millions of ways, but it involves no truth.

Man lives through the desire for life. <u>That</u> truth is a far more important realization. People can use our books, but the greatest use is a kind of mental, spiritual, and psychic acceleration that allows them to use all of their abilities better—but they must decide how they will use truth.

Ruburt's feelings after his nap involve the material given earlier, primarily on two lives in one, but also are based upon old feelings you are now handling in your pendulum work, that are in the process of being resolved but the strong time elements are strongly involved.

Now, I want hot towels on the knees. And I bid you a fond good evening.
("Thank you very much, Seth."
(10:29 PM.)

DELETED SESSION
MAY 17, 1978 9:42 PM WEDNESDAY

(Jane said that yesterday and today she's known "more profound changes" in her body than she has for many years. These have taken place throughout her system. With some of them has come unsteadiness and disorientation in vision and walking, as new groups release, and so forth. Yet walk she did, at least to some extent. We asked that Seth comment.

(I might add that her bodily changes keep taking place in the rhythms that

Seth has mentioned often. Today, for example, her stomach muscles haven't bothered her at all, as they had so much last Monday, as described in the session then.... Jane said that she thought tonight's session would be a short one.)

Now: another Doctor Seth session.

Ruburt's body has been repressed. Everything was working, but in a very restricted fashion as far as <u>locomotion</u> was concerned. The body was repressed rather than expressed. It was inactive, in that it was operating, but nowhere near a good efficiency level, again, as far as <u>locomotion</u> was concerned.

Your pendulum work, your determination, and the sessions have aroused Ruburt's determination to act physically, rather than to retreat, and your suggestions concerning safety are important. The last page of your pendulum material is excellent.

You might add very briefly to that material, one or two suggestions following what you have—that stress expression: "Do I feel safe to express physical vitality?" Or questions as to whether or not Ruburt and his "subconscious" feel safe enough to progress, generally speaking, into an area of psychic, creative, and physical expression.

Give us a moment.... Other questions before the last page, however, might be, does Ruburt equate being out of condition with modesty, or humility? Does he equate flamboyancy with showing off in a negative fashion, showing that being physically retiring could be construed as a virtue. His body <u>is</u> resilient, and it is responsive, or it would not be reacting so agreeably and definitely to your new suggestions and its activities. The very changes are proof of its powers of recuperation and resiliency.

Certain muscle groups were very tightened, and tended to bunch. This also tightened ligaments, and inhibited joints, affecting of course even other areas. The bunched groups are releasing. Some cause various sensations as released muscles try to catch up. The entire head and neck area was restricted. The body has set up its own rhythms of recovery, since it is now sure that that <u>is</u> what Ruburt wants, and his attitude toward his body has greatly changed for the better.

That rhythm includes some very gradual changes in important areas, so that other portions are not restrained. It also includes accelerations of releases as the time is ripe. Ruburt should not be overly concerned at his locomotion, walking, in any given day. For one thing, his overall increased activity chairwise provides an overall general increase of strength and flexibility. Even when he brings the chair into the bathroom, he must for example get up and down. More, however, on some days he will feel actively like walking, and then he should do so, and even in a day when he does have difficulty, there will almost certainly be some periods when he will feel the same urge. The important thing is not to worry, and also Ruburt's condition now is such that the body <u>seeks</u> more and more activity.

The eyes have annoyed him because the motor activity of the neck is increasing so. With that, however, he has been able to paint and type. Checking with the pendulum, when any possibly annoying events occur, is excellent.

Your pendulum work is at the point where you are lulling fears, and in the process of dissolving them to a normal level. Now you want to begin to encourage through your questions the repressed feelings also of hope, of expression, even of natural flamboyant behavior. Does Ruburt feel safe enough? That is how your questions can run. Ruburt feels safe enough in your lovemaking activities, and that exuberance and response is excellent, so again, make sure that such events become a part of the normal expression of your lives.

(10:07.) Give us a moment.... I want to stress that Ruburt's body is responding remarkably well, and that it is not a matter of operating better in a restricted posture, but a much more significant response, in which the body is, quite simply, straightening itself out. Without that, normal walking would be most difficult. At this rate, it will not be long before the muscular activity makes Ruburt's walking operationally better, for the muscles are incredibly strong and resilient, despite restraints they had been held in.

The ankles were strong enough, despite their poor position. Work on the feet progresses along with the knees, and all of that largely originated from the head/neck area.

Give us a moment.... Ruburt will be relieved, and quite joyous, when he does start up his active writing again. The most important thing, however, is that he trust and follow his impulses. The three-hour period <u>may</u> include painting if he prefers. I simply wanted to make the point that time be allowed for it. The feeling of creative pleasure as he paints, and follows the impulse, relieves his mind, takes it off his body, and automatically regenerates other creative impulses. He will go through several paintings and then tire of the activity, and <u>want</u> to write.

He received excellent ideas the other night, for *Seven*, after painting all day. Desire is important. At times now he will feel conflicts, because he wants to do several things at once. But a month or so ago he did not <u>feel</u> those desires.

His natural desire to write will quickly return full blast when he stops worrying about it. The concentration, again, on ideas, dreams, and suggestions for out-of-bodies will be quite helpful.

The Neuman adventure shows the high activity in Framework 2 for *Oversoul Seven*, but is also an offshoot of your own new feelings of hope regarding Ruburt's situation. That adventure alone is rearousing Ruburt's feelings toward *Seven*, and his anticipated renegotiation of the *Seven* contract is a direct result of your pendulum activity and understandings.

I told you a long time ago that *Seven* would be a movie *(probably at its time of publication in July, 1973).*

I have a suggestion, though you may not be ready to follow it as yet. As you talk to each other in the bedroom before sleep, since you, Joseph, fall asleep so quickly, remind yourselves together that as you sleep you will attract from Framework 2 the very best events in all areas of your lives.

I want to reassure Ruburt in this period that significant areas of recovery are now indeed being accomplished, and he can indeed proceed to normal locomotion if you continue as you are doing.

"*Unknown*" Two will indeed almost immediately bring about an excellent increase of sales of volume 1—and when the two books are out they will give you an excellent additional steady income. Creatively, you have already made certain decisions that you are keeping from yourself, in terms of a book of your own in the future.

(With a wry, quiet look:) I would like Ruburt to soak his knees following the session, and Ruburt wanted me to add that he is most appreciative of your efforts in his behalf. You are each at a turning point, however, of a most beneficial nature.

I bid you then a fond good evening.

("Thank you, Seth.")

I have said all I need to say.

("Okay."

(10:29 PM. For the record: Tuesday last, Alan Neuman called Jane to tell her that he had decided to make a movie of Seven *himself, instead of trying to interest others in doing so. Presumably this means he will try to arrange financing, etc. He told Jane a lot of technical and legal details she didn't very well understand, but he is certainly sincere, she thinks, about* Seven. *He told Jane that he would have some news for her "within a month"—which would be fast service indeed. He stressed that he wanted Jane to have good legal protection, and a say in quality control. Jane told him in her subsequent letter that we are relying upon Prentice-Hall and John Nelson to tell us what to do about legal advice when the time comes, if it does.*

(The next day Jane called Tam, got the info from him as to his screen treatment of Seven, *then relayed the word to Neuman.*

(I think Seth commented on Volume 2 of "Unknown" *because of all the returns Volume 1 is getting these recent weeks, after initially selling very well. I have no ideas at all about doing a book of my own.)*

DELETED SESSION
MAY 22, 1978 9:43 PM MONDAY

(As Jane and I worked with the pendulum on Thursday morning, May 8, I thought of two questions for Seth that we'd never asked him before. 1. Since he is presumably dead by now, what does Dr. Instream think about psychic phenomena? Does he remember Jane, etc? 2. What about the young psychologist we met at Oswego during our visit to see Instream? What does that individual now think about psychic phenomena: Does he remember Jane, etc? Has he heard of her? Why did I get to talking with him in the conference room on campus, then take him to our room, where he proceeded to so upset Jane?

(Last night Jane had a dream she didn't like. She couldn't recall it clearly, but it featured her talking to a man, objecting to him that he'd told her something he'd given her would be painless—but that it was instead quite painful: a suicide pill, or something like that, she said. "You told me it wouldn't hurt..." I was there as a bystander. Jane had agreed to do something that wouldn't hurt, but it did. I asked that Seth comment.

(This morning Jane and I worked with the pendulum on the question of inspiration, and discovered that there was much there to be learned and clarified in her attitudes, and mine too, for that matter. The three pages of questions we devised are on file. We learned among other things that Jane felt she had to hold off on new inspiration while we fulfilled existing commitments—schedules and contracts, etc., and that she wanted to help type "Unknown" Reality, Volume 2, presumably, I thought so that she could get it out of the way so she'd be free to go on to other things. I hadn't anticipated her doing that kind of "work," though. This afternoon she did type on the first session for the book, though, and said she felt much better. We asked that Seth comment on the whole idea of inspiration for her, beyond material he's already given.

(As we waited for the session to begin we got involved in a near-heated discussion of the question of inspiration. The material we covered is indicated in Seth's material immediately following, so there's no need to recap it here.)

An excellent discussion—and quite apropos—for it shows how your working methods differ. It also shows considerable misunderstandings on both of your parts.

Ruburt "works" intuitively. The results appear quickly sometimes effortlessly. He uses a different kind of organization. That organization is holistic, so that it deals with large issues. He begins there, and the details necessary fall into place. You might quite properly say that much "work" is involved, but it is of an interior, concentrated, intent and largely invisible nature. Often only the results show.

When Ruburt becomes consciously aware of those results, then he is inspired. That is, he encounters a fresh flow of new perceptions, or of perceptions suddenly appearing in an original manner, so that he is seized with energy, and has merely <u>then</u> to let the intuitive information flow. That is the way he operates. The same applies—in different degree, now—in his painting.

Inventions often come in the same fashion.

I have given information on this before, but you settled upon the idea of work, as you think of it, because it was the only way at the time that you could justify art to yourself. Naturally, however, your working method is different, and is built up of an intricate series of quite complicated logical judgements involving spatial relationships—in for example particular kinds of immaculate gradations. I am speaking of your painting now.

Ruburt has always rather envied your approach. His, relatively speaking, is a fiery approach. He is quite unaware, consciously, of doing any work for these sessions. He does, of course, for our communications do not just happen, and my voice *(much louder, briefly)* like his, is an inspired one.

Inspiration, however, is not predictable. The fact that these sessions are predictable says much, however, for the longstanding nature of such unpredictable events.

Inspiration, however, in its appearance is spontaneous, and those who possess it have their problems if they want to make such inspiration available to the world. There are those who can go from one spontaneous inspiration happily to another equally spontaneous one, and feel no desire to form any kind of art from it, or to order it along the ways of the world.

You were quick to <u>intuitively understand</u> the nature of such inspiration. You were quick to nourish it. You helped give it form, so you do understand inspiration. It is not a luxury, but the nature that sustains each individual and the world. Ruburt has more than appreciated your support, and in fact you have indeed inspired him, so your conversation earlier upset him considerably.

The world thinks that inspiration is impractical, and you have both made unfortunate distinctions between inspiration and work. You can afford to do so more than Ruburt, since your natural working method falls more easily into that kind of context, where the effort shows in time. Ruburt cannot afford such distinctions.

(10:05.) Give us a moment.... Ruburt has tried to pace himself to you, because it seemed your way was the more practical. He does not think of jobs to be done. The use of the word means one thing to you and one thing to him.

Now let us look at the dream, and also at today's activities. The dream told him that he had agreed to deaden himself to a certain extent, and that he did not think deadening yourself would be painful. He would just slow everything down. He was confronting the part of himself that decided upon the course to which the other part agreed, while you stood by, watching. He discovered that trying to deaden yourself is quite painful.

The dream initiated your pendulum work on inspiration, for to Ruburt to deaden yourself is to deaden inspiration, which to him is the quickness of life. Now he did this because of his ideas of work, and of jobs to be done, and effort.

When he thinks of work in that fashion, then feelings of responsibility, respectability, scorn or criticism emerge, to thicken the picture. He felt that inspiration was providing so much material that it could not be handled in time. He also felt that his inspiration threatened you with more work, which, it seemed to him, was not particularly pleasant for you, since you often spoke about your difficulties in doing the notes, and only lately have you begun to say when you are doing well.

Often my sessions are meant to lead him somewhere, or to stimulate him in certain fashions. Today he felt like acting actively with *"Unknown."* Both of you there have concentrated upon impediments, and suddenly, finally, his desire led him to begin typing the book. He began thinking in terms of what he could do, so that now we see that he is not only physically desiring to do more, and trying it, but also mentally stimulated, and with a new sense of purpose as far as *"Unknown"* is concerned, and a desire reawakened to play with *Seven*.

The body responded rather immediately with further loosening in all areas, and greater circulation and loosening, particularly in the arms and fingers.

The physical situation is a good one. All areas are further releasing, but the inner impetus is far more important.

Take your break.

(10:18—10:36.)

Your desire to know has always inspired Ruburt to go further in his own explorations.

You must free your own rhythms so that they work together smoothly, as indeed they can, for they complement each other. As I have said before, Ruburt can indeed handle details quite well, and is an excellent logical thinker.

You underplay your own intuitional abilities and spontaneity. The lines are not all that finely drawn. You are both coming along quite well now, but yes, you should cut Frank's visits to every other week, for you need to concentrate now upon your own approaches. Many of Frank's ideas are appallingly short-sided, and while you are working with your own beliefs a visit every other week is enough for now—without courting Frank's opinions, as can happen when

Ruburt wants Frank, in conventional terms, to acknowledge improvements that are definitely occurring, but that Frank is too slow to perceive.

Ruburt can use a particular though brief encouragement in the morning immediately upon awakening, but overall the body is responding beautifully. He can perhaps try to walk a bit more now.

Your time concepts are particularly limiting, because they lead you into a particular focus in which you concentrate upon impediments to your desire. This bothers both of you considerably, so that Ruburt in particular will anticipate distractions a week in advance.

I would like you to try something—and give it a reasonable try. Make an effort to alter your focus—just your focus—so that you concentrate upon what you want to do. If you do that, then distractions will seem to minimize almost immediately. Not only will you react to them differently, but the distractions themselves will vanish in a considerable manner. For one thing, your focus will automatically serve as a new point of organization in your own lives, so that you will automatically begin to sidestep many distractions of your own making. Life will indeed automatically seem simpler in that regard.

Your pendulum sessions can go for three-quarters of an hour now at the most, but regularly, and when you are done the two of you should briefly discuss your goals for the day. That individual and combined intent, stated, can be most effective.

Very briefly: Instream is astonished at his own opaqueness in life, and the chances that escaped him. The younger man was, when you met him, afraid himself of schizophrenia, and had a great need to establish his own sanity at the expense of anyone who showed any but the most conventional characteristics.

I believe he is teaching, or taught, in a midwestern university. You approached him because of your own quite conventional feelings, that because he was comparatively young he would be broadminded. You also sought to form a contact with someone more or less a contemporary, who was in the psychological field.

You thought that if the Instream affair did not work out, this might be another point of contact. That desire led you to disregard conflicting feelings, urging you to leave the man alone.

You also thought two opinions were better than one, and you hoped that the man could provide some information about Instream himself, so that you would know better how to deal with him.

That is enough for this evening. Please take the change-of-focus material into consideration, both of you. And I bid you a fine, inspired good evening.

(*"Thank you, Seth."*)

(10:58 PM.)

DELETED SESSION
MAY 24, 1978 9:30 PM WEDNESDAY

Good evening.

("Good evening, Seth.")

Now: the present is the point of power. You make your own reality.

Your civilization has decided upon certain beliefs of a quite contradictory nature, however. Animals know that the present is the point of power, of course. They do not have any other kind of time to contend with in the same way that you do.

I do not want to go into the complicated reasons why your civilization chose such beliefs, but you are everywhere presented with their effects. In your historical times, no civilization has been based upon the precepts I have given you. Children also know that the present is the point of power, and that precept is a biological truth, for the physical body in your terms cannot act in the future or in the past, but only in its contact with the present moment.

We have been involved in a re-educational process from the beginning, then, and wherever you have not succeeded it has been because on those areas you were not able to fully accept those precepts, and apply them effectively. In those areas where you have not been effectively successful, you often <u>seem</u> faced with evidence to the contrary—and that evidence can appear to be quite concrete, because it is of course reinforced daily.

Such evidence can be of small or large measure. For example, it is a statement of fact, my dear Joseph, that when you leave your work on *"Unknown"* you must then spend much time reacquainting yourself with the material, struggling to assimilate material, regaining continuity, and so forth. I know of your trick with the crossword puzzles, so that words later come to your mind at your suggestion. That is also a fact, and you constantly reinforce that fact whenever you have difficulty with puzzles—so that difficulty is most usually turned into an enjoyable challenge, with resulting triumph.

You have an excellent grasp of *"Unknown" Reality*, and of all the material contained therein. You have, however, reinforced the difficulty through accepting it as a fact, and then treating it, of course, as a fact that must be dealt with on its own terms. You do know, however, that your mind can have such material on hand. It can deliver it to you in the same way as your crossword puzzle exercises, but you have not thoroughly understood, in that regard, that the point of power is in the present, and that you do there also create your own reality.

You have often allowed old beliefs to the contrary to inhibit the exercise of your own mental acuity. You can indeed change that, but you must realize it, and want actively to do so. You must stop reinforcing the negative suggestion, and instead when you leave your desk tell yourself that when you return you will pick up your work where you left off easily and naturally.

The same sort of thing appears when Ruburt gives himself poor suggestions. It is highly important now that he add a new emphasis, encouraging relaxation, which brings along with it always greater freedom to move and respond.

Your society teaches that it is almost virtuous to worry. I would not go so far as to say that it is <u>immoral</u> to worry, but worry is a biological impediment. It increases the concentration upon whatever problem is involved, for one thing, and it has a self-hypnotizing effect. Not to worry in your society can seem quite impractical indeed. Yet a refusal to worry as such will often show remarkable results by freeing the creative mechanisms, relaxing the body, and therefore allowing solutions and resolutions to occur naturally. Worrying impedes your reception of Framework 2 activity.

I want Ruburt in particular to take one day at a time. I want him to do the best he can in that day, to refuse to worry about anything. That takes a firm decision. Instead of Star Trek's "I will not kill today," have him substitute "I will not worry today." This is to be followed with a focus toward relaxation. Simply keep relaxation in mind.

(9:57.) Give us a moment.... Overall, you have been doing well. Remember the change in focus I spoke of at our last session. Your intent to put these ideas to work builds an inner psychological support, and the more you act upon the beliefs the more that support grows.

Ruburt's trunk has been in a constant state of change. Both of the suggestions that I gave him this evening will be most helpful if followed, for they will allow the physical processes of healing to continue with less strain.

You have been changing the beliefs of a lifetime, and you are helping others do the same. Such desires and the challenges mean that you <u>are</u> provided with additional energy and support in Framework 2, but you must have the faith that this is so, and that faith will allow you to draw upon it.

This is a brief session, to be followed by Ruburt soaking his knees. What I have said tonight, again, can be most important if you allow yourselves to really let the significance of the words sink in. And above all, remember what I have said in the past about self-approval, for when you allow yourselves to disapprove of yourselves, you automatically darken your day and its accomplishments.

End of session. Three-quarters of an hour is plenty for the pendulum, so that you do not have more to deal with than the "subconscious" can easily handle in one sitting.

A fond good evening.
("Okay."
(10:06 PM.)

DELETED SESSIONS
MAY 29, 1978 9:38 PM MONDAY

(Today Jane did well, walking about the house quite a bit more often than she has been doing lately.

(Before the session we talked about some questions we'd written down for the pendulum work tomorrow morning. They had to do with inspiration, Jane's attitudes toward me as an authority figure, and so forth. This noon she'd made a very revealing remark, to the effect that her being out of condition was of service to me, also. I agreed, of course.

(We hoped Seth would consider some of the questions this evening. In past days Jane's rhythmic alterations between soreness and comfort in various part of her body continued, almost as though on a schedule.)

Good evening.

("Good evening, Seth.")

A talk about attitudes.

In the largest terms you cannot really call attitudes good or bad, though they certainly seem to be one or the other often in your experience. They can be better equated with colors—some dark, some light, but all in all beyond such classifications as morality.

Let us for the moment forget where or how each of you chose certain attitudes. If you did not have some trust in yourselves, some appreciation of your own characteristics, you would not have allowed yourselves to develop and use your abilities at all—or, for that matter, you would not have been able to form a vital long-term relationship with another person.

If you doubted yourselves and feared for the basic goodness of your beings, Ruburt far more than you, then this doubt was still <u>relative</u> and not absolute. By the time you met, however, certain attitudes were already paramount, regardless of your diverse backgrounds.

Though Ruburt was a good-looking young woman, with much vitality, he had no children, and indeed had been determined not to, for writing was the overwhelming interest in his life. He also needed love, however. Though you were in your thirties, you had not married, and your sex life was rather controlled. You both had at that point decided not to concentrate upon family life.

You had furthermore decided, and separately, before you met, to avoid conventional long-term relationships in the world of business. Neither of you wanted conventional jobs, regardless now of any prestige or security they might bring. In that regard you saw yourselves as like spirits. You believed in the importance of developing your own abilities, because those abilities so naturally manifested themselves as strong elements of your personalities.

You both felt that the development of those abilities must be protected, lest the need for financial security lead you into full-time work on a long-term basis. You felt that you must to some extent allow your love for each other to nourish those abilities, and yet not jeopardize them lest it lead you into parenthood.

You felt that you must to some extent at least protect yourselves against your neighbors—who as both of you said often "Would take up all of your time without a qualm"—neighbors or friends who you felt would not understand your goals, however good their intent. You must then jointly protect your time.

I am describing attitudes. Years ago, when it looked—generally speaking, now: I am simplifying—as if you might be swallowed by Artistic, you rebelled and became ill. You made certain readjustments, the sessions began, time went on. You were not selling paintings to any considerable degree. Ruburt knew he would not take a full-time job either. You may sometimes forget now how vehement your joint ideas <u>were</u> in those years, against the ordinary individual's prospect of working eight hours a day, year after year, in the same place, doing the same thing. So Ruburt added the necessity of money to his creative goals, in a strong fashion.

(10:00.) This often stimulated him to new accomplishments. The addition, however, brought with it a new sense of responsibility—not just to make money, but as his writings continued he wanted his creative work to be "responsible" and he began to discover that others, so it seemed, were all too ready to latch upon what he almost considered magical inspirational productions, and to follow them with very literal minds. So then his creative endeavors not only had to bring in money, but they had to be good, moral, responsible, for they were becoming part of a body of work.

The creative abilities, of course, do not think of bodies-of-work. They create out of the joy and natural necessity to do so, and their productions also exist in a realm far too large to be so easily categorized.

Your other attitudes, mentioned earlier, continued, and the more the world seemed to knock at your door, however gently, and the more the mail came, the more convinced you both became that your solitude must be protected. The attitudes mentioned belong to some extent to each of you. That is why, for example, you went along as long as you have with Ruburt's condition. Neither of you liked it. <u>To that extent</u>, Ruburt does speak for both of you *(as Jane said this noon),* and in your own way both of you rewarded him for creative material, and withheld approval for any tendencies that ran counter to those mentioned attitudes.

The same sort of situation operates in millions of families, and the rewards that you gave each other for your creative endeavors were excellent, and worked beautifully. They still do. There is nothing <u>wrong</u> with the other attitudes. You did, however, both for years believe most firmly that your creative endeavors were dependent upon the need for protection from others, the world, from time, and even from any of your own characteristics that did not seem to fit into that overall pattern.

When Ruburt really became worried about becoming pregnant, he simply stopped having his period, and <u>that took care of that</u>.

When, as time progressed, the need for constant decisions to speak here and there, to see thus and so, to do housework or write, <u>or whatever</u>, Ruburt simply began to cut down on the body's availability to action, <u>and he felt that that would take care of that</u>.

You were each for some time relieved. These are patterns of attitudes of long standing, and at different times, as Ruburt improved, and new decisions came to mind, he backtracked, and you largely went along. With the continuation of the physical restraints other problems grew, and Ruburt would become frightened that his body could not indeed heal itself, and you feared the same. The past "failures" seemed indisputable evidence.

I realize your predicament, so do not think I am being unfeeling; and yet, my dear friends, on other levels those <u>failures</u> were considered <u>successes</u>. You finally got it through your heads that something had to be done, and something <u>is</u> being done. In the process, you see, your views of life are changing, and that change is showing that your creative abilities, if expressed, <u>will</u> automatically allow you to express your natures—your <u>natures</u>—and will lead you into your most advantageous way of life.

Before, you did not believe those abilities could protect themselves, but needed you as stern parents to protect them from the world, and even from their own spontaneity.

Take a brief break, and I will continue.

(10:23—10:34.)

Now: Ruburt felt that you were more naturally disposed toward solitude and so forth, discipline, more naturally opposed to distractions than he was.

He felt he responded to people more emotionally, and so he took steps to see that artificial restraints were applied, so to speak, for those tendencies, he felt, could jeopardize not only his own work, but yours. And if that happened, he feared that you might retaliate, either by becoming ill, or by becoming eventually cool to him.

All of this meant he was left with body beliefs, so that he believed his body could not respond normally. Again, the evidence gave seeming confirmation, so that his confidence in his body was lessened. You both used his condition as an excuse for not doing certain things because you believed an excuse was necessary.

Your attitudes of course affect each other, so Ruburt looks to you for your reactions. He is somewhat afraid of mentioning any improvements, for fear either that you will not approve of them, or that you will, and then be disappointed on the following day. Your encouragement of his walking is excellent.

The soreness lately at night will pass, but as he sleeps this week the shoulder blades and rib cage and neck area have all been stretching. The sensations are one thing, and again the bodybuilder has his coach, but if Ruburt awakens sore, with you asleep, he can feel isolated.

In all such cases, some reassurance on your part will greatly help, and often can cut such episodes short. The body beliefs need to be tackled regardless of the attitudes that gave them birth, and your reassurances of his attractiveness are important—for he convinced himself at least to some degree that because of his condition he was not attractive to others.

"It is all right. You are getting better. Any soreness is caused by the body's new activity."

If you remind him of that when the circumstances warrant it, it will be most helpful.

I do not expect either of you to be saints, so certainly do not expect it of yourselves. If you hear Ruburt grunting, et cetera, try to recognize the event, and try to reassure him, when possible. That is important. On the other hand, he should begin to definitely tell you when he is feeling better, when he feels releases, so that that new evidence can begin to more effectively take over from the old.

Let him do his walking or whatever so that he is free to just sit and write before or afterward—you follow me. You are doing well, though, and also any change of routine or pattern in your lives within the general context is good, for you need the variety.

I would like the hot towels applied. End of session, and a fond good evening.

("*Do you want to say something about his dream with Gert Bustin last night?")*

I want the hot towels applied. Tit for tat.

("All right."

(10:55 PM. And guess what? Jane did apply the hot towels to her knees after the session.)

DELETED SESSION
MAY 31, 1978 9:55 PM WEDNESDAY

(For the last several days Jane's arms, shoulders, hands, rib cage, and related parts have bothered her tremendously—more so than ever. Presumably, muscles and ligaments are still stretching, but the process has been very painful for her, making many movements she used to enact very difficult. Her walking has been impaired also by the extreme sensitivity of her upper body. Her stress relieved itself to some degree today as the hours passed, although she was still quite uncomfortable, still unable to walk as much as she had been doing recently. I asked that Seth comment on all of these developments, and why they were so painful for Jane.

(I also wondered when Jane would show some improvement in walking for there's no doubt about it. She's walking considerably less these days than ever before.

(As we waited for the session Jane felt a little better. Even this morning, she said, hadn't been "as bad as yesterday." This morning, we'd asked a series of pendulum questions about material in Monday's session, concerning work, inspiration, protection, and so forth, and obtained some illuminating answers.

(Shortly before the session began, Jane made a remark about her hands feeling better after her nap. For whatever reason, this seemed to trigger an insight on my part. I found it quite difficult to describe to Jane, for I always felt unspoken, unverbalized connotations in the background that, I thought, represented new ideas for both of us. My words made the insight sound more prosaic than it really was, I'm afraid. I tried writing it down so that I could read it to Jane: "Why did the personality adopt a course of action—being out of condition, say—that eventually came to assume such proportions in life that the focus upon it equaled, or even surpassed, the hours spent in the creative actions of writing that the personality said it wanted to do each day above everything else?"

(The above isn't an accurate definition of what the insight was about, and I do think it was a valid one; it may be as good as I could get it in discrete words, I told Jane after I'd read it to her. I was after an understanding on various levels of the fact that Jane had created something that certainly assumed equal billing with her other creative work—that the personality may have been quite aware that this would

happen, and was willing in some sort of terms for the situation to exist for a number of years.

(*Jane only said that the insight, if accurate at all, was depressing, after I'd read it to her.*)

Now: some people who are very wealthy cannot truly enjoy their wealth in their need to protect it.

They imagine that thieves will steal it away. They might wear imitation baubles instead, while leaving their real jewels hidden in a bank vault. The greater their wealth, the more some such people struggle to protect it.

In some cases the individual's money or jewels are not even available to them themselves, but hidden in the bank's deep vaults, behind all kinds of barriers and hidden time locks that must be cared for by bank attendants. Such people do not want publicity, for someone might find their address and rob their valuables—those that remain at home.

Now, <u>to some extent</u>, you and Ruburt felt enough the same way to make the analogy feasible, only Ruburt was the one who constructed the edifice that would protect his own abilities, first of all, and yours as well. Beliefs are the attendants—not strangers at all. With such an edifice, Ruburt can only use his abilities under certain conditions, and he imagines all kinds of impulses, situations, or whatever, that might steal them away, or steal away the <u>time</u> necessary to express them. Just like our millionaire, who everywhere imagines in the most innocent face the gluttonous look of the thief-to-be.

The millionaire checks all of the locks, perhaps, or has the bank president show him the latest security measures that are being taken—and <u>to some degree, now</u>, Ruburt, and you to a lesser degree, have checked Ruburt's security system. Was it secure enough to keep you from accepting invitations, to allow you to avoid distractions, or emotional complications that might arise from any considerable contact with others in, say, "professional terms?" Ruburt built the edifice, but you looked on, for though you disliked the building blocks, say, the symptoms—you thought until very lately that it did serve its purpose very well.

This is a partial answer to your question, voiced earlier. One thing does not depend upon the other in what I am about to say.

You have both built an excellent edifice of a different kind, in Ruburt's books and mine, and in the sessions themselves, an edifice most admirable, and one that is composed of a kind of material that on its own possesses, among other characteristics, automatic self-protective ones. Not trusting that, however, or understanding this, Ruburt constructed a security system of his own, and with the best of misguided intentions.

Unfortunately, the system itself began to impede the very abilities it was meant to protect. Such abilities must have freedom, and insist upon it, and so the security system itself always felt in jeopardy. The body kept insisting that it was being put upon most severely. Our last session should also be read in context with this one.

(10:18.) Now give us a moment.... As given in the last session, the cost of running the security system was finally becoming too great, and at different times strong efforts were made to dispense with it. The old beliefs were still there, however, and between the two of you, at the first hint of "danger" Ruburt hastily put the system back together again.

The dilemma between expression and protection is a paramount one in your world, and people handle it differently. Ruburt began to feel hopeless about his condition, more and more dissatisfied with it, yet no longer certain that he could dispense with it even if he made his mind up to do so. And you often felt the same way.

Your household situation was set up with Ruburt's *im*mobility, relatively speaking, largely uncontested. As it became harder for him to navigate, it became "easier" for him to stay at home. Now you are contesting the issue, and *(in)* doing so, some patterns should become apparent. It takes your time, and his now, to encourage his walking, and if this is in "working hours," both of your old beliefs are directly challenged.

His body's improvement directly challenges those old beliefs, and brings them into the open. I do not want to overstate, but it is as if, for example, the upper portion of his body had been held in a vice. That vice is indeed breaking up. I have largely explained this before, but the position of the arms, trunk, neck, jaw, head, and ribs were all related. The arms were not just shortened, but only worked in certain restricted positions, where they were relatively reliable. All of that is changing, and must for the further release of the walking mechanisms.

Some discomfort is involved, and that discomfort instantly brings up feelings about belief in the body. Ruburt's faith in his body is growing, but each such situation, right now at least, can and should be a new learning process.

You have seldom assured him that one day he would be walking normally, because, of course, you are also caught in the same dilemma. Often in your society you are afraid to hope for the best, because you have been taught so long that misfortune is in one way or another the natural course of events.

In that light, faith or hope seem tricksters. Ruburt in particular, and you also, must understand that he can indeed recover normally, that he can indeed walk normally again—and moreover that normal walking is the body's natural tendency—his body's as well as anyone else's.

You must realize that expression and not repression is the natural complement of creative abilities, and that in freeing his body, in encouraging physical mobility, he also encourages and frees his inspiration, his psychic awareness, and creativity.

(10:35.) Give us a moment.... Your joint determination is very strong, and is working for you. Definitely encourage his walking as you have planned to together. The disorientation leading to lesser walking for a while was simply the body's way of protecting itself during periods of initial imbalances. Enough of that is over, however, and Ruburt is determined enough, now, so that whatever you decide upon can be followed through, though the distances might vary. You will see an overall improvement, however.

The whole area of work, time, inspiration and protection should be explored, and kept in the open, and Ruburt should write some kind of statement that expresses his understanding of the matter thus far, and states his questions. Try to arrange it so that the walking periods still give each of you, say, a certain amount of time between for your creative pursuits. I will have more at our next session. The important thing to remember is that the edifice was created, and can be torn down. Again—Ruburt's body <u>can</u> perform better. End of session, and a fond good evening.

("Okay." 10:43 PM.)

DELETED SESSION
JUNE 3, 1978 9:30 PM SATURDAY

(I told Jane at suppertime tonight that she was having a session this evening. The reasons were obvious, I thought: This morning she'd awakened with her neck, back, and so forth in a very rigid state—so I wanted to know what had happened yesterday, or recently, to bring about this state of affairs when we'd thought we were making at least a modest kind of progress. There had been a number of developments in the past few days, and the session that follows outlines some of those as they apply to Jane's condition, so there's little need to repeat them here.

(We had attempted to find reasons for her rigidity this morning through using the pendulum, with some success, we thought, but as the day passed there was little response physically on Jane's part.

(Through the day Jane herself received periodic insights from Seth about the condition, mostly having to do with her fears that she wasn't walking enough, and not trusting the body to do its own thing in the recovery process. The gist of the impressions seemed to be that she ought to ease off walking while the body recovered

—*a very strange state of affairs, it seems to me, and a situation that has bothered me often before: Why should the body give up certain functions if it's in the process of recovering? I doubt if I for one will ever be able to fully comprehend that kind of reasoning—whether from Seth or anyone else—since I think that as the body —any body—recovers, its range of activities expands correspondingly instead of shrinking. Yet Jane said the material from Seth blamed her panic-stricken attempts to see if she was walking enough each day.*

(Jane asked me not to read any of my original notes to her before the session, since she was trying to get herself in a quiet mood so that she could have a good session.)

Now: I know what I want to say, but sometimes with you two it is difficult to know the best starting place, so we will begin thusly—dealing with yesterday and the details you wanted. No interruptions or questions, for now, if you will.

Now yesterday Ruburt told Frank that he would see him every other week, and he told a white lie to cover the real reason. Frank had brought him flowers. On the same day he called your friend Peg, already wondering if he might have hurt Peg's feelings the week before. He invited Peg and Bill for the evening, but Peg had made other plans. Ruburt felt he must have hurt Peg's feelings, and this made him also feel somewhat abandoned, fearing that the friendship might simply lapse.

Beside this, he received a letter in the mail, reporting the worst kind of nonsense, saying that the correspondent and his wife had heard that I was holding back *"Unknown" 2*, because the information could not be handled by the populace.

The letter re-aroused several states of feeling: time taken for *"Unknown" 2*, for one thing, but also Ruburt was struck by the gullibility of the correspondents, who were saying in effect that <u>they could not lead their lives properly</u> unless Ruburt could deliver the material. The character of such nonsense reminded him of the worst elements of the psychic field.

Now: you worked with the pendulum yesterday. You did not work with the pendulum however regarding those specific events *(since they all took place after our morning pendulum work)*. A good portion of the session will deal with such issues.

When you and Ruburt begin such a program as the pendulum, <u>for example</u>, it is valuable <u>because</u> of your joint initiation of it, and it served several excellent purposes. The best was probably the opening of fluent communication between the two of you, and Ruburt's understanding that you would go full steam ahead to help him recover—his understanding that you did indeed want him to recover. That was highly important.

The pendulum sessions have also served to bring issues out into the open. I watched you both with those sessions, and tried gently to monitor how you handled them. With the best of intentions, you have made a few errors there.

First of all, many of the questions reinforce the idea of fear, for example, or lack of safety, each time they are asked. Am I afraid of the world? Am I afraid of my neighbors? Am I afraid of inspiration, or whatever? Do I trust the world or inspiration or whatever?—but your questions themselves are now loaded with built-in negative suggestions. Besides this, in an odd fashion, they lack a certain specific nature, as I will shortly explain, and there are too many of them by far to be handled at one session. That is, their number precludes any one single clear path, specifically noted. I want to stress the purposes they have served, and their general nature and so forth did help to bring up a variety of important issues. You now have too jumbled a variety of material to effectively handle.

The negative aspect of some of the questions has not helped. I would like to suggest a different approach, and one that would have greatly benefited the situation yesterday, say, and today, had it been used earlier.

(9:52.) Give us a moment.... a long one.... You said yourself I believe once that life contains elements of each other reincarnational existence, and that each day did also. The problems and attitudes that bother Ruburt also appear—one or another of them—in each day. The pendulum can best be used to deal with specific events, with specific attitudes. I want to suggest a different kind of program, that is, a version of what you have, and that will bring better results. I am aware of course of your conversation this morning, and I must state that it is difficult for me to try to explain what is so clear to me, and obviously unperceived by either of you a good deal of the time.

The body is full of sensation. The most pleasurable of bodily sensations prolonged overmuch, or concentrated upon unduly, can appear quite painful. In your latest attempts to remedy the situation, and in your determination to do so, you have ended up concentrating upon the problem, putting it foremost in your minds, searching for the reasons, and giving yourselves no rest.

Ruburt usually has a variety of bodily sensations, often simultaneously: some pleasant and relaxing, while others may be unpleasant. Again, with the best of intentions, the focus of your pendulum sessions has not been of the best lately. And you yourselves felt swamped by so much material. I am aware that often neither of you thinks Ruburt is improving one whit—and of course that is part of the difficulty. It is not the other way around, however it appears to you. Ideally, Ruburt could completely recover with no discomfort. Practically, he is indeed experiencing more discomfort than he needs to.

That is because of the concentration upon the problem, the concentration upon the unpleasant sensations, rather than any pleasant ones, and also because you have indeed determined to settle the problem, and opened up so many issues at once.

Shortly after Ruburt began using the chair, for example, he decided that he would try to walk to the end of the living room. He had you put a pillow on a chair so he could rest there if he did not make it. He felt a sense of accomplishment, and some delight with himself when he walked to the end of the room and back without needing the chair. Spontaneously he began wanting to walk more, and again was quite pleased when he made the circle for the first time.

The next two days his hips were going through considerable changes and it hurt him, so he did not walk nearly as much, and you both became frightened—Ruburt more than you. Following this he instantly decided that he must walk considerably more—at least 3 or 4 times around the circle—and at the last count, once an hour whether or not he felt like it, and particularly when he did not feel like it.

Now walking is obviously good for him, and I have encouraged it. I realize now that I simply cannot expect either of you <u>at this point</u> to trust Ruburt's body to know what it is doing. There are times, according to the changes occurring, when naturally it would not walk, say, for a good part of the day, and often left alone, it might suddenly want to exercise new positions. But you both become frightened, adding to the body's stress further.

So for now I simply suggest that Ruburt walk gently three or four times a day to whatever degree seems natural at the time. Otherwise, my position is this —and here I repeat—because overall changes in position and balance are necessitated in order for normal walking to occur, one portion of the body at this point is not going to right itself so that, for example, Ruburt's arms are suddenly straight while his knees are bent. All portions of the body are stretching. The arms <u>are</u> longer. The legs have straightened. The knees are looser. The neck areas are releasing—but at any given day or period, right now, one or several areas might well be stiff or uncomfortable.

Last week Ruburt's legs again were <u>more or less</u> of equal length. The left leg has straightened further, so now the right side is newly stimulated to stretch some more. Ruburt feels that stretch. The sensation itself is a strange one—quite active rather than passive.

You do not trust that beneficial changes are occurring in the body until you <u>see</u> what you consider are the proper results, particularly in better performance.

The fact is, of course, quite unapparent to you both, that there is better performance, in that the legs are lengthening, the ankles are loosening. They are not becoming tighter. The main fact is, however, that you still do not trust the process, and that you concentrate upon the poorest aspects of physical evidence and therefore continue to perceive it.

(10:25.) I cannot change my stand on that issue, regardless of your opinions of it, the two of you. Everything that I am saying tonight is an effort to minimize Ruburt's discomfort, and to quicken the healing. I am going to suggest a program, and regardless of what you think of it, the two of you, I would like you to try it, and urge you to do so. I do not expect that you will approve of it entirely, but I can assure you that it will be beneficial if you try to place trust in what I am saying.

After breakfast, use the pendulum to insert positive suggestions of a specific nature—not about the world, but psychological supports and directions for the specific day. Such suggestions do direct your focus psychologically.

Do this together. The suggestions should be clear and to the point. Ruburt has two old lists of such suggestions that can be used as a model—and those lists worked well, incidentally, at the time.

Now: instead of dealing with large issues, Ruburt is to write at least a page about his feelings that day, with particular emphasis upon any issues that bother him at all. Over a period of several weeks, for example, he will have dealt with specific incidents and his reactions.

I do not know how you want to handle this, but the two of you should go over that page of feelings together. According to the day, the situation, you may then want to work with the pendulum, considering some specific event or issue from that day—but this need not be a lengthy session at all. With your discussion, perhaps 10 minutes with the pendulum would be sufficient, The pendulum also can be used when any event occurs—again, when specifics apply.

The set of the day in the morning, however, should consist of positive suggestions that automatically reassure the subconscious of its energy, strength, and safety—for those reassurances automatically help alter beliefs that have been built upon countering feelings. That is, you *are* then adding new information upon which the subconscious will then act.

Ruburt's writing down his feelings will assure that not only nothing goes underground, but will take care of current issues as they happen.

(10:40.) Give us a moment.... The physical reasons for Ruburt's eye problems are as I gave them. Psychologically, they began when Ruburt became worried over two issues. He began to feel hopeless when he knew he needed more dental work, and became afraid he could not make it to the office. He looked

too ungainly, he felt, besides, even if he could make it. He also began to worry about helping with *"Unknown"* at that time, and about *Psyche*.

Give us a moment.... Writing things down is excellent for Ruburt in particular, and so again on those days when no specifics events occur, to be included in his notes, then I want him to write down his feelings about 1: inspiration, 2: work, 3: *"Unknown" Reality*, 4: *Psyche*, 5: *Emir*.

It is most likely, however, that those subjects will come up, you see, in any case in his daily writing down of feelings. The writing down allows for the immediate release and expression of feeling that becomes impossible with so many pendulum questions. The pendulum can also be used quite effectively, for only a few moments, but habitually, before bed—the two of you together—with Ruburt suggesting that he will rest comfortably and awaken refreshed in the morning, that he will have a therapeutic sleep.

Give us a moment.... I am aware of the fact, of course, that you both want Ruburt to walk more and better—but you must also not <u>judge</u> his body's walking by usual standards. Allow it a sense of accomplishment as it progresses. It does know when it is ready to try out new positions, when it needs rest—and while I see your concern, do allow it to express some variety there.

The program I have outlined should allow you to take more advantage of Framework 2, but you must both remind yourselves of the good intent of the body, and the power of your own intent. Do not anticipate impediments. I said this before, and you have never really followed through, but if Ruburt would note down whatever feelings of release he has, or whatever improvements he senses, and if you would both recognize those as accomplishments, they would greatly improve in number and quality. You believe that or you don't, but the fact remains.

End of session. Now prepare questions if you want for our next session, but read this one over carefully, first. The only hint I can give you for your benefit is one, again, that I have given you often before: try to imagine Ruburt's complete recovery as a creative endeavor—a creative venture, in which all kinds of inner events occur even before, and way before, the completed picture shows itself.

Again—*Cézanne* did not show in any way on the outside, yet the "work" was largely prepared before the first line was written. You trust the creative process in art. Only in dealing with Ruburt's body do you both become so literal, so determined. It seems you cannot trust the creative abilities' biological translations—but the body is certainly as creative as the mind, in those terms. Whenever the two of you manage to free your creative abilities, and set them to work on the physical situation, you do see some results.

It is as if you have page 5 of a book, and glare at it because the entire manuscript is not there, and fuss and fume at what might happen to prevent the next page being written. End of session.
(*11:05 PM.*)

DELETED SESSION
JUNE 5, 1978 9:32 PM MONDAY

(*This morning, following the suggestions Seth gave in the session Saturday night, Jane and I embarked upon a new program of suggestion through using the pendulum, writing down feelings, and so forth. All material is to be accumulated in a deleted notebook for study. Jane has already written her first page of feelings; among other items, it concerned her feelings about the delays on* Emir, *and her sleeping for a couple of hours this afternoon.*

(*But the whole thing seems like a good plan. and we plan to do the best we can with it. Above all, it appears to be vital that we have faith and confidence that the body knows what it's doing, and that Jane's healing processes continue. It seems that this attitude is the key to everything else. We wanted Seth to comment this evening.*)

Now: a few comments.

I want briefly to explain a few more reasons why I suggested a change of program. There is nothing wrong with asking "Are you afraid of thus and so?" of the pendulum, for example—particularly when specific events are involved, and where action is possible. For example "Am I afraid of the implications in this letter?" and then, according to the reply and circumstances, Ruburt answers the correspondent in a particular fashion, states his feelings, or does not answer at all.

Such incidents serve as important lessons, for in each case Ruburt will be able to see that the fears are unjustified—that a fear is based on anger instead, or that the fear exists but is exaggerated in degree.

In any case feelings are thusly encountered, understood, and acted upon. Practically, you can only react to the world as you encounter it through specific experiences, and you cannot escape it, for it will come to your door. The earlier questions about fear of <u>the world</u>, for example, reinforced <u>to some extent, now</u>, generalized fears, without for example specific incidents connected to them.

I did not mean to suggest that words like "fear" should not be used, but the day should not be begun by reminding the self of generalized fears. Beginning the day with the positive suggestions will, as time progresses, reinforce Ruburt's sense of personal energy and power, and trust of the self. This does indeed insert necessary new countering information, and also allows for the expression of fears—for Ruburt will feel safe enough to express them.

I said I must deal with the situation according to your individual and joint understanding at any given time. In some periods, for example, certain methods will work better than others. It is natural enough in stressful situations to fluctuate, so that when you have been largely in a Framework 1 reference, I often give you advice geared to it, while allowing you avenues out of it into Framework 2. The morning suggestions are Framework 2 openers, so to speak.

Now: in Framework 1 you often use too much force to get what you want. You often ignore imagination, and believe in <u>making</u> things work. You try to force events. That is what Ruburt was trying to do, say, several days ago. Understand that <u>per se</u>, basically, Ruburt has nothing against walking. Not walking well in the past served certain purposes. One was to avoid distractions, as you know—distractions often being things he would otherwise like to do.

Sunday was somewhat of an example of the advantageous way to handle things. He felt the impulse to do the floors with your sweeper *(while I was mowing grass)* and because of our Saturday session he ignored the arm difficulty enough to do the kitchen. That stimulus naturally led him to do the bathroom, and to plan to do the bedroom. For that time, he enjoyed the activity. Several times he felt like walking, and he walked for brief periods three or four times. Sunday is not considered a "workday," however, so it was easier for him to follow through on those impulses. But the body was overall stimulated, enjoyed the activity, and felt accomplishment. His mind was refreshed. He felt somewhat physically competent.

(9:57.) That kind of activity would automatically and naturally stimulate him to further walking. He gets upset and irritated with the chair, because now he <u>is</u> getting around the house more, and realizes that walking would be the natural way to do so—where before he was content to be in one place.

The impulse to do the floors, however, creatively stimulated Framework 2 activity. This is very difficult to explain, so that you avoid contradictions, <u>but in the larger sense</u> (underlined four times) no effort is required.

Now when you believe that much effort is required, and you let go the effort, you can become only more frightened. Ruburt must gradually try to understand that in that larger sense no effort is required.

I remind you often of the behavior of muscles, and so forth, so that you will not be suddenly upset when Ruburt has bad days, or discomfort, because I realize that that has been largely your framework of reference, and it is of no benefit for me to ignore your beliefs in that matter—and what I have said applies. You are dealing with—in a way, now—two separate sets of "facts," and each work, so when you insist upon emphasizing the facts of Framework 1, then there is apt to be soreness as muscles readjust, uncomfortable periods, and rules that must be followed, like walking every hour, or walking at least once a day or face feelings of hopelessness, or whatever.

I do not expect you to suddenly switch all of your orientation in this situation to Framework 2—yet again I have hope *(louder)* of gently enticing you both to take great-enough advantage of Framework 2, so that you have more confidence and experience with its qualities.

Framework 1 always concentrates upon impediments. There is something to be conquered, and force must be used. Early man's identification with the natural world so led him to feel a part of it that he did experience a kind of being-with the universe in a personal manner or context. He did not think of impediments in that manner.

Now Ruburt is a part of the world. Our books are a part of the culture. There are differences in the world, but those differences merge together to form its character. A sense of identification particularly with the natural world lessens any feelings that you would need defenses against it.

Ruburt's body <u>can</u> perform better. There are no impediments to prevent it. His arms can comfortably release themselves, and his trunk, and in perfect rhythm with his legs, knees, and feet. These ideas, <u>accepted</u>, work automatically, though some time in Framework 1 would be involved necessarily; but the releasing ease and the gradual overall improvement would be quite perceivable.

Your pendulum exercises—and again, they were helpful—were still largely Framework 1 references. The pillow pounding was simply meant to allow physical expression that would vary on different days, and would open the body to the idea of the normal exertion of such energy. When you number the number of times, and so forth, then you are dealing with something else, with Framework 1 reasoning. All that can spread over into other activities.

When you do the morning suggestions then, keep Framework 2 in mind, for you are placing your intents there. The writing-down of feelings and any subsequent pendulum follow-through on specific feelings or events allows you to deal with necessary Framework 1 activity.

Ruburt's feelings about his nap: he finally remembered what I told him some time ago—<u>to relax is to let go</u>. Relaxation makes action possible. It is not lax, does not mean laziness. Relaxation allows the body to rest securely in the source of its being, and refreshes the mind and spirit as well.

The feeling, of course, was based on lack of trust. He followed the impulse to nap, but when he did not instantly find a perceivable "good result" afterward, he began to doubt himself again.

I want you to keep Framework 2 in your minds—for that reminder alone can help you understand that your needs are being met in Framework 2, and the physical results will indeed appear. If you do not believe that, then you must deal alone with the set of Framework 1 facts. At the end of a week, say, as you look over Ruburt's feelings, you will find that they do fall in several categories, and then I will discuss those categories.

Remind yourselves of Framework 2 in *all* areas of your lives, particularly that spontaneous psychic experiences, inspirations and insight are readily available.

End of session, unless you have a question.

("I guess not")

I bid you then a fond good evening—and I look forward to your progress.

(10:29 PM. There are several excellent points in the session that we can integrate with the previous one – especially those about using the pendulum to check out specific fears, etc. In larger terms, Seth's admonition to "let go the effort" is very important.

(I've written down a couple of questions for Wednesday's session, and will list them there. They have to do with the way Jane reacts to the world through her mystical nature —something we seldom consider, if ever; and any possible inhibiting factors in her behavior that might have been set up after the psychic business started. I found myself wondering if she wanted to be more active in the world —through tours, speaking, classes, or whatever, but that she'd inhibited such desires because she felt I wasn't interested in them, didn't want to spend the time on them that would be required, etc. I wondered if Jane's sitting on such desires, unexpressed, could have resulted in some of her fears of scorn and criticism, etc.

(Later in the day, Jane said she'd received some very interesting insights—possibly from Seth—about her mystical nature as it reacted to and with our world. She described them to me at the time, but I cannot recall her material clearly enough to note it here. I did suggest that she might write something about it herself, and at least before tomorrow night's session.)

DELETED SESSION
JUNE 7, 1978   10:07 PM WEDNESDAY

(As noted at the end of the last session, I had two questions for Seth:

(1. Does Jane's inherently mystical nature give rise to conflicts with the <u>non</u>-mystical world she finds herself in this time around? She may be so different in basic ways from most of her fellow human beings that conflicts may be almost inevitable—

at least until later in life, when the personality has learned what the situation is and can make adjustments. Jane said that she never thinks of mysticism, herself, yet I think such factors could operate easily enough in our world. My question is based upon the environment and situations she found herself in as she grew—not upon any questions about why she <u>chose</u> such circumstances in this life to begin with.

(2. I found myself wondering if my own attitudes might have strongly influenced Jane's early psychic behavior in ways neither of us suspected—that she may have inhibited certain elements of her abilities because she feared my own ideas about distractions, time, failure, etc. Perhaps, Jane had <u>wanted</u> more physical and psychic activity all along, I thought—more tours, TV, publicity, fame, money, whatever—but all those things she held back on because of my own negative attitudes. I speculated about whether her sitting on such desires, not daring to admit them, say, might have surfaced as fear of scorn and criticism, and so forth. If such factors operated, they'd be the opposite of those we usually hold accountable. I do know that Jane has the abilities to perform all of those activities, and this almost idle realization recently may have triggered the more concrete question.

(Yesterday evening after supper I received two pages of material from my deceased mother—accomplished by my familiar thrilling sensations, similar to my reaction to the Jack Wall data in the dream notebook. I note the event here because Seth comments on it this evening.

(Jane has written down her feelings each day since we began the new program, and we've then discussed them. The system seems to be working very well. We also use the pendulum before bed, with very good results. She hasn't walked a great deal lately, but our emphasis is now on trusting the body's own wisdom as to when it wants to perform, and what it wants to do. We seem to know a new kind of peaceful understanding, at least to some degree. Jane reports a continuing series of physical changes throughout her body—from the legs and ankles to the shoulder blades, elbows, ribs, etc. As Seth remarked, nothing is tightening up.)

Now: the creative abilities deal primarily with Framework 2 orientation.

Man painted, thought, dreamed, sang, and so forth from the beginning. People are creative whether or not their particular kind of creativity happens to fit in with their cultures, and whether or not their creativity can fit into economic contexts.

<u>In a way</u>, then, in certain terms, work as conventionally <u>understood</u>, and creativity, are indeed basically quite different. Creativity is a kind of psychic play, an exploration of reality, and an individual reinterpretation of it, and of the events of Framework 1. The artist might need to know technique and certain methods, and so forth. He may or may not sell his paintings, but the difference between the artist and other people is his or her way of being—a difference in

the style of existence.

In your society, work has many connotations. It usually involves spending a certain amount of time at a job, for which you receive financial payment. Most work involves consecutive thinking, in terms of time. If you do not have a job you are lazy—so that work becomes of course a virtue, as well as, usually, a necessity.

Ruburt's creativity is highly individualistic—and not, however, narrow in scope. As given in some old sessions, certain difficulties began when Ruburt tried to make his creativity fit the conventional work patterns. The creative person often is not wanted at a job, because their creativity by contrast with others' behavior shows the vast difference between what I will now call <u>joyful work</u> and the usual variety.

The paper Ruburt wrote was excellent. He should do a follow-up on it. For some insights in this area I would like to come through his own experience of direct feelings. The entire issue, however, involving both questions, I would like to save for our next session. Hopefully, Ruburt himself will have insights in the meantime that will make my material pertinent.

(10:20.) The creative self, however, is not nearly as specific in nature as Ruburt once thought, when he considered himself a writer only. The attributes of the creative self are those of the personality, so that these attributes cannot be accepted under certain conditions and repressed otherwise, without difficulties resulting.

Ruburt always did realize he was quite different from other people. The initiation of psychic experience deepened that feeling. You both felt he must be very careful. To be creative in Ruburt's particular way, you need a variety of characteristics that will allow you to probe alone into the nature of your own experience, and yet abilities that will also help you relate to the world—and Ruburt has those necessary abilities. He believed, however, that one set was opposed to the other. Therefore, to keep things orderly, one set would have to go. This is very simply put for now.

Your own ideas suited your temperament, but many of them did not particularly suit Ruburt's. Again, I will elaborate on all of this at our next session.

This one will be brief. The pendulum suggestions are, as you supposed, too bulky *(in the morning)*, and Ruburt should reorganize and cut them to some degree. Main points should be the trust of the body—that is paramount—and the expression of the creative spontaneous self <u>in all areas</u> of daily life. You helped him considerably today by reminding him to trust his body.

Drunks often need someone to reassure them, so they will not drink, and your reminders when you think Ruburt has forgotten can be most helpful.

The body itself is further changing, and in the most beneficial of ways, so that reminder is important. The evening suggestions have been shorter and to the point—and to some extent took effect almost immediately. I do, however, want some material from Ruburt before I cover that material myself.

Add to your question, to read before our next session, the implications of private creativity and public distribution of creative work. I will also have something to say about Ruburt's own insights involving the secret aspects of his nature.

(10:35.) Give us a moment.... There are, as Ruburt supposed, learned patterns superimposed upon his basic nature. This is of course natural with each personality. The creative self, however, left alone, and being in a Framework 2 reference, will take all aspects of life into consideration. It lights up all aspects of life. When Ruburt hampers it by trying to make it too specific, and ties it into distorted ideas of work, then divisions occur that need not occur.

Mysticism itself involves, basically, encounters with the art of being—a kind of creativity that in usual terms may produce no product at all, creative or otherwise. Such experiences may be translated into poetry or art or whatever, but initially they involve a spiritual encounter with reality. This encounter promotes a heightened state of creativity, even though, again, a creative product per se may not show.

Ruburt got so he wanted such encounters only if they fell into his ideas of work. I wanted to begin this material this evening. The main point for now that I want to make is that Ruburt does indeed perceive the world differently, and he cannot try to force that vaster kind of perception into the narrow confines of ordinary work ideas.

He is not just being creative when he is writing. He is being as creative when he contemplates the kitchen table in his own fashion, and is enjoying then a state of consciousness that is to some extent uniquely his own. The creative state of mind cannot be shut off and on, yet Ruburt has approached it only as it related to his ideas of work.

I simply wanted to get the material started—get an early start for our next session. Continue your program, and when the suggestions have been pared down into a clearer kind of statement, then Ruburt should indeed—alone this time—read that material after lunch.

End of session, and a fond good evening.

One note: your encounter with your mother was, as you know, quite valid. It was closer on her part to you than on your part. That is, she was more aware of you than you were of her. Speaking to her mentally at times could be quite helpful, particularly during, say, your naptime. End of session.

("Thank you." 10:49 PM. Seth commented on my Stella Butts experience just as I was about to ask him to do so. I'd forgotten to remind Jane about that experience before the start of the session. A copy of the experience can be found in my dream notebook.

(We've already reorganized and condensed the morning suggestions, as Seth recommends our doing in this session, and find that they're now much more effective. Jane has been sleeping well.)

DELETED SESSION
JUNE 12, 1978 9:15 PM MONDAY

(Today we were visited —unannounced—by a young man named Jim Poett, who has been assigned to interview Jane for The Village Voice. *We talked to him for at least a couple of hours. This wasn't an interview: he is to call Jane in a couple of weeks about that procedure, after he's read more of her work. Jane gave him our unlisted phone number. The* Voice *is a New York City newspaper.*

(Numerous questions were raised by the event, of course, but Seth doesn't go into them this evening. Jane and I have started our own list for Wednesday night's session, instead. It can hardly be a coincidence that this "opportunity" materialized shortly after we began our new program suggested by Seth, and what we've learned about our attitudes toward publicity, scorn and criticism, and go forth. Perhaps our handling of the affair will show just where we're at, as they say. No commitments have been made, and I'm anxious that Jane consider whether she even wants the interview, as well as the questions that would then arise, should she answer yes.

(Jim Poett said that we would see the article before it's printed, at our insistence; I'd find it strange indeed to cooperate with a venture that would end up taking us apart in ways we didn't approve of. But Jane says she trusts him, and I'm willing to go along with her feelings on the matter.)

Now: there are gradations, of course, to creativity. Certain important kinds of creativity demand incubation periods, during which the conscious mind cannot follow the inner processes. It goes its own way, concentrated in day-to-day reality, while the inner portions of the self amass great information, perhaps, try out new organizations, and utilize the inner senses. The "results" then emerge to the conscious mind, and you have inspiration, and a creative "product."

Ruburt's creativity not only involves that kind of behavior, but the mystic elements of the personality, meaning that the inner activity is very intense, so that Ruburt learned from a young age to develop a <u>certain kind of</u> secrecy. His poetry was largely mystical poetry, and though he did not dwell upon the fact, he realized that this vast inner reality of his was quite beside the point of living as far as other people were concerned.

To some extent, he tried to emulate their behavior—that is, to behave the way they did, while at the same time he intently pursued a rather adventuresome inner psychic existence. That existence was expressed in the personality, but not in the normal conversation with the boys he dated, or with his friends. In early years, the church did serve as a structure. When he left it, however, he was without such a structure, and when he did discuss such matters with the priests, they often had more pragmatic sexual interests in mind.

He became quite good at expressing this inner life regardless of other circumstances, and the situation at home, and he understood that it was at odds with what was expected. It was the most vital area of his life, so quite on his own he decided that he would forgo motherhood and a conventional family life.

A good deal of the time, he hid his own decisions from himself. His nature is open—basically trustful, and direct in its dealings with the world and others. He began to find, of course, that the world could react quite differently to openness and trust. He has great powers of concentration, as indeed all mystics do, and everything in his environment becomes charged and important.

The strong private nature leads to personal discoveries, and his basically direct way of dealing with the world means that he wants to share those discoveries. He often feels that he needs protection against that same world, for while he shares so much with his fellows. He still feels basically apart from them in important ways.

You shared that kind of feeling to a considerable extent. As contacts with the world are lessened, however, there is little feedback, so that the "dangers" of the world can easily become exaggerated—and little experience is gained in dealing with the far more mundane aspects of such contact.

(9:35.) Give us a moment.... If you recall, Ruburt could chatter quite well, and carry on in a more or less normal manner while brooding deeply about something, and saying nothing. He was bound to publish his work—any kind—but equally determined to protect his private nature. The secretness meant that he could hide his intent from himself for some time. Most people, as I mentioned, experience their contacts with the world through many prepared structures—that of church, community, clubs, professional organizations, family affiliations, academic affiliations—and these frameworks serve automatically to cushion such contact, and in a way, while permitting contact with the world, also blunting it to some extent. In that respect, most individuals do not stand alone, and, in that respect Ruburt feels that except for you he does, and

must meet the world "head-on" when there is such conflict.

Do you want a break?

(9:40. "No, I guess not." Seth asked because the storm that had been threatening for several hours was finally in the process of breaking. We had most of our windows and both doors wide open, but since all seemed rather sheltered from the wind anyhow, I decided to see if we could ride out the storm without shutting up the house.)

He did not want to be put in the position in which he felt he had to put his self-respect on the line. He did not like the public aspects that he <u>felt</u> confronted him. There was no ready fellowship in the psychic field, in which he felt he could take part. At the same time he felt that he should indeed go abroad—out into the public arena, and that he was cowardly for not doing so.

He is quite gifted in dealing with people, however, and in that respect he is a born teacher. To some extent that kind of activity gives his conscious mind something to concentrate upon during creative periods of incubation.

Both of you see the foibles of others rather clearly. Ruburt began to concentrate upon them, however, and also feared that the classes might turn into more public endeavors as they became better known—one of the reasons for dropping them.

His fear of the spontaneous self originally developed simply because that self seemed so different from other people that he tried to keep it within bounds. He tried to tie it to writing alone, which was the closest approximation he could make to creative conventional activity, while still allowing himself expression. His own abilities, again, kept working through all of the frameworks, however, and none of them could content him.

The mystic is primarily concerned with a one-point relationship to the universe. Ruburt used to feel as a child threatened by crowds. He did not like to sit close to others. The two of you maintain a psychic distance from others, even your closest friends. In a way the symptoms are a statement of the distance Ruburt wanted to maintain from public life, because he felt equally that he should go out into the world in a public manner, and "tackle it."

If he were free of fear, it seemed to him, he would do so. Ruburt, however, deals well with individuals, as in class; while preserving his privacy he still extended it. He enjoyed radio, even on your tours, because he spoke from a concealed viewpoint, where his person was concealed. The secret elements of his personality rise up against the public connotations of standing before the crowd. This is not necessarily a fear, say, of performing inadequately, nor a fear of exposure in ordinary terms. It is a distaste for being surrounded by the public emotions.

Ruburt did begin to feel more and more apart from the ordinary world, and both of you concentrated upon that feeling of apartness.

Take your break.

(10:00. Now the storm was going full blast, but we left the house open to the wind, thunder, and lightning. Very refreshing, although I had to ask Seth to repeat a word or phrase every so often because of the noise. Resume in the same manner at 10:12.)

Now: in a way the mystic's goals are eternal—that is, they involve comprehensions sought for whose validity is in important ways independent of historical time, even though the comprehensions may be couched in certain frameworks.

In other periods, for example, there were acceptable frameworks through which mystics expressed themselves, and most cultures have such avenues. In times of transition the old avenues no longer serve. Ruburt has no exterior framework to judge his subjective experience against, for even when he was in the church his experience did not fit the mold.

Your society teaches a basic distrust of the self, but even then from their organizations people look for a sense of approval. While relying upon himself, Ruburt still had no guidelines, and to some extent he felt that he had to rein himself in, to go cautiously, and he began to doubt himself. Even science fiction was not large enough, imaginatively, to contain his abilities, and when those abilities did indeed flower he was afraid he was more of an outcast than ever.

While trusting himself enough to use the abilities—and in a largely uncongenial social atmosphere—he still found it necessary to be highly critical, and not to rely upon the abilities too much, lest he was unknowingly as deluded as many people would certainly say he was. That meant, however, that to some degree he cut himself off from solutions that the abilities themselves could provide.

Give us a moment.... Once again, of course, there were no guides in the exterior world, and the two of you determined to explore the nature of reality to the best of your abilities. You also decided that you must use great caution while you were doing so, in your dealings with the world.

The pendulum suggestions are meant to reinforce the basic trust in the self, and in the self's abilities to handle experience without enforcing artificial armor. Both of you chose to do what you are doing, and accepted your historical period.

Give us a moment.... Ruburt acted as naturally as possible today, reminding himself to be spontaneous. Your natural way of dealing with the world is also one of trust *(to me)*, but you also feel that the world might betray such trust.

True trust, however, is your greatest protection, and you cannot be betrayed, for you will not attract deceivers. It is far better to trust, for you open up Framework 2 so that benefits become available that might otherwise not be—and even if it seems that a trust is betrayed in an individual case, the overall picture will prove to be far different.

I will continue at our next session. And answer any questions that you might have.

("Okay.")

End of session.

("Thank you.")

(10:32 PM. The storm was still in good progress, although weakening a bit. The air was much cooler. We could hear the gutters running full. Softer lightning flashed occasionally down in the valley.)

DELETED SESSION
JUNE 14, 1978 10:10 PM WEDNESDAY

(Tuesday night. Jane wrote her feelings down for the day, as usual. They're on file. We went over them this morning. Their contents are embodied in the two papers that are reproduced below; the first one, from the library, she received before placing a call to The Village Voice; *the second, from Seth, came through after she made that call, and called a few people about visiting us next Friday night.*

(Jane's Tuesday paper on her feelings is evidently a very important one, representing some excellent insights on her part about her repressed impulses, her fears about my reactions to various events, her private nature and public appearances, and related topics. I'd say that to some extent at least its content flows from the proposed interview with a reporter from The Village Voice, *a contact made with the business manager at WELM in town, and so forth—hardly accidental, we think, that these events connected with publicity, her work, etc., come into our awareness at this time. They seem to be like small test cases, meaning that our reactions to them, how we handle them, will show rather clearly where we're at these days, as they say.*

(First, from the library, after we'd done our thing following breakfast today:

("Despite the beliefs and teachings of religion and psychology, impulses are biological and psychic directional signals, meant to nudge the individual toward his/her greatest opportunities for expression and development privately—and also to insure the person's contribution to mass social reality."

("On a biological basis, impulses are like [or can be compared to] emotional instincts; individually tuned, so that ideally *impulses are stimuli toward action—*

that results as a consequence of complicated inner 'unconscious' computations. These computations are made by drawing upon the psyche's innate knowledge of probabilities on a private and mass basis."

("Impulses have a life-serving, life-promoting, creative basis, and possess a spontaneous order—though as we will see, that order *may* not be immediately apparent since the orderly pattern is larger than our conscious span of events."

("The authority of the self has been eroded by religion, science, and psychology itself, so that impulses are equated with anti-social behavior, considered synonymous with it, or with individual expression at the expense of social order."

("It should go without saying that impulses are the basis upon which life rides—and that they represent the overall motivating life force."

(After finishing the library material, Jane called The Village Voice on impulse, but ended up feeling she didn't do well: She didn't get to speak to Jim Poett, who was not there, or to his editor. She asked a friend of JP's to have him send her tear sheets of his last two articles, which I thought an excellent idea. The friend, also a reporter, mentioned the Middle of Silence people to Jane, which she didn't like, although she learned things. Jane also gave the reporter our phone number, which she regretted doing later. I said I thought it better that she did follow the impulse, though, since anything, any action, was probably better than sitting immobile.

(Then Jane received the following material from Seth through writing, which in itself is quite unusual. I was painting, or mowing grass. Either way, here's what she wrote down:

("If you listen to your impulses and keep them clear—each one [in *your* sequence] will clear your path further. You both *did* wonder about the Silence Gallery affair, and decided not to mention it [to Jim Poett]. The *call* [which was action, a creative synthesis of your joint feelings], gave you information you didn't have before—that The Voice [as an entity] knew of the Silence Gallery in a confused way. This means you can mention it and insist that they not be mentioned. It also means that you have additional knowledge to use in making your decision [about the interview]."

("Your impulses work in a *specific* manner, dealing with each individual or event, and based upon information that exists in Framework 2—which may not be consciously available."

("Working with your impulses will *always* get you off dead center. *Some impulses* are cautionary also–and steer you away from potentially troublesome events. Some are urgings *not* to act in specific cases."

("Important steps:

1. Learn to recognize and identify impulses, to separate one from the other.
2. Realize the impulse means something.

3. Sometimes one impulse will automatically lead to <u>another</u> action. Its purpose is to lead you someplace else [beside itself].

4. Impulses are impetuses from Framework 2.

5. Impulses are <u>not</u> disruptive. They <u>are</u> directional signals that clear your path and make it smoother.

6. Some impulses are simply educational, bringing hidden intents to consciousness.

7. <u>Remind</u> yourself that the best possible events are being brought about from Framework 2.

8. Your impulses will automatically provide you with the proper balance of solitude and company, private and public activity, exercise and rest—<u>for you</u>!

(*After supper this evening, Jane had a rather strong reaction, a new determination that had arisen from her encounters with the idea of impulse and inspiration. Making ready for the session, I discovered that she was quite vehemently going over and expressing [to some extent] what she'd learned today. She didn't know whether she'd have a session or not. We talked about it all. She was "agitated, yet half-relaxed," she said more than once. I thought it all a very good sign that some of our new thinking was beginning to take hold. Certainly the events were healthy and positive, compared to our earlier ways of thinking and reacting. I can't describe Jane's reactions too well from the observer's viewpoint, except to approximate them here. Her stomach was queasy, she said, as it sometimes gets when she deals with very personal material that is also very accurate.*

(We sat for the session to see if it would develop after all.)

Now: the new policy of writing down Ruburt's feelings is beginning to pay off, and is leading him to an <u>understanding</u> of the feelings, to a recognition of his impulses. And toward some understanding as to why some impulses have been largely buried in the past, and why others, while recognized, were denied a hearing.

The material on impulses was indeed from me this morning, and in a way that material, coming through as it did, was the result of Ruburt's dawning understanding that his own abilities can indeed help him solve his difficulties when he allows it. The morning material is important, then, and should be appended to the session.

There is something I want to tell both of you, and I hope you can see what I am trying to say. Ruburt does not need to apologize to anyone for his less-than-perfect physical condition, nor feel that his physical lack of mobility—relatively speaking—casts aspersions on the sessions or on our work. Nor need he feel that in contrast to our material his physical performance is woefully inadequate. The wording of that last sentence is important, for obviously his condition is inadequate—but he owes no one an apology in that regard.

Neither of you should feel embarrassed—or, rather, ashamed—of his physical condition either, nor consider it more reprehensible because of our work, than you would consider it otherwise. This entire material is important and vital.

Original thinkers, creative innovators, often have their difficulties with their fellow men, even if their careers are backed up by academic credentials, organizations, or whatever. Again, Ruburt has none of those frameworks. He was also to some extent blighted by those same errors that our material is trying to correct, as each person is to some extent in your world.

His feelings, as stated to you this evening, show a new emotional as well as intellectual insight into the situation.

(10:25.) Give us a moment.... Briefly: Ruburt has always felt the strength of his abilities, even before he recognized consciously the areas into which they would lead him. From many sources—literature, psychology, religion, biography, he felt that creative or artistic people, those highly gifted, were persecuted by others, hunted down, misunderstood, and poorly equipped to deal with the social world. On the other hand, he felt that they were beset by errant impulses, extravagant, destructive behavior, the taking of drugs, overindulgence in alcohol, or even by suicidal tendencies.

Such gifts he felt were quite odd presents indeed from the gods. Those who possessed such gifts knew it at once, but they must walk a cautious path while still allowing the abilities expression and insuring their development. The ideas about the creative personality are erroneous. They <u>seem</u> to be factual only in periods when the goals of a society do not fully include the arts or philosophies in the larger organizational structure of the community.

Be that as it may, Ruburt began to withdraw from the world, and in important ways denied himself the experience of dealing with others in those respects. He is gifted in dealing with people. He has the capabilities that allow him to hold his own very well, blocked only by fears and hesitations. He <u>does</u> have a very strong private nature, along with an ability to communicate to others—and as my material stated this morning, a greater understanding of his impulses would lead to a natural balance. He might not want to see anyone for months, in which case his impulses would be to refuse any interviews or whatever. Then the impulses might change overnight, leading to a more sociable time.

One important issue is to forget "the world," and instead deal with specific instances. The world is made up of individuals. Ruburt's position <u>has</u> been conciliatory, and encouraged protection <u>above</u> expression.

As long as you rely upon Ruburt's physical condition to say "no" for you, then Ruburt is still using it to avoid facing such issues or making decisions in that regard.

(10:41.) Give us a moment.... The material I gave this morning is especially important, and should be studied. The medication *(a stronger aspirin)* is all right for Ruburt. He is using it as an aid. The soreness that he experiences at times is a physical result of mental ideas, generally, that it will hurt to face the world, for example, and this new knowledge of impulses, and of his feelings, should help there.

Give us a moment.... I have never wanted to dwell negatively on what might have happened in terms of probabilities, and have mentioned it very briefly only—but Ruburt's psychic initiation, and your own, represented a breakthrough of the most important kind in this life, and automatically shunted aside, for good, many other serious difficulties that otherwise could have occurred.

That was important privately. But in your own searches you are literally leading millions of people, many who will never write you, and effectively inserting ideas into the society, that will in their time come to flower also.

That challenge was difficult, but offered, and still does offer the opportunity for a kind of personal exploration of reality to which few have access. In certain terms, such new understanding can also bring its own stresses and strains, simply because such individuals must of necessity find themselves ahead of their times, and in a different position than they were in before with their normal accepted reality.

They also of course <u>must</u> to some degree still bear traces of their society's official errors. So do not have Ruburt knock himself too badly, and do not feel hangdog in your attitudes about his condition, when you think of it in relationship to our work. That change in attitude alone can be very beneficial.

All of this information should help accelerate his improvements. It is significant that he has of late felt like standing unsupported, even if only briefly, for this means that he is beginning to sense a point of balance. He should encourage those impulses whenever possible, of standing unaided, even if the time is brief.

(Today, also, Jane walked around the bed—although touching it—on two separate occasions.)

Your own communication with each other is becoming clearer, and can still be improved upon. The other material he received <u>was</u> from the library.

Give us a moment.... Ruburt should not disapprove of <u>himself</u> because of his physical condition either. He can quite rightly disapprove of the condition, however. He should, again, perhaps with your help, now write a new list of his accomplishments, and also of his positive characteristics, so that he keeps self-approval in mind, and your compliments when he does look well are always helpful.

That will be all for the evening, unless you have questions.

("Well, it's certainly no accident that the interview thing with The Village Voice *came along at this time.")*

Of course not.

("Or the radio program hints with WELM.")

You should use both events to learn from them. What you do is not as important as your attitudes toward your decisions. Fears are understandable. They are natural, but it is not natural to be ruled by fears.

End of session, and a fond good evening.

("Thank you.")

(11:01 PM.)

DELETED SESSION
JUNE 21, 1978 10:28 PM WEDNESDAY

(No session was held Monday evening; we worked late instead, and did so on Tuesday night also. Jane did pick up some bits of information from Seth on Monday night, however, and her version of them is attached.

(Questions had begun to accumulate since last Wednesday's session, of course, and I made notes on a few of them. I suppose they could be summarized in the one I wanted Seth to consider above the others. It stemmed from his material in the session for June 5, when he said that "letting go" could have its frightening aspects for Jane, especially when she relied on such actions to improve her physical abilities like walking. Since she hasn't been walking much since we embarked on Seth's new program on June 3, I wondered if her attempts to let go had *resulted in some fear on her part. I wondered about whatever beliefs Jane might carry still, that much effort was required in order to accomplish anything worthwhile in Framework 1, even though we might agree that the help we needed must come from Framework 2.*

(Tonight Jane said she thought she'd "done a damn good job" of keeping her mind off her condition, especially while painting and writing—all the time except when "something hurt quite a bit." I saw her remarks as correlating with my primary question for this evening, since Seth has told us that her feelings of distress at such times result from her mental attitudes as much, or more than, physical circumstances.

(In any event, through our conversation before the session, we felt sure that Seth knew what we'd like him to discuss tonight.)

Now: you are, of course, taught that any meaningful endeavor takes a great amount of effort of a certain kind—the exertion of the will, the utilization of the time in an organized fashion—and this can promote a tooth-gritting determination in some people.

In a sense, to "give up all effort" is almost blasphemous in the light of predominating beliefs to the contrary. Eastern religions are the only ones that even remotely try to approach such a principle, and they do so in highly distorted fashions. Western religion and science promote the ideas of competition, effort, the <u>emphasis</u> upon the will, divorced from the imagination, so that to "give up all effort" can be read as an abdication of responsibility, an indication of laziness and sloth; or in fundamental Christian terms, the devil finds work for idle hands.

In a strange fashion desire promotes action seemingly without effort, or the effort seems so natural, so spontaneous and so joyful that it is not recognized as effort in the old fashion. The great artists did not use their abilities so much through the utilization of will and effort as they did through following their own natural impulses, desires, and intents. These form a true sense of purpose, so that the aspects of the will and the effort fall naturally into place to bring about the desires.

Parts of original Christianity did indeed speak of this "letting go of effort." In a curious fashion, such letting go of effort might well result in an increased abundance of creativity, for example, but the mental and psychological set allows an individual to become more aware of the basic motivations of the personality, that show themselves quite clearly through the impulses, and through desires—particularly when they are not overlain by layers of "I must," "I should," or "I must do <u>this</u> or <u>that</u>." Such thoughts cut down on both impulses and action, by setting up invisible barriers.

For example, Ruburt might think "I must make up my mind, go out into the world, do lectures and tours, state my case, be an excellent example of the material, not only in normal physical condition but in glowing health." or "I must stay at home, hide from the world, keep myself restrained lest I give into images of self-grandeur." Either course, a true letting go of effort, leads to the realization that the impulses of the personality innately know if the self's best paths. <u>And only when someone begins to doubt those impulses and their validity do difficulties arise.</u>

The letting-go of effort should be also a mental and psychological stance applied not only to Ruburt's physical dilemma, but to his—and your—relationships with the subjective and objective worlds. Again, such letting go will indeed always promote action, and get you off dead center, so to speak. This is not a statement of passivity in conventional terms, but a creative releasing of the basic personality from the restraints of hampering beliefs.

Now recently that phrase has been introduced into your suggestions. Because you are so used to the belief in exerting such effort, in the beginning, as I mentioned, some fear can be involved as you begin to let the effort go, while watching to see that you aren't backsliding instead, or being irresponsible. This letting-go happens naturally just before the initiation of any creative endeavor.

Ruburt did experience some fear, but overall has handled it well. I do want to make the point that that state of mind should be applied whenever possible to all areas of your lives. Now physically, the burning sensations are the results of stretching. Often, say, the back areas of the leg will be loose and comfortable while the topside knee portion might be sore. This means that the relaxation of the back muscles and ligaments is allowing new stretching of ligaments connected with the knee, and the condition might be reversed the next day, or in an hour.

The same applies to the arms. The feet are coming along excellently, so that they will be flexible enough as Ruburt walks more—that is, they will be able to manipulate in concert with the changed positions that the legs are now beginning to achieve.

It is true he has not been walking much. And it would take a saint to ignore that fact. The body is making necessary changes, however: the chair activity keeping the knees limber enough while undue strain is not placed upon the body at this time. The change in chairs is excellent, and shows that the hips are changing also. Whether you have noticed or not, he has begun to gain weight again, and there are multitudinous small new motions, particularly in the bathroom, that he is scarcely aware of as yet.

The material he received from me *(Monday evening)* was from me, and his suggestion that you work late that evening was the result of a creative impulse on his part. The material on variety is rather important, and also is connected with the fact that I suggested he forget the work sessions for a while. It is quite effective to read such sessions regularly, then to drop them for a week or so for other material, and go back to them. The unconscious, in its own way, digests the initial material in the interim. In your situation, variations are important, since they exist in an overall stable framework.

The body utilizes both energy and chemicals differently at night. When you are awake for periods of time during those hours, very refreshing conditions exist mentally and physically. You might, in parentheses, put that this is connected with the waking-sleeping patterns prevalent on earth, to which you referred some time ago.

(And about which I've always wanted more information....)

It was natural enough for a while that Ruburt be quite aware of bodily sensation when he tried to "give up all effort," but he is beginning now to sense the body's pattern of activity, its relaxation, its stretching periods, and so forth. One important point: he gobbles experience, emphasizes it, studies it—and that quality also means that his bodily sensations are treated in the same manner. That is why the concentration upon the moment, upon his writing, upon, say, meals, immediately helps to take his mind off of his body. Remember desire in terms of Ruburt's <u>wanting</u> to vacuum a rug, or whatever, and encourage those desires rather than an attitude of "I must do something physical today."

The letting go of effort will indeed more and more release such desires. Ruburt has to a considerable extent largely disposed of the habit of negative projections, though he still catches some now and then. Except for the point of power, he has not actively promoted his desire to walk normally, and this was <u>relatively</u> wise, for as he begins to let go of effort he was not tempted to think of contradictions, as he might have had he more actively encouraged those desires.

So now we come to imagination and desire. When these are utilized properly you do not need effort, for effort becomes effortless. It is and it is not. When Ruburt feels he understands this, without taking any special time, let him think of using desire and imagination together, purposefully <u>disconnecting</u> them for this exercise from willpower or effort, and seeing himself shopping with you in a store, or walking a beach in Florida, or anything else that automatically comes to mind.

Now the will can be used, but when there are divisions then the impulses and imagination should be released in such a fashion, and they will then mobilize the will, in such a way that action is united.

Do you have questions? I tried to cover the most important points.

("I guess not.")

The session should be read carefully, and the sessions given to trust of the body emphasized, now, instead of, say, the work sessions—again for now.

I add a humorous note: the north-south orientation of the bed does have advantages. End of session, and a fond good evening.

("Thank you."

(11:20 PM.)

JANE'S NOTES
JUNE 19, 1978 PM MONDAY

(*Out on the porch tonight off and on I kept getting stuff from Seth but so normally and smoothly that only something Rob said later made me remember. I decided to read* Seven *tonight instead of having a session. Rob said, "You must want a break in the routine-" and his remark brought Seth's material back, though now I know I don't remember it all. These are the main points:*

1. *The body likes extremes now and then. Any changes in routine for me are good.*

2. *I did get fleabites Friday from the Blumenthal's dogs and the body used the situation to accelerate the… natural immunization? processes… anyhow, to hasten healing process.*

3. *Many physical conditions have an allergic connection—the person "allergic" to certain portions of the self— so that kind of stress can be overall quite beneficial.*

4. *Some humorous remarks about changing bed to north-south position.*

5. *Drop work sessions for a <u>while</u> – read once or twice a week.*

DELETED SESSION
JUNE 28, 1978 8:50 PM WEDNESDAY

(*No session was held Monday night.*

(*Much has taken place since then. Jane has withdrawn* Emir *from consideration at Prentice-Hall, and in back of that decision lies a story too complicated to recite in detail here. Tam's letter of today catalyzed her action, however, when he told her that Prentice-Hall had decided to publish* Emir *through the children's department. Jane feared the book, which she regards as the beginning of* Oversoul Seven, *would be lost in a tiny printing. The advance would also be very low.*

(*Jane relied on her impulses and Framework 2 for her decision—actions that she would have probably found very difficult to carry out earlier. "I still can't believe I called up a publisher and told them to send back a book they wanted to publish," she said more than once. "You can't say I wasn't spontaneous," she added, "or that I was cowardly or wishy-washy…." Actually, a string of events, evidently out of Framework 2, were involved, and would make a most interesting study of how Framework 2 aids one in making decisions or bringing about events they want to see happen.* Oversoul Seven *is also involved in some fashion, especially the movie aspects*

—*for when Jane called Eleanor Friede to offer her* Emir, *Eleanor told Jane she was about to call <u>her</u> about* Seven, *the call having to do with possible motion picture connotations, through a well-known screenwriter; that is the kind of event intertwined with the whole affair; nor have Jane and Eleanor contacted each other for probably a couple of years.*

(All in all, the whole affair is proving to be quite instructive in a number of ways. Eleanor is to see Emir *for possible purchase. Jane's ability to deal with others is obviously better. Her physical condition continues to show beneficial changes. I don't think it any coincidence that Jane contacted Eleanor, who is the editor for Dick Bach, who is a counterpart of Jane's. [Jane first called Pat Golbitz, but Pat was out of her office—so Pat doesn't get to see* Emir *first.]*

(More developments took place today, before I began typing this session. Tam called Jane to inform her that Eleanor called John Nelson [which Jane already knew] —but that Eleanor and her screenwriter friend had the money to do a movie for Seven. *So we'll see what develops in this continuing saga. Clare Townsend of 20th Century-Fox called Tam today and asked about seeing the manuscript of Jane's second* Oversoul Seven *book, which Jane has just begun typing. Townsend is involved with Alan Neuman, of course, who also wants to do a movie of the first* Seven *book, etc. A chart made of all the events to date would show an interlocking pattern of lines, I believe, like a spider's web. Hardly a "coincidence" that it all begins to develop at relatively the same time.)*

Now: I would like to clear up a few misconceptions.

Ruburt is not an extremist—nor, on the whole, is he given to extremes. He has at times taken some <u>comparatively</u> extreme measures, and they were taken to some degree because he felt he could be an extremist.

His early background was <u>relatively</u> different: an invalid mother, no father, on welfare, et cetera, so his environment alone to some extent placed him in a different light in the eyes of his contemporaries. Added to this, from the beginning he did indeed –relatively, now— stand out. His unusual vitality, abilities, and intelligence were apparent, but they were not conventional abilities. The ability alone did not win friends and influence people.

Ruburt's intelligence was not one to follow blindly, and so his marks were not outstanding. Even in school, both religion and science teachers found him troublesome in that regard. Writing poetry is hardly extremist behavior. Neither did the circumstances surrounding his college dismissal come about as the result of any extremist behavior.

By then, however, Ruburt began to fear that he was headed for trouble— that he was too impetuous, headstrong and impulsive. Leaving Walt for you on a moment's notice, so to speak, was not extremist behavior either, for he had spent three years in that relationship, and gave it indeed all the trial period it deserved. And though he loved you, he did not "plunge" into marriage with you either. In not wanting children, a good amount of discipline was used by both of you—the kind of discipline that simply would not be possible for people "driven" by impulsive desires. Ruburt finally did put an end to his menstrual cycles a good deal earlier than might have happened otherwise. It is easy enough to say that that was extreme, but many women have hysterectomies for the same purpose.

You are both apt to say that Ruburt goes to extremes, and several times I used the word myself, and Ruburt never forgot it—but I did not use it with the same implications that it carries for him. A sense of purpose steadily applied, the continuity of feeling and work, the steady application over a period of years, these are not the marks of an extremist.

I want to make these points because Ruburt's physical condition in part was the result of his feelings that left alone, in good condition, he might resort to "extreme behavior."

Now, what would that extreme behavior consist of "at its worst?" He felt that if he were a person given to extremes, then to use his abilities he must apply due discipline so that his head was not turned, so that he did not become a victim of fame, as many other writers and artists did—or so it seemed. It certainly should be obvious to Ruburt now that his personality contains some quite conservative aspects—a marriage going into two decades and more does not exactly make one worry about promiscuity. So many old fears were based upon misconceptions on the part of the personality that in younger years found itself to be quite different than its contemporaries, and gradually began to set up defenses against them.

When the psychic development began, Ruburt was triumphant, for his abilities were flowering, and intuitively he sensed that direction, but the part of him that also dealt with the world was somewhat appalled, for again, such behavior was not conventional, and it was not particularly "the way to make friends and influence people."

He wrote poetry as a child because he is a poet. He never consciously asked himself why he did something for which there was so little practical reward in the childish world. As he grew older it did put him in the papers, as he won poetry awards, but it was not a thing that others understood.

In the past, Ruburt didn't realize fully that his nature was both flamboyant and conservative—that his nature was protected by a natural inner caution that would make the path for his flamboyancy clear. He did not need disciplinary methods that led to physical restrictions of the body.

(9:15.) Now. Give us a moment.... Ruburt is definitely building up a good and dependable sense of trust with the body, and under conditions that were admittedly not of the best. Your own attitude has been excellent—I congratulate you on it, and I congratulate Ruburt on the mental changes of attitude that he is now in the process of setting up.

This is particularly important since the body itself is now working with improvements involving the relationships of motion between its various parts, and the quickening of nerve impulses connected with motion. I am aware that much of that <u>does not show</u> as yet. Ruburt's balance, however, while standing, has definitely improved. The body has gone through several complete processes of late, and as these occur each time the discomfort has been less, and of less duration.

The feelings of trust are definitely taking hold. There will be no problem with the walking, and in a short time these complete processes will be at a point where he will consistently want to do more walking on a day-by-day basis. Thus far, his impulses have been correct, and <u>forcing</u> the walking at certain times would not be advantageous.

The alterations of sleep patterns are also of benefit.

The business decision today is in its way an example not only of Framework 2, but of Ruburt's growing trust in himself, and in his willingness to act on his own behalf.

Your own attitudes, however, have changed more than you realize, and the inner changes in Ruburt's body will begin to show themselves in <u>exterior</u> improvements in performance. Ruburt knows he stands easier in the bathroom, for example, but did not realize that was significant.

The soreness that he does experience sometimes at night is of less intensity than before, and it happens when the body is in the middle of one of those overall processes, so that a large number of muscles and joints are being exercised at one time.

The personality is always pleased with its abilities. If those abilities are extraordinary, or if they do not fit into the social structure, a personality can approve <u>and</u> disapprove, use the abilities, and yet feel the need for protection. I want to erase, however, any ideas that either of you might have that Ruburt is an extremist. He is far too tolerant, for one thing. Extraordinary ability may seem extreme behavior when compared to the mundane lives of many people. A mountain-climber is not necessarily an extremist; an extremist goes from one kind of extreme behavior to another.

I do want you to find the sessions on self-approval, and to read them—both of you.

Do you have questions?

(I asked Seth for his interpretation of my dream on Sunday morning, June 25, in which I was highly upset to see my father careening backward in a truck, down Pinnacle Road. A copy of Seth's comments is attached to the dream.)

Ruburt's interpretation was correct.

("At the moment I don't remember the interpretation.")

He interpreted it thusly. It was a statement of fear, and fear's resolution. Your father was the symbol of yourself. You were afraid that you were doing everything backward—specifically with *"Unknown" Reality*, and that the affair would be a disaster—or the car would crash.

Mixed into this were feelings about your age, and that you were spending too much time on the project. Instead, you discover the car does not crash—and not only that, but your father is much more vigorous at the end of the dream than he was in the beginning. You still had not quite recovered from your fear, however. Your father was used as the main character, of course, because he is referred to in your notes, because you planned photographs of him in the beginning, and because in the dream he represented the disapproving portions of your own personality.

The dream was meant to do two things: point out the fears that were still present, and to show you that though present, they were groundless. The car, which was the vehicle of expression, would not crash. It was not going backward. The backward motion referred to time, and how much time you felt existed between the book's dictation and the delivery of Volume 2.

Now *(humorously)*, I am here, more or less in a recording or in the original, whenever you want me—but I do want to reassure you both that you are indeed doing well.

End of session, unless you have further questions.

("Well, I was going to ask why we're getting all those returns on Volume 1.")

Tam's answer is generally a good one. Many people rushed out to buy the book at once, and are impatiently awaiting Volume 2. Many booksellers ordered *"Unknown"*, sold many copies, and then returned large numbers. Reasoning that when the second volume came out, they would reorder and have both together.

A second-volume book can often work in such a way. But Volume 1 will do excellently as soon as Volume 2 is in the offing. And before that there will be other spurts, as those people who are now reading the earlier books will begin to look for Volume 1. There is a lag there.

("What do you think of Prentice's reaction to the Emir *thing?")*

I am letting Ruburt handle that for his own experience—not that I do not tip the scales now and then at other levels.

("Okay.")

Now I bid you a fond good evening. And feel free with the sessions. If you want to write, and it happens to be a session night, as far as I am concerned there is no difference. Your Wednesdays or Saturdays are meaningless to me.

End of session—and a fine good evening.

("Thank you. Seth,"

(9:45 PM. Jane started the session a little earlier just because things worked out that way—hence the earlier ending. The activity on the telephone excited her—a good reaction all the way, I thought. I also thought Seth's description of the bodily changes taking place very good, and hopeful besides. This is just the way she's been reacting lately.)

DELETED SESSION
JULY 3, 1978 9:35 PM MONDAY

(On two occasions within the last week—Saturday and Sunday—Jane walked for the first time in at least a year. She took a few steps without the aid of her table or chair each time—very encouraging progress for her, and fitting in with what Seth has had to say recently about her coming spontaneous urges to begin walking again. Almost each day we reread some of the late sessions doing with letting go, trust of the body and impulses, and similar concepts; they have been a great help. The last session is particularly good in that respect, dealing as it does with the stages of the healing process, the gradual lessening of discomfort each time such a bodily process takes place, etc.

(Before the session Jane said she thought Seth might discuss some of the ideas in a book by Fred Hoyle, the English astronomer that she's reading, on the ten different universes of man. To our considerable surprise, much in the essays has turned out to be not what one might expect, and Jane disagrees with a number of points therein. She's found Hoyle to be, in an odd way, more "unimaginative" than she expected, and strangely idiosyncratic and even dogmatic.

(I mentioned that it would be interesting to get from Seth sometime information about the counterpart—families of consciousness concepts as pertaining to other than human creatures. Seth hasn't gone into the ideas as related to insects, say, or birds or the animals—or viruses or bacteria, for that matter—at all, and I'm sure there is a wealth of fascinating information there. I came up with the question the other day, also, because I'm working with his counterpart material for Section 6 in Volume 2 of "Unknown" Reality.*)*

Now: your scientists, endlessly it seems, pursue particles, theorizing about them, so that you have particles with certain kinds of characteristics, propensities, and leanings.

They "unite" to form, of course, the larger particles in the physical world. These particles are invisible to the human eye, and do not appear in the mundane affairs of daily life—that is, you do not meet a quark on the corner *(with amusement)* and say "Hello, how are you, state your name and business." You are familiar then with the idea that matter is composed of a conglomeration of particles that reach seemingly infinitely "beneath" the physical stuff of the world. *(Rob: re particles & elements, created without end, distortive instruments, etc.—see session 19, January 27, 1964. Excellent.)*

The varieties of consciousness—the inner "psychological particles," the psychic equivalent, say, of the atom or molecule, or proton, neutron or quark—these nonphysical, charmed, strange forms of consciousness that make experience go up or down *(all with amusement)*, and around and around, are never of course dealt with.

If physical form is made up of such multitudinous, invisible particles, how much more highly organized must be the inner components of consciousness, without whose perceptions matter itself would be meaningless. The alliances of consciousness, then, are far more vast than those of particles in any form.

The atom, the molecule, the proton and neutron, the electrons, the quarks and other families of particles represent aspects of consciousness itself, which man then projects into the world of physics.

I have mentioned counterparts in a very gentle fashion, and families of consciousness, as these are related to mankind. These are the "largest" psychological particles in the terms of our discussion. The problem is, again, that while you <u>are</u> focused in the world of matter, you are allied with only one aspect of your entire consciousness. <u>In a way</u>, you perceive your consciousness almost as you perceive the smooth surface of the coffee table *(indicated)*. You even relate to your consciousness in an objective fashion.

Many people feel that they have a consciousness in the way that they have a car. You perceive events in the same fashion, almost surface-wise. There are particles that move faster than light. There are portions of your consciousness that move faster than light also—but while you conceive of your consciousnesses as a kind of psychological particle, then your experience of it becomes limited to the world of matter in which you believe it must exist.

(9:56.) In a strange fashion, of course, the word "invisibility" only has meaning in your kind of world. There is no such thing as true psychological invisibility, and basically consciousness can perceive without light in physical terms. Matter seems composed of mosaics of particles, interacting in electromagnetic fields, but the mosaics of consciousness interrelate in ways almost impossible to verbally describe.

The physical world is dependent upon the relationship of everything from electrons to molecules, to mountains and oceans, from cultural organizations to private dreams, and in the scheme of reality these are all interwoven with exquisite order, spontaneity, and a logic beyond any with which you are familiar.

The counterpart idea is merely a small attempt to hint at that interrelationship—an interrelationship of course that includes all species and forms of life. Ruburt's idea of the four-fronted self is also an attempt to hint at that complexity in human terms.

The so-called laws of cause and effect operate at <u>a certain level of consciousness</u>. The level of consciousness itself creates the experience of cause and effect. Other portions of your consciousness are quite actively, vitally engaged at other levels, yet there is no division between you and them. There seems to be only because of the beliefs that cause you to limit perception. Those beliefs, of course, include the experience of time as a steady progression from past to future. Time, in those terms, is simply part of another kind of event.

You do not simply have, say, one past self, or one future self, but many—for your consciousness <u>shoots out</u>, so to speak, in all directions "faster than the speed of light."

The consciousness of all species interact in that fashion also, as do of course the consciousnesses within atoms. Such communication takes place constantly, and for men and animals it is particularly apt to in the dream state. The organization of the world would not exist otherwise, in any terms. Basically, then, your consciousness and your perceptions operate faster than light. For that matter, this of course applies to many important communication systems within the body itself, and to the constant alteration of cellular tissue and genetic material that would never be perceived through physical means.

For that matter, the consciousness that you recognize and call your own is the result of this faster-than-light capacity for communication that is a natural attribute that is the main source of your being. Energy is constantly sent into the physical universe through such means.

(10:10.) Give us a moment.... I see that our friend walked unaided. The impulse to do so, of course, is always present. He is beginning to trust the source of his being. Further changes are indeed happening, as I said they would. There is direct and instant contact between yourselves and the source of your being. There is an intimate relationship between you and that portion of the universe that spawned you—that divine particle of consciousness *(softly, amused)* that constantly grows into your being that grows into what you are.

You should understand that we have been talking about Framework 1 and Framework 2. Ruburt felt, and so did you to some extent, that it was easier to experience Framework 2's spontaneity in the mental realm of imagination—but you each felt that the physical body was tied somewhat more rigidly to the dictums of Framework 1, to cause and effect. In that area Ruburt found it difficult to free himself.

A thought, in those terms now, is as physical as a foot—and a foot is as mystical as a thought. The physical body must be born and die. Within that experience, however, there is full freedom, and regardless of any ideas Ruburt might have had, the body <u>can</u> right itself in a moment—regardless of how long, in your terms, it has been in difficulty. That is why I have stressed the importance of impulse, and Framework 2's activity, for there you are not confined to cause and effect.

Ruburt is progressing well with his psychological experience, and that is allowing the body's continued release.

He should have a taste of a higher level of consciousness again, which further lifts him out of the cause-and-effect sequence. Some dreams he has forgotten have already begun to acquaint him with new developments. Change in sleep patterns are beneficial also, because quite without knowing it you automatically tune your consciousness to the time of day, relating to it in a certain fashion, and the night work offers a releasing pattern, an alternating current almost.

I will have more to say, broadening the concepts of counterparts, though most probably in a different way than you might have supposed.

End of session, unless you have a question.

(I took a long pause while I tried to recall a couple of questions that I knew I wanted to ask, but couldn't recall. Actually, Jane had originated them, and I'd asked her to write them down – which neither of us had remembered to do. Very vexing.

("I guess not." I finally told Seth. "I had a couple in mind, but I can't come up with them.")

A hearty good evening—and congratulations to our friend.

("Thank you."

(10:26 P.M. "I got such good information through," Jane said, "that I thought the session lasted much longer—I felt way out, as though I was transcending time, like I was tuning in to a nugget of information that seemed endless. That was a great feeling....")

DELETED SESSION
JULY 5, 1978 9:52 PM WEDNESDAY

(We had two questions for Seth, since we're trying to get into the habit of writing such down as they occur to us: 1. Jane wanted Seth to comment on why he'll take off on something she's read, and reinterpret it his own way, or carry it further; her question came up because he did this Monday while she's reading Fred Hoyle's book, Ten Faces of The Universe; 2. Jane wanted Seth to give information on her "significant" dream of last Saturday morning, July 1. She couldn't remember any details from it, but has talked about it often; she thinks it had something to do with health.)

Now: Ruburt feels a strangeness in the air this evening.

Several important projects are clicking together in Framework 2, and Ruburt feels as if some dimensions in space-time are warped. The effect of events in Framework 2 is constant, but there are moments in your terms of particular acceleration, where "work" done there seems to quiver the edges of your reality in Framework 1. This is such a time.

This is particularly true in terms of Ruburt's physical condition. His dream did inform him of that, but this also means that the mental conditions of limitation are being released enough so that other areas of your experience are now ready to come together in newer fashions.

It is very difficult to try to explain the nature of any event, or the ways in which any given specific mental attitude can release or inhibit the expression of any given series of events. Probabilities do not operate alone, isolated, but largely in terms of conglomerations, so that, say, like does attract like.

In your cases, changes of attitude have begun to alter Framework 2, so that a corner is turned. In other terms, this can be likened to the discovery of a new world or land that has existed, of course, but whose existence was unsuspected. It has still to be explored. So those kinds of changes are in the air, so that many of the connections you have made in many areas will click together in another fashion, more beneficially, and more purposefully.

Ruburt's standing and walking seemed to happen suddenly. The inner work had been going on. He will of course have other and more extensive such experiences, but overall the mental work is now beginning to be strong enough in your framework, so that more and more results, in your terms, will show themselves.

Ruburt has been remembering the idea of effortlessness, and that is all-important.

Those changes automatically, again, and quite effortlessly, reach out into those other areas of your lives, for fear does not then hold back beneficial developments.

I have a suggestion. It cannot harm either of you to try it, and it is this: try to take it for granted that distractions have a meaning in Framework 2 that is not as yet obvious in Framework 1. Oftentimes events that seem distracting, annoying, or that happen out of context, actually are parts of other patterns, larger ones that are part of Framework 2 activity. I gave you one example that you understood clearly, when I spoke about the individual who wanted to catch a plane. All of his plans went wrong. His efforts seemed to be challenged at every turn. He was beset by difficulties. He missed his plane—the plane crashed.

If he <u>knew</u> later of the plane's fate, he thought "How lucky for me that my plans were thwarted." If he never learned of the crash, he might think that he was simply beset by distractions, and that his efforts went nowhere. The same thing can happen, however, where no crashes or disasters are involved, and no dangers are implied, but where events that do not fit into your implied pattern intrude into it.

Each such event, again, is indeed connected with <u>your own</u> overall intents, and may be working toward them, but in a way that appears disruptive. An encounter, for example, that is a nuisance today may suddenly spark a new insight tomorrow, or appear in your own work in an entirely different form that you do not recognize, simply because you are not used to looking at such distractions in this kind of creative light.

(10:14.) The benefits of such distractions do indeed, I admit, seem quite invisible to you, and in your joint experiences they often appear simply as nuisances. Therefore, you are hardly ever able to follow them through so that you can connect any particular insight or auspicious event with the "originating" distraction. I can quite honestly compare such distractions with, say, the distracting thought that might take you from a familiar train of thought into another new mental territory. The distracting elements are exaggerated, however, because of your joint misunderstandings on the subject. The visitors, for example, are not numerous. In many cases, however, the contact alone opens up different aspects of your own consciousness in response. It is almost as if you were able to look at our material from your own viewpoint, and yet at other levels to perceive it from your visitors' viewpoints. That adds to the richness of the material, for you bring to the sessions not only your own experience, but the sensed experience of others.

You must understand that I am not telling you not to limit visitors. I am telling you that creativity often parades under the guise of disruption—and the word is "parades."

Ruburt read Hoyle, and Ed Young called *(this evening)*. Ruburt felt the call was disruptive, though he likes our friend. Ruburt's concentration so briefly upon Hoyle's book was picked up by Ed Young, and Ruburt's opinion of Hoyle's world was picked up by Ed Young, who has the same opinion of the scientific establishment. There are endless points of organization, intent, and interest that unite events. Many of your distracting events have uniting qualities that escape your joint notice.

The ramifications of Framework 2's activity of course require great reorientation on your part, and necessitate a changed view of daily events. In that view, it will be seen that all events work toward your purposes—<u>when you realize</u> that they do. Otherwise you run into the old problem of contradictions, and if you believe that distractions are simply that—distractions—in competition with your work, then they will certainly seem to be in your experience.

With a changed attitude, however, you will be able to follow those distractions' "transformations"—that is, you will be able to glimpse how this distraction ends up in that insight, or how that distraction actually initiated a beneficial event, when in the past, everything seemed unrelated. Events fit into each other. They are composed of a psychological thickness.

(10.30.) I hope to give you more sessions on the nature of events, in a package, so to speak, though Ruburt will have to be at his best since the concepts are so difficult verbally.

Give us a moment.... The simple event of Ruburt reading Hoyle's book: Ruburt began reading certain ideas with which he is not yet consciously familiar. Some of those ideas, however, were picked up in California. My last session was in a way—<u>in a way</u>—the result of Ruburt's begrudging decision to "take time out to read the book." It got his attention. I am aware of his emotional ideas, of course, and to an important degree I am free of his prejudices, but more than that, <u>in certain terms</u>, my consciousness is not limited, so that I can take from Ruburt's understanding his good comprehension of where science is, and then tell you where an enlightened science might go.

More important, I can tell you that atoms, for example, are primarily consciousness. Objects are the result of a specialized perception. I can perceive your objects as objects, or not—but the true nature of reality must come from a study of consciousness.

End of session, unless you have questions.

("I guess not.")

And I have plans of my own—through the years *(whispering)*—so that all the material will be produced that will be of most benefit—with your willing help. A hearty good evening.

("Thank you. The same to you.")

(10.40 PM. I would imagine that Seth made his last remark because Jane and I were speculating about the fate of the material after our deaths – getting a literary executor, etc.)

DELETED SESSION
JULY 12, 1978 9:28 PM WEDNESDAY

(No session was held Monday evening, since Jane was enjoying a very beneficial relaxation.

(Last Wednesday, July 5, we mailed Emir *to Eleanor Friede at Delacorte. This morning Eleanor called Jane to say that she "loved it," and made a Jane a firm offer for its publication. Jane accepted the offer. Eleanor is to call again Friday after conferring the production manager about costs, etc., but in the meantime is preparing contracts. The production manager has the script with him in Albany, New York.*

(At about the same time Emir *was mailed, Jane sent Richard Bach "a crazy poem" that she'd written a couple of days earlier. Sunday, Richard called us from either Nevada or California. He gave Jane the excellent news that wherever he went the Seth books were known, and that Jane truly was changing our society through her work. This sort of news always surprises us, I guess, because we must be more isolated than we know; also, the sales aren't all that great, so I always wonder just what the person bases such statements on when making them. But Dick's message was certainly a heartening one, and one I'd say that Jane could really use to good effect.*

(Certainly the Richard Bach-Eleanor Friede affair is reactivating a probability that was available, of course—or one could say that Jane decided to draw from Framework 2 those certain elements to work with in Framework 1. Interesting to see what happens.

(I had three questions for Seth. 1: Jane's weight, which I'd realized recently, had dropped without my noticing it. Seth's recent remark, that she was beginning to gain weight again, had alerted me to it, although I'd noticed in recent weeks that Jane was much too thin—when I helped her put on a shirt, take a bath, etc. 2: What's going on generally with her, physically, or as Jane put it "Why is it—her recovery—taking so long?" 3. At least a few words from Seth generally on the whole Emir *thing.)*

Now: good evening.

("Good evening, Seth.")

Ruburt's impulse to take *Emir* from Prentice—his impulse to call others, his call to Eleanor—all of these events represent a change of mood, and inner decisions of which Ruburt is not as yet aware.

He is moving out of one house. He is no longer on dead center, wondering what kind of treatment he might receive at another house—and so he is moving at important psychological levels. He was willing to take a chance, therefore he was not quite as determined upon safety above all. He allowed the impulse to surface initially, and then he allowed himself to act upon it, <u>in a sense</u> "throwing caution to the wind." That is, he was not going to have *Emir* cut in two, period, even if it meant, as he hoped it would not, that he must ship it around to many other places.

The impulse allowed Framework 2 to operate, pulling in new probabilities. They are not "old" probabilities. No probabilities are old. No matter how far into the past they may seem to go, they emerge freshly and newly at the point of activation. For Ruburt in a way it was an expression of daring, partially the result of your suggestions, and his growing understanding that he had become not too spontaneous, but too conservative. Our sessions also helped.

No one in his childhood, in his 20's, or in your early relationship, ever warned him that he could become too conservative. It certainly did not seem that he was being overly cautious in any regard, and yet when his sexuality was perhaps <u>most</u> noticeable, he made sure he took up with a man, Walt, who could not take advantage of it—a very cautious step for all of its unconventional overtones.

People expect conventional behavior, so his spontaneity was then more apparent, and often frowned upon. The conservative behavior that, for example, kept him a virgin into his mid-twenties, was never understood by others—no one, for example, would have thought him at that time a virgin.

The desire to write was <u>not</u> conservative, but in many ways his attitude toward it became so. His attitude toward his publisher has largely been the same. Ruburt is certainly not considered conservative, and yet a need for safety and security certainly added an overly heavy hand in his approach to life—particularly of course where the world was involved.

So the affair with Eleanor is significant, particularly since the book was assured publication with Prentice. He has been concerned about *Emir*.

Physically, the situation is thus: the vital areas of the head are now largely being concentrated upon with healing activities. That activity is carried downward through the body, gently changing the rib area, shoulders, arms and hands. The greatest work is now concentrated in those areas.

The sore periods—and Ruburt should remember this, again—<u>are</u> of less intensity and duration. The legs, in contrast, are resting, in that quieter activity is occurring there now, as the ankles very gently are beginning to regain greater mobility. The upper portion of the body and its posture is extremely important in his walking, and again in general—in general—the upper or the lower portion of the body has the greater activity in healing at a given time, while the other portion is <u>relatively</u>, now, at rest.

(9:49.) There are different periods when he <u>will</u> suddenly feel like walking without support, and will do so, and much more easily than before. His impulses will tell him when. In between, the healing process still continues, but the overall stage of development may not be such that will allow the kind of overall posture needed for walking without support.

The main issue is, again, maintaining the trust in the body's processes, and in its intent to heal, and in its ability to do so. It is natural enough in your positions to become discouraged now and then, as Ruburt in particular does. When he feels that he is generally in such a mood for a day or so, he should definitely tell you about it. He is very seldom however in such a mood for any period, for each day now brings some definite feelings of release to his body.

It is only when a particular period of soreness bothers him *(as now)* that he falls prey, and even then he largely catches himself. The change in the point of power is also highly significant, for he is doing it now with a good sense of motion and imagery, and without any feelings of contradiction.

I told you that he was beginning to gain weight, and so he is. This does not mean he cannot gain more. The back area in particular is somewhat more noticeable, since the muscles are beginning to work more. The circulation is improved—veins and so forth show more—but he has begun to gain because even in the chair he moves his legs more, which has increased his appetite.

The body will gain naturally as he is able to handle more weight. Some additional arm exercise, for example, will also help, for the muscles simply then demand more food.

(9:59.) Give us a moment.... The most important point is to cultivate your faith in Framework 2, and for Ruburt to realize that the releasing feelings in his body signify the fact that his body is indeed releasing.

I realize it is very difficult not to question how much longer, or when will the healing be observable enough so that there is no doubt of its most positive outcome. The answer is up to you. The faith that the outcome is assured brings it about. I realize, again, that that is asking a bit much of you—yet if you continue even as you are there can and should be some very definite and tangible "proof."

The release of a muscle in the neck, the release of these muscles above Ruburt's eyes *(gesturing)*—those are also observable "proof"—but only if you accept them as such.

Some excellent healing took place Monday evening, and Ruburt was right to relax. That healing is making possible some other improvements <u>that have not yet shown</u>. Again, the stress should be upon self-approval and acceptance for both of you.

The Eleanor decision, made in the area of work, also activates physically important healing elements as far as Ruburt's health is concerned. It is almost as if you hit one bell in Framework 2, and three or four others also begin to ring.

As far as the weight issue is concerned. Ruburt's mental attitude is highly important, and the suggestions you are giving <u>are</u> helping. When you relax in the moment, when you do not worry, then you do not use energy needlessly. Worry and anxiety have often kept Ruburt's weight down. Relaxing in the moment and enjoying the beauties of the day, as per your suggestions, is vital in that regard.

Beyond writing down his feelings, for a while at least let Ruburt make a list each day of the good things that happened, or the portion of the day he enjoyed. Have him see how many such things he can note, and this will automatically help him focus his attention in beneficial ways. It would not hurt to go over Ruburt's notes once a week together.

Except for the obvious physical limitations, Ruburt is healthy, however—small boned—he should be for example wiry. And while he can indeed use more weight, your cultural idea of proper weight is somewhat exaggerated. So remember that also.

Dick Bach is correct: you are affecting your times far more than you may suppose—else how could you be so <u>imitated</u>, or how could there be so many instantly manufactured Seths? It seems that I spring like a genie out of each and every Ouija board. The quality of such material should show Ruburt by contrast the extent of his abilities, and he should not concern himself with any such matters, as far as worrying about them is concerned. They fall by the wayside because they do not have the strength to survive.

(10:15.) I may have some surprises for Ruburt, and in the meantime I close the session, having, I believe, covered your questions.

(Seth, above, referred to a manuscript we received today, in which the coauthors claimed that Seth would do the introduction, and so forth. The book also contained much Sumari and speaker material.

("I have another question," I told Seth before he could say goodnight. "It's about my dream last Sunday morning, when I was climbing the church steeple that reached way above me into the sky. Only I couldn't do it and came back down.")

The dream is self-explanatory. You represented yourself, and yet you also represented your idea of the species in its relationship to the acquisition of any ultimate knowledge. For one thing, the dream represented an attitude, of course, that truth was something apart from man, hopefully to be acquired, and definitely involving an ascent.

The church symbolism was also obvious, but the situation itself exists in an intellectual framework. Intellectually known truths are the goal—truths almost like some exotic product to be attained by man, as man searches through science or religion for ultimate answers.

Such a quest, indeed, seems almost impossible. In the framework of the dream, then, you and mankind seemingly could not succeed. Truth does not exist on the vertical. No particular structure of knowledge can lead you to it. This does not mean that truth is unavailable. It simply means it is not structured in the usual way—and it even means that in Framework 1 it cannot be proven—for what can be proven in Framework 1 must always be relative.

In a strange fashion, the dream process in which your dream occurred was truth. The creative energy that fashioned the dream was truth—though the questioning kind of attitude you had in the dream of itself would make truth seem always unavailable.

(Heartily:) End of session—unless you have another question.

("No. That was very good.")

Then I bid you a fond good night. It was very good—it was your dream.

("All right. Thank you very much.")

(10:28 PM.)

2 killed, 5 hurt in Pennsy crash

JULY 17/78

MANSFIELD — James Moore and Amanda Bock, both of West Falls, N.Y. near Buffalo, were killed and four members of their family were hurt in a head-on collision on Rt. 15 near here Sunday.

John N. Simcox, 20, of Williamsport, identified by Mansfield state police as the driver of a pickup truck that struck the Moore family's station wagon, also was injured and is hospitalized.

Simcox was formally charged this morning with two counts of homicide by a motor vehicle, operating under the influence of alcohol and passing in the face of oncoming traffic. Dist. Magistrate Eleanor Trask signed the warrants for his arrest.

Three of the injured are in critical or serious condition.

Simcox, Mr. Moore's wife, Shirley, 49, and three of their children were taken to Soldiers and Sailors Hospital, Wellsboro. One of the children, Diana Moore, 14, later was transferred to Packer Hospital, Sayre.

Mrs. Moore and Paula Moore, 10, were listed in critical condition at Soldiers and Sailors Hospital this morning. A hospital spokesman said the mother and daughter had chest injuries, face cuts and possible broken right legs.

A Packer Hospital spokesman said Diana was in serious condition with a fractured skull and cuts around the eyes.

Mark Moore, 18, was reported in stable condition at Soldiers and Sailors Hospital with a chin cut.

A hospital spokesman said Simcock was also in stable condition with chest injuries and a cut right elbow.

State police said Simcock was driving a pick-up truck south on Rt. 15 about a mile north of Mansfield and was in the process of passing another vehicle when the truck collided head-on with a station wagon driven by Mr. Moore, 47, at about 8.35 p.m.

The truck broke into three pieces and the station wagon with its six passengers left the pavement and traveled down a 50-foot embankment, troopers said.

Tioga County Coroner Dr. Harry Williams pronounced Mr. Moore and Miss Bock dead at the scene. The cause of Mr. Moore's death was a crushed chest, while Miss Bock died of a crushed skull, Williams said.

Trooper B. L. Norton said Miss Bock, 77, was believed to have been an aunt of the Moores'.

Twenty-five Mansfield firefighters and 10 firemen from Tioga responded to the crash. Firefighters used a jaws-of-life device to free one of the survivors from the wreckage.

Accident victims improve

7/19/78

MANSFIELD — A western New York mother and daughter who were critically injured Sunday in an accident that took two lives, were in improved condition in the hospital today.

Mrs. Shirley Moore, 49, of West Falls, N.Y., and her daughter, Paula, 10, were reported in fair condition today at Soldiers and Sailors Hospital, Wellsboro.

They are still in the intensive care unit where they have been treated since being admitted in critical condition, a hospital spokesman said.

Mrs. Moore's husband James, 47, and Miss Amanda Bock, 77, believed to have been an aunt, were killed in the accident on Rt. 15 a mile north of here.

Another daughter, Diana, 14, has also improved and is listed in satisfactory condition at Packer Hospital, Sayre.

She had been in critical condition when she was transferred from the Wellsboro hospital shortly after the accident.

A son, Mark, 18, was released from the Wellsboro hospital Tuesday, a spokesman said.

John N. Simcox, 20, of Williamsport, remained in fair condition today at the same hospital.

Mansfield state police have charged Simcox with two counts of vehicular homicide, operating under the influence of alcohol and unsafe passing.

DELETED SESSION
JULY 17, 1978 9:30 PM MONDAY

(*Today Jane heard from Tam that Prentice-Hall had signed a contract with a Dutch publisher for a translation of* Seth Speaks *into that language. The news was a complete surprise to us. Because of paper problems, costs, et cetera, the edition is to be in two volumes, and there's a two-year time limit. Tam told Jane that at our request he'd checked with John Nelson, who in turn had checked the contract with the Swiss publisher, to the effect that the German-language translation of* Seth Speaks *is definitely not to be cut, as that particular publisher had wanted to do a couple of years ago. So the two foreign-language editions of that book are certainly good news —the kind that Seth wants Jane to list daily, as he suggested she do. But the <u>Dutch</u> language? It had never even remotely occurred to us.*

(*Today I mentioned to Jane that I'd like Seth to discuss any beliefs she might still have that might reinforce feelings that it still wasn't safe to recover fully. We've given up using the pendulum to check out such things, and I wanted to know what might be operating to either slow up Jane's recovery—which, after all, is still moving along—or perhaps to delay it indefinitely. Jane agreed. Last night in bed she was very sore and uncomfortable in the head, neck, jaw and shoulder areas especially—so much so that she slept late this morning, when finally she did get to sleep after 7 AM. She felt better as the day passed, though, which seems to back up Seth's contention that her periods of acute discomfort are a good deal shorter these days, and not as intense. A good sign, of course, and one we're well aware of.*

(*I hadn't read today's local paper until I had a minute to scan it while we waited for the session to begin. Jane had read it, however, yet missed the article I called to her attention. It's attached to this session as page 302 and describes what seems to be in ordinary terms a senseless and horrendous story: A 20-year-old drunken driver crashed head-on into another auto, killing two people, the father and an aunt, and putting the other five passengers, all members of the same family, into the hospital. Since the article is attached, we can pass up the details here. Jane and I talked about the feelings of guilt and blame that are fated to surround the survivors for the rest of their lives, particularly the teenage children and the drunk driver. It seemed that they would carry a heavy burden for perhaps half a century, say. For my part, although I believe Seth's contention that there are basically no accidents, I was still torn between understanding of that premise, and outrage that a young drunk could wreak such havoc on a seemingly innocent family of seven people. I didn't know whether to attempt to forgive him or demand life imprisonment, for example. In short, I thought it grossly unfair that the cause of the accident was still alive—although hospitalized —while two "innocent" victims were* *dead, with a whole family damaged beyond repair, for life. It seemed too much to bear, and quite unexplainable in ordinary conscious-mind terms. I thought it a classic example that <u>could be</u> explained in Seth's terms, though—the type of new information that at least could try to make sense out of such seemingly random happenings that we see as so tragic. In that way, then, my discussion of the event touched upon pretty basic premises of the Seth material.*

(However, neither of us had the slightest idea that Seth himself would use the account—which Jane hadn't read, don't forget—as the subject matter for his first delivery tonight. I'd say he did an excellent job of it. And his work in turn led me to what I think of as an exceptionally good idea for a book, which I'll describe at first break.)

Now: there are no accidents.

You form your own reality or you do not, so let us look at your newspaper story.

First of all, a few necessary preliminaries with which you are acquainted. In a manner of speaking, your conscious mind, as you think of it, is a psychological convention. In that regard your society, your civilization, your way of looking at reality—all of these at that level also represent highly conventionalized behavior and learned responses.

You organize experience in certain highly ritualized patterns. Your conscious mind perceives these clearly, while you pretend that this official version is all that exists. Your conscious mind, generally speaking, interprets reality according to your private beliefs and those of your civilization. As long as the civilization maintains certain beliefs, then events must be perceived in a complementary fashion.

For example: when you believe that the universe itself is meaningless, and the accidental result of chance, then of course you must also believe in automobile accidents, and all kinds of <u>chance</u> encounters with fate.

While you believe that death represents the end of personal consciousness, then death must indeed seem the ultimate tragedy or surrender. While you believe in conventional ideas of cause and effect, and can discover none in a particular instance, then that event can certainly appear meaningless—perhaps cruel, and certainly the result of an accidental behavior in which all good intent has vanished.

In larger terms, much larger terms, <u>all</u> events are creative. Physical life is a fantastic event, in which all kinds of preferences, feelings, beliefs, desires, and experiences are possible—within of course the physical level.

I mentioned before that some people court exciting and dangerous sports, living quite purposefully on the edge of death, and choosing to taste life spiced exotically by the ever-present sprinkling of ashes. Others might say that such behavior is neurotic, but in larger terms such a phrase is meaningless. In the same way, however, some people do live their lives so that its light is experienced in contrast to death in a different fashion—so that the rest of the years' experiences are seasoned by that earlier taste of death.

In the case of your newspaper story, the same kinds of events happened several times in various ways to all of the people involved. At unconscious levels the results were known, and the seeming accident was a planned event—a play ready to happen when all parties involved found the circumstances apt.

The father *(a Mr. Moore, killed at age 47)* had other difficulties. He did not want to die of a long illness. He felt trapped. He wanted to leave his wife *(who is 49)* and yet could not bring himself to do so. The older woman *(an aunt, killed at age 77)* also wanted a quick death. The wife, however, also unconsciously aware of the events, would therefore share in them.

The children were also obviously involved, and the accident would give them a new lease on life, for they had sensed an overall pervading sense of despair that lay at the family's center stone, so to speak.

Relatively speaking, they had become spiritually listless. In their own ways they felt that perhaps life had no meaning. Brought so close to death, their own youthful strength rose, and while the tragedy will haunt them, still they will wonder that they were spared—and therefore seek for the meaning of their existence.

(9:49.) In a way they will feel special—saved from the "clutches of death." In perhaps a manner that appears strange, they will experience a new sense of their own validity, for if they were saved from death, then <u>something</u>—if only the fates—must have found them worthy. This does not mean that they will not feel guilty also at their good fortune, but it does mean that their lives will for them have a special brilliance and a contrast, in whose light they will experience all the other events of their years.

The "victim car"—or rather its inhabitants, and the driver of the "killer car" had alike reached out into probabilities, seeking circumstances that would in fact occur. The children were not to be killed, for example, and in some near encounters in the past, their deaths would have been involved.

The father in many ways wanted to save face, so that his death should indeed appear accidental, and the result of someone else's fault beside his own. He did not want to live into an old age—but more than that, life had lost its flavor for him. He had sired his children, loved as well as he could, done his job—but there was no contemplative life to look forward to, no greater love than the one with his wife—and that love while conventionally sound enough, did not content him.

He was looking for someone like the young boy, someone whose actions would result in his death, but in a death without malice, a death that would in its way serve an important purpose. For the "accident" saved the young man's life, and this was our father's final gift to the world. The boy was inclined toward suicide. He would not have taken anyone with him. He wanted to die, but also in an indirect fashion, in that he could not consciously shoot himself, while he could kill himself in an event that seemed to be accidental.

The boy was filled with guilt, but a guilt that had no name, no label—a psychological guilt that was the result of his upbringing, and that perhaps involved the existence of a brother. He felt inferior to a sometimes terrifying degree.

He had nearly killed himself before in the same fashion, and also when not drinking. The accident gives him a specific event upon which to lay his guilt, but coming so close to death, his own instincts for life were rearoused, so that he is literally given a second chance.

(10:11.) Now all of those motives and feelings were well-known to the participants. This does not mean that they arose often to the conventional conscious mind, yet even then there were fairly frequent-enough thoughts, for example: What will happen if I hit another car when I'm driving? Or how can I get out of this predicament—on the father's part—while still saving face? How can I die without becoming ill, which I abhor, or without having my death labeled a suicide before my children?

The conventional conscious mind pretends, and pretends well. It pretends that accidents are possible, that death is an end, and it tries to ignore all of the great threads of feeling and intent that do not fit into that picture. It is a game of hide and seek, for emotionally all of the participants in that "accident" were aware of the approaching event, and at the last moment it could have been avoided.

There is nothing in man's nature that makes such behavior essential. A true realistic exploration of the nature of experience would automatically study that kind of emotional interrelationship, but while your society delineates the inner particles of matter, it avoids the inner psychological "particles" that form the most intimate experiences of your lives.

(Amused:) It is a good accident that you read the article. Take your break.

("Thank you.")

(10:15. Jane's delivery had been fast and sure throughout, the material unexpected but excellent. It would be most interesting, I told Jane, if eventually we could manage to check out some of Seth's material on the surviving members of the family discussed this evening—after the wounds had healed, and provided any of them would be willing to talk about what had happened. Personally, I'd not try it for fear of prying, nor do I think Jane would.

(Our conversation about this during break led me to what I think is an exceptionally good idea for a book—one done even in conventional terms. It would be for the author to conduct a survey of the surviving members of families involved in such accidents, to study the after-effects, see what changes the tragedy had brought about in their

lives, their habits, ways of thinking and looking at life—in short, the detailed study of each family case history would comprise an intimate, in-depth probing of all the complicated effects that had resulted from that single tragic event.

(I told Jane that the farther back the author could reach for his studies, the better, so as to have more room for study as far as the passing years were concerned —say that he interviewed a man of 40 whose father had been killed while the boy was 19, say. The idea actually embodies several ideas, or books. A detailed study of one large family group so involved in a tragedy could easily take up an entire book. Another approach would be half and half: First the family story in usual terms; then that same family story studied with Seth's ideas in mind. The insights that could result, Jane and I agreed, could have excellent psychological and social implications toward understanding of such seemingly senseless accidents. I think that Seth's insights into the accident discussed this evening are a good capsule case in point, and much more penetrating than could be arrived at in usual terms.

(So I felt a keen regret, actually, that the idea, one of the best I've ever had, will probably never be used. Neither Jane nor I have the temperament for it, or even the time if we did want to do it. It could be developed as a novel. We talked about the difficulties that might be involved in getting family members to talk openly to strangers, too, about what had happened to them. Some we thought would be glad to, others most vehemently not. Also, how would one explain to a family that with Seth's ideas in mind certain other family members had <u>chosen</u>, or <u>planned</u>, their deaths? Not an easy thing to do at all, unless lots of time was available, and perhaps an exceptional willingness to learn on the parts of such families. I suppose that part of any such survey could also go into the <u>refusal</u> of certain families to restudy what had happened to them in the light of Seth's ideas.

(Jane wanted some material on herself for the balance of the session, in line with my comments recorded at the start of this session. Resume at 10:35.)

A small point I wanted to mention: we have used Monday evenings for a certain kind of healing process, which is why sometimes no sessions are held then.

Apropos of your remarks: you should do your work, as you used the term, first of all because you both want to do it. As you know, in a fashion you are appealing to portions of peoples' minds that exist "beneath" the conventionalized version of consciousness that they take for granted. The words are perceived consciously, but the concepts run directly counter to many usual beliefs—not just scientific ones, but to the beliefs that underlie the accepted establishment of the world.

The books reach people in many fields of endeavor, and they strike a strong chord. They begin to play new notes of consciousness that change reality to whatever degree from the inside out.

Our work, in those terms, may have turned into a career, but not a career that you can equate with others. You are writing new rules. You are not good lawyers, or physicians, or whatever. You purposefully, while speaking to your times, speak to those beyond your times and to the future. Instead of children you send ideas into the future.

You both decided—and insisted upon—adding this timelessness to your lives. You avoided other roots that might allow you to fit into the times in an easier fashion, for those very roots would tie your imagination and ideas to the times, however invisibly.

There are many new affiliations that will be developing in the future, new fields of endeavor. It is far more important that psychology understand our work, for example, than that your current physicists do.

I want to give a fairly thorough session Wednesday on your current circumstances, and Ruburt's condition, so I will do that then. I would suggest, however, that you again begin to do the library together for a few moments each day. I will discuss your attitudes Wednesday, jointly, and make the points that will be beneficial currently.

Your discussion at break was beneficial—for both of you expressed feelings, and fears. Fears should not be concentrated upon, or anger, but they should be expressed. Not enough attention has been given by Ruburt to his feelings in his daily records.

I will go into all that, however, and for now will merely state that the improvements are continuing, and that his trust in them is paramount. I will discuss all of that in detail.

Your dream contest idea is excellent. I bid you a fond good evening, unless you have questions.

("No. I guess not. Thank you."

(10:51 PM—At break we'd also expressed our fears about Jane's progress, beside talking about the book idea. Jane was especially concerned that every time she improved so far she'd regress because she'd touch upon certain hidden fears that she'd adopted as protection against the world. I added to the discussion by noting that I was deeply concerned that she'd reinforced her own self-doubts through what I said about the world myself, over the years. Sort of a vicious-circle idea.

(Also during break, I'd told her I'd found myself stewing rather often about the reception of Seth's material by the world at large, and science in particular. This had even showed up in one of my dreams. The dream contest simply represented seeing which of us could remember the most dreams within a week. I won by one dream according to Jane.

(Late last week Jane received her first copy of her book on William James, and this noon we received the additional 11 copies that were due us from Prentice.)

DELETED SESSION
JULY 19, 1978 9:27 PM WEDNESDAY

Now: a few remarks before I get to Ruburt.

I meant to point out at our last session the multitudinous ways in which our sessions are related to the events of the world. Sessions are initially mental, and yet many of them result of course in books, which are read by others.

You wrote recently that to some extent or another your daily reality was being changed by your dream recall—an excellent point. Perhaps that idea can give you some glimmering of the ways in which the daily events of your readers' lives are changed as a result of our sessions. They see the world differently, and in one way or another they communicate that difference to friends and associates. That is a kind of qualitative event that in its own way cannot be judged or ascertained, and it presents a certain kind of emotional evidence—a living knowledge—that is transmitted to others, and is <u>in its way</u> more valuable than any scientific treatise that might validate our work.

If many of your letters are from those in need, this also shows that people, who were previously in despair at finding any methods to help themselves, now want all the information they can get. Often the contact is really enough, and the reply, whatever it is, for it assures them that someone, somewhere, is trying to operate within a circle of knowledge and sanity.

(9:35.) 1. Now: the main issue with Ruburt is the building up of self-trust. This is highly important, and can be done by following the precepts I have mentioned. Impulses should be acknowledged, and according to their nature acted upon—<u>or not</u>—but expressed.

The impulses will automatically lead to Ruburt's greater understanding of himself, and each one in its way will be a signal to act or not to act from Framework 2—all in line with a greater pattern that seeks Ruburt's full physical recovery <u>and</u> the fulfillment of his abilities.

The acknowledgment of such impulses in the procedure just given will automatically help build Ruburt's trust in himself, and it is a good idea for him to note such impulses, for later on certain occasions he will be able to see how such and such an impulse, followed on its own, led him to such and such a beneficial event—an event that at the time was completely invisible or unforeseen.

2. Another important way of building his trust is the following—and, in parentheses, (I have given you this material before, but I am organizing it for your current use). The second way, then, is for Ruburt to concentrate upon those improvements he senses daily, either in performance or in feelings of ease, release,

or relief. For no day passes without some of these.

3. Thirdly, he has begun lately to sense how this is done, and that is to remind himself of the mysterious effortlessness behind his life, so that he does not try too hard. This trying-too-hard has caused him some distress.

4. The next way is to make a definite attempt, again, to live in the present, or at least to live one day at a time. This is highly important at this stage.

All of these ideas can be put to excellent use now. Along with them, however, again, Ruburt should remember the playful, spontaneous attributes of the creative self. Preparing *Oversoul Seven* gives him a good point of concentration, yet beyond that he should allow himself the leisure and pleasure of playing with concepts, with poetry, and even with painting. I suggested you do the library together again for that reason—and your dream contest is good for that reason.

Your ideas *(about seeing people)*, mentioned earlier, should definitely be acted upon—that is, you do both need <u>some</u> personal communication with others. Planned distractions *(with amusement)* of short duration, but more numerous than your present habit allows. Your work even requires that give-and-take with others. Only your habits and attitudes have prevented this, but the idea should be practically put to work.

The ideas I have just given will help Ruburt build up self-trust, and in the main that is all that is holding him back right now. The body is responding, and his trust is growing, but it must be built up considerably.

Your own attitude has been highly beneficial, and has helped him in countless instances. He enjoys it when you play with ideas, and this also stimulates his own activity. Many people do not trust themselves, of course. When you are building self-trust, and your body <u>is</u> in any way impaired, then you are learning to do something that you did not do when your body was operating beautifully.

The suggestions are of benefit. You should discuss any daily issues that seem troublesome when they occur, or check them with the pendulum—one or the other. The building up of trust, however, will automatically accelerate Ruburt's improvements, minimize his discomfort, and hence add to his confidence and performance. He should also read the last few of our sessions, and I have listed my suggestions this evening for his more convenient use.

(Louder:) <u>I think you are doing beautifully on *"Unknown"*</u>—but then I <u>always have</u>.

I have given you the most practical suggestions that I can, and unless you have questions I bid you a fond good evening.

("Well, how about his response to the hot weather?")

Give us a moment.... He attributes hot weather to laziness, leisure, lack of vigor, fruitless activity, and it annoys him. It is not invigorating. Except for a few occasions he has not begun new projects in the summertime. He equates it with vacations and the world's playful activity—that is my answer.

("Okay. Now why can't he get settled in his new room?")

I would not dare to comment, if it were not that he is curious enough to court my response.

Large or not, expensive or not, the room has only one window. He thought ahead of time that the size of the large window would more than compensate, but he carries some of his grandfather's old ideas that the wind should be able to blow through a room so he has been uncomfortable there. That is the only answer I will give for now.

("Okay.")

You can, of course, always use the pendulum, as you used to, both of you, to indicate what portions of the house you each personally prefer to use for certain activities. Remember, however, that your responses may change at different times.

I have personally mentioned often the bed reorientation, which would help both of your dream activities, and add to your general well-being also. I have nearly given up, but since we are speaking of such issues I mention that also.

End of session.

("All right. Thank you."

(10:05 PM.)

DELETED SESSION
JULY 26, 1978 9:52 PM WEDNESDAY

(A few days ago I wrote out a "new manifesto" of beliefs for Jane and me, to replace the suggestions she's been using in the morning after breakfast. She likes them better, she said, and so do I; at this time they seem to fit our situation. I wrote them because I've been becoming increasingly concerned about the slowness of her progress—or, to put it another way, because I felt that beliefs must still be operating in the background to account for the slowness of her progress. I also talked about resuming use of the pendulum to see what beliefs of a negative sort were still active there.

(No session was held on Monday night. Instead, on Monday and Tuesday nights Jane and I were interviewed—on tape—by Jim Poett of the New York City Village Voice. *Seth spoke at the end of last night's final interview, and did very well as usual. JP is to send us a transcript of the session, as well as an advance copy of his interview..*

(This Saturday evening we're to be visited by Scott and Helen Nearing, who are spending the day at programs for a homecoming festival at Mansfield.

(I missed having Monday's session delayed, since I had a couple of questions for Seth. They

represented my recent, and growing, concerns about Jane's progress. I've found myself waking up early in the morning, stewing about her condition; usually I get up and eat breakfast alone, then call Jane by ten AM. I've noticed that the worry interferes with my appetite—something most unusual.

(My questions were, roughly: 1. What beliefs might still be operating behind the scenes, still interfering with Jane's recovery? 2. What about her lack of activity walking?

(Before the session I explained that I didn't think feelings of hopelessness had much to do with it, since if the background fears were dispensed with the body would automatically right itself, and those feelings would vanish. I asked Jane if she had given up using the typing table as a help in walking, and if so, why? She too expressed concern over the points mentioned here. At the same time, she said she'd felt pretty good today. I said I needed reinforcement myself over my fears about her condition, and she answered that she might have to initiate a program of walking with the table, soon, if she didn't spontaneously start doing more walking.

(I would add that much of my present concern seemed to have been brought to a conscious focus by an even that took place last Saturday evening, when Jane spontaneiously asked the Bumbalos over for a drink. She's written her own account of the event, so I'll just note here that at the end of the visit, she spontaneously felt like standing up and walking normally—an impulse that she hasn't been aware of for a number of years, but is so normal to most people.)

Now: you both handled the entire interview situation well.

Ruburt allowed himself to act according to his nature, in the circumstances as they were presented. This was highly important. Your added encouragement at the end of the evening, resulting in our session, was of great benefit. I want to discuss some of these issues, because they are related to your questions.

When Ruburt does not see people, his reasons are sometimes much like yours, topside. In effect, of course, he becomes afraid to see people. He sees himself at such times in an inferior physical situation, so that it seems to him that physically "he is not a good specimen," but obviously flawed. So it seems to him that he does not see people because he is ashamed of his physical condition.

When no effort is made now and then to encounter strangers, or guests of that nature, in any position of relative authority, then Ruburt does not question his feelings or beliefs directly. The fact is of course that the feelings existed before the physical condition.

With the interview, Saturday's planned visit, and even with the connection with Eleanor, you both decided to be a bit more open in that regard. The encounter with the reporter, for example, on quite practical levels represented a shot in the arm, in that it quickly showed Ruburt that he is quite able to deal with such situations, that he handles them well, and that sense of confidence can then be used as new information to help break down old beliefs of inferiority.

This does not mean of course that you must helter-skelter have a burst of interviews of visitors—but after three or four encounters with people of any supposed authority, Ruburt is then in a position to make new decisions on such matters, based on current knowledge and his own preferences: and he will no longer avoid such adventures out of fear.

He yielded to the impulse to say yes for the interview, where earlier he would not have. His fears would have prevented it. Any new such experiences give him not only new confidence, but allow for a give-and-take with other portions of the self, which will be quite aware of the changed status, so all of that is important.

You yourselves, through following your impulses, changed your suggestions, and this was because the flow of experience directed you so that you followed the changes in Ruburt's psyche. You are as good as anyone else (#1 of 11 suggestions): a simple enough statement, yet behind it there are other issues. Ruburt needs the free time, meaning relaxed time, in which to allow the body's continued healing, and your new suggestions tuned into all of the reasons behind the slowness of progress, as it seems to you. The grim determination, for example, by itself tightened muscles.

The event with your company *(Bumbalos)*, however, points rather dramatically toward important changes in Ruburt's mental patterns, and he has had reminiscent experiences since. I have told you that the changes are first mental, and therefore let me briefly give the reasons for Ruburt's ease and sense of freedom the evening that your neighbors were with you on the porch—you know what I am referring to.

Ruburt felt like neighborly contact several times earlier that day. He felt that you would go along, but on your own would prefer no company. That evening he followed his impulse. He felt proud of himself, at ease with the company, and he spoke of matters he considered important. A feeling of peace filled him as he enjoyed the evening, and he forgot his physical problems. The drinks did further aid in the relaxation—but there was a freedom of expression, a trust of the self, a concentration away from the body, and a self-acceptance.

These factors triggered that brief moment when Ruburt thought he could get up normally. That instant was important neurologically.

(10:15.) Give us a moment.... The arms and legs have been activated this week, the ankles and hands also. Ruburt has exercised often because separate portions of the body were ready for certain motions, while the overall balance for walking, for example, was not present, since various areas of the body were changing at different rates. There will be periods when he feels like walking often, and shortly, and they well may be followed by periods when separate portions of the body may want to be exercised, say, alone.

The suggestions you are using now, however, are in concert with the current stage, and that means that if the two of you can stop worrying long enough you will be met again by some vastly reassuring new walking attempts.

You were quite correct last night, incidentally: the knees have changed. So have the ankles. In the past two weeks, however, in particular, there were periods when the arms and legs were both changing in their own fashions, so that Ruburt did not feel like walking, while he did feel like exercising. He had difficulty with this *(left)* leg, and became upset—but the back leg muscles were exercising themselves. Nerve impulses between the spine and toes were being regenerated, and that is further loosening the knee.

Your new suggestions, however, are more potent than you realize, for you geared them yourselves to specifically cover those issues that have still bothered Ruburt, and also added to your own concern.

Take the break or end the session, as you prefer.

("Take the break. It doesn't matter."

(10:25 PM. This actually represented the end of the session. It was one of the most difficult sessions I ever recorded; I told Jane that by its end I was barely able to write Seth's words legibly. In spite of the very reasonable tone of the material in it, to me it seemed to fly in the face of all of the accumulated fears that had been bugging me, and Jane also, I thought. As soon as Seth mentioned her feelings of inferiority at the beginning of the session, it was all downhill for me; I thought we'd done a reasonable job on encountering those with our pendulum work, but it seemed that they were still as present and active as ever. Nor could I take any comfort from Seth's remarks about encountering strangers, or even friends, I said, since it seemed that whenever any outsider was present we were both constantly worrying about whether they would notice Jane's condition, whether she ever got on her feet, and so forth, until it seemed that those episodes were hardly worthwhile. Jim Poett told us that the Voice *will send a photographer up for pictures, so I'd figured we'd spend time worrying about* that, *too.*

(No need to go on with the barrage of negative things I said after the session, I suppose. Naturally my feelings of being ashamed at the whole deal stemmed from my much deeper fright at the situation, and my growing fears that we weren't getting far in coping with the situation. As I see it, our only hope lies in getting our minds off the whole thing, as happened last Saturday night. Jane received from Oversoul Seven *last February 20th a page of material about techniques, methods, and concentrating on doing "what's right," that I think is the best information we could possibly get, no matter what the source. It's already helped me in my painting. Each of us has a copy on our workroom wall. If we apply what it says, it will be our salvation.*

(Note: The next day, even though she's mad at me, Jane walked a few steps with the table on two occasions, and did very well.)

DELETED SESSION
JULY 31, 1978 9:55 PM MONDAY

(As referred to in the last deleted session, Saturday evening we were visited for a half hour or so by Scott and Helen Nearing, who were participating in homesteading workshops at Mansfield State Teachers College for several days. They are very nice people. He is 95, she is 78.

As Jane said, "Scott conserved his energy, but he seemed to do well enough, although his movements were slow, especially walking and sitting down. But he appeared to have the use of all his faculties. Helen was very agile. Scott Nearing was quite interested in how well the Seth books were doing, whether any of the "leading magazines" had interviewed Jane, and so forth. The reasons behind his interest are brought out in tonight's session, and in Jane's own brief summary of the visit in her notes.

(Odd notes: Today Jane received the contract for Emir *from Delacorte, but is not about to sign it yet. She wants to talk it over with Tam. And Tam was interviewed today by Jim Poett who is still tracking down witnesses relative to the article he's doing on Seth and us for the* Village Voice. *Tam is to call Jane following the interview, or if it's too late Jane will call him Tuesday morning—which she did. She learned much about both the contract and the interview.*

(This evening we watched a movie on HBO before settling down for the session. Jane was very restless, and had been so for much of the day. She wanted action, was full of nervous energy. Several times today she walked a few steps, with either the aid of the kitchen counter or her table, and did well.

(She felt pretty relaxed by the time the movie was over, but wanted to have the session because she thought it would contain material on Scott Nearing.)

Now: Few people would see any connection between William James and Scott Nearing, and yet both were in their own ways peculiarly concerned with "the American soul."

Nearing was born into the world just left by James, and he saw the industrial developments that at one time William James had anticipated with such vigor and optimism.

(I should note here that SN was evidently born in 1883, and that WJ died in 1910—which leaves a period of some 27 years during which their physical lives overlapped. So either Seth is in error here, or his words carry a symbolic meaning. But SN never met James, he told Jane in reply to her question.)

Your country, far more than others, has been a country of individualists, do-it-yourselfers—a country of enthusiasts—and of course some fanatics, but a country of pioneers in one fashion or another. As a young mean, Nearing, as he told you, was aware of spiritualism, and of those very aspects that were so explored by James, and he was fascinated. Spiritualism exists with such fervor in your country because Americans like the idea of a communication with the dead on an individual basis, minus the intervention of priests, and hence the pioneering spirit was early tuned to do-it-yourself séances and the like. Americans would explore the spiritual world as they pioneered the physical continent.

Emerson, Whitman, to some extent Thoreau—these were men who spoke of self-reliance, either in the natural or the spiritual world, or both. Gifted young men of Nearing's period had to some extent then two lines of endeavor.

Nearing is fascinated by mediumship and the like. He enjoyed the thought of mediums defying organized religions, and of women in such a position putting scientific establishment investigators to shame. For all of that, such endeavors, he felt, could not really be brought to any clear resolution in a clear-cut, literally perceived fashion.

He became aware of the growing inequalities of government, and again saw in actuality the early industrial world perceived by James. But James was a gentleman by class, almost in European terms, and Nearing picked, say, the individualism of Whitman or even Thoreau over Emerson's "inner independence."

Nearing then wondered how democracy could operate, when—as he saw it then—capitalism kept the poor poor, and added to the gains of the wealthy. He grew sore with the worker's plight, and felt that thoughts of art, spiritual merit, or pretensions were meaningless if men were ill-fed. Therefore, he turned his efforts to bettering his fellow man's physical state. He butted his head against the government. In a fashion this involved old Christian principles, of course, as pure socialism does—so that a man shared his goods with his fellows, and all land belonged to the people, so that private property—in those terms—would not exist.

(10:14.) He was too spiritually violent for the socialists or the communists. He was too socialistically inclined by far for the establishment, and when he turned finally to the land, it was a proud and yet defiant retreat. He would show how the individual could operate as divorced as possible from government. He was an esthetic in workingman's clothes, despite himself, espousing the old Protestant virtues of diligence, hard work, and no nonsense and no frills.

These were all exterior versions of his inner spiritual journeys, for he now looked to nature for support, sustenance, and strength. He looked to nature's virtues. It was not greedy, nor would he be. He revived within himself, and within others, the American pioneering spirit, with its distrust of government, its individualism, and its eccentrics.

As he grew older, however, he remembered more and more that scent of spiritual exploration, the encounters with spiritualism, and he began to wonder if after all it were possible that spiritual nourishment of itself would better man's state. Had he put the cart before the horse? And what good was the most equitable arrangement of land or property, of food or goods, if the ordinary worker was still somehow basically discontented?

Nearing had to admit that while inequalities still were rampant, the basic conditions of the workers had vastly improved during his lifetime. There were indeed goods for all—yet those goods seemed to produce little peace of mind, and the workers, through strikes and so forth, demanded more and more a cut of the pie—as if to assuage some inner hunger.

Nearing had turned away from such goods and products, yet he had in his earlier years thought that these if were only distributed equally the world would be changed for the better. He is a symbol of the frontier spirit, and many youngsters through the years have been helped through his efforts. He began to understand, however, that more could be offered, that the inner realities of mind, in some fashion, caused the exterior realities of experience. He wanted to meet Ruburt to make sure that someone was embarked upon that search. And that it would continue after his death. And in his own fashion, he passed on some energy to Ruburt as a gift to help him in that endeavor. Take your break.

(*10:28. A note: The next day, Jane and I saw the Nearings in color on a national TV broadcast from the festivities at Mansfield. It might also be of interest to note that the younger man—with wife, whom none of us met—knew in Mansfield of the Jupenlasz family. They were probably my parents' closest friends in Mansfield, and the Jupenlasz girls, Matilda and Gertrude, used to baby-sit for Loren and me. I learned to my surprise from our chauffeur that the father, Fred Jupenlasz, whom I remember well, had only recently died at the age of 85. For some reason, I'm not sure of the first name of Fred's wife, whom all of us liked very much. In later life she was severely crippled with arthritis. In vivid memory is a picture of her attempting to get out of the family car in front of 704 N. Wilbur Avenue, in Sayre, after Fred had driven the family over to see my parents for a visit—probably on a Sunday.*

(Interestingly, my informant about Fred, who was probably connected with the Mansfield College in some way, had been in the town only since 1971. I described to him the house in which I was born, situated directly across Route 6 from the old college buildings. My informant also mentioned the Jupenlasz harness shop in Mansfield, which I recall well, and talked of a Jupenlasz cousin, who runs it now; and there are still customers....

(Resume at 10:35.)

Now: briefly and emphatically: there is no reason for either of you to feel ashamed of Ruburt's physical condition.

(This of course as a result of my outburst following the last deleted session; see the notes.)

You make your own reality—and few people are trying to understand that principle as you are. This involves a learning process—a whole new orientation, not only of thought but of feeling, and necessitates a different kind of emotional reality.

It is very important that your readers also do not latch upon "you make your own reality" in such a way that they reinforce old beliefs about poor self-worth, sin, or iniquity. Your joint reactions last week, following our session, are perfect examples of two things. First of all, of course, you both voiced the fears and beliefs that were still causing the difficulty. And secondly, because of your progress the affair was instantly turned into a creative one.

You personally expressed feelings that both of you had had, and then both of you were appalled by the feelings and used them as springboards. Ruburt realized that he had been afraid to try walking again. He recognized fear, challenged it, and found himself surprised. The expression of feelings was therapeutic, and a part of the entire healing process, as far as it involved the both of you.

Symbolically, a boil erupts and the flesh cleanses itself. As a result of the increased walking, motor activity is quickening. In a fashion the body is being massaged from the inside. More circulation is demanded. The ankles are changing to a considerable degree, and they will continue to do so.

Ruburt's motions—some of them—have quickened since last week, in walking. It was an excellent idea "not to hide" when company comes—but any remarks should be made as statements of facts, simply and quietly, and not as apologies. The ideas of shame are simply new versions of old religious concepts, or of scientific ones: if there is something physically wrong with you, it is either a sign of inner sin or of incompetency in terms of survival of the fittest. Neither concept has anything to do with the basic merit of a personality.

I expect some quickened activity on several levels—and now I bid you a hearty good evening—unless you have a question.

("I guess not, thank you."
(10:50 PM.)

DELETED SESSION
AUGUST 2, 1978 9:44 PM WEDNESDAY

(I had four questions for Seth. 1. Why does Jane often feel blue when she wakes up from naps? 2. Why does she have trouble typing manuscripts—as with Seven *currently? 3. A couple of days ago I wondered aloud if part of Jane's difficulties might stem from her blocking out impressions that she may be picking up at random from those around her, as well as from the environment. The idea being that she may fear something like invasion, in exaggerated form and so has set up a rigid system of physical, symbolic protection. Such a need wouldn't have developed, of course, until she became aware of her psychic abilities to begin with. 4. As we discussed those questions before the session, I wondered whether the poor results of her daily predictions concerning the mail might have a similar basis, whether she told herself or not that she wanted such impressions to work out.*

(Yesterday Jane sent Tam a copy of the Delacorte contract for Emir, *so that he could study it for her.*

(Jane continues her improved walking habits, mainly in the kitchen, and sometimes with the aid of the table.)

Good evening.

("Good evening, Seth.")

Now: Ruburt's irritability is partially physical of late. The body wants to move. Irritability is indeed in its way a sign of life and vitality. It is not <u>passive</u>, for example. Physically Ruburt is nervous. The nervous system is being activated. He wants to walk—and is being driven toward motion, even though his <u>present</u> capabilities as yet only allow him to go so far. The irritability then is a healthy, nervous reaction. The nerves are physically urging him on—hence of course the walking in the kitchen, the impatience in the chair, the odd nervous sensations in the legs and hips, and behind this, your decision again not to hide —not to be apologetic. His body is already less apologetic.

On the other hand, the decision to have the interview *(for the* Village Voice*)*, to take up with Eleanor, and so forth—these events catapult old beliefs to the forefront of Ruburt's mind—an excellent reaction, by the way—for when those beliefs are voiced and discussed then they can be understood and eventually dismissed.

There are periods of rest necessary, so for a while Ruburt did not write down his feelings. He was tired of dealing with them. Now they are coming to the forefront again, and Ruburt is tying them into your early springtime pendulum sessions, so that some new benefits now can come from that old work.

The decision to have the interview of itself meant that Ruburt was less afraid. The event of the interview showed you both, in concentrated form, how much you hid from others, and led to the further decision as described in our last session–not to hide Ruburt's condition, and not to be apologetic about it either.

Now in answer to your question about impressions.

Let us briefly discuss the past. You both considered yourselves fine intellectuals, and at that time advocates of science and of the mind. You, Joseph, were particularly distrustful of the emotions, particularly of course of any raw emotion, and you preferred, if possible, to discuss emotions intellectually while feeling them as indirectly as possible. Ruburt was more emotionally demonstrative, more open to people, while frightened of them at the same time.

When he danced, he often felt that he was dancing out the emotions of others. When our sessions began I spoke to you in an intellectual rather than emotional manner. In the beginning the two of you experimented more or less together, with your psy-time and so forth. You did not allow yourself to be moved by people to the extent that Ruburt sometimes did.

He grew afraid of drinking, lest his inhibitions be dropped, and he began getting impressions about other people, and telling them. Several affairs frightened you both: the woman in labor, for example, and the affair in which Ruburt banged upon the table. You both felt that considerable caution had to be used. Ruburt drank considerably in class—yet always with one eye watching the other. He had to show that he had psychic abilities, but that he was in control of them. He had to prove that he was a reasonable person. He felt that you would disapprove of many class events, in those classes you did not attend—that you would think he went too far.

(10:05.) It is very possible that you would have found the emotional aura at least vaguely unpleasant on some occasions—so Ruburt always tried, because of his own feelings as well as yours, to be intuitional and intellectual <u>at the same time</u>. He was also afraid of making errors, because unlike other psychics, he could not simply conveniently forget them or make up a story to cover them.

Since his psychic abilities did not show themselves in a conventional fashion in his early years, he did not learn to trust them as he might have otherwise, yet this was part of the entire picture. What he is trying to do is to turn on the "high intellect," or "spacious mind." The high intellect or spacious mind is a combination of what you think of as psychic or intuitional, and intellectual qualities—only raised to a much higher degree, and united.

This happens when the intellect is in your terms strained to the utmost, and it finally opens up within itself to form what is in those terms a new faculty.

Ruburt has emphasized the intellect's critical qualities, so that they serve as an impetus to lead him to this opening that he knows exists, though he only senses it so far, and has experienced it but briefly. It would carry him where intuitively he knows he can go.

It is for this reason that he has stubbornly resisted other areas of help in his physical condition, and it is the reason that you have gone along.

(10:13.) Give us a moment.... This does involve you practically in periods of discontent, a discontent that is in its way a constant reminder that prevents you from being satisfied with lesser answers along the way. Ruburt is being led to discover that the answers to his intellectual questions about his abilities, my existence, life after death, the solution to his physical problems, can only be discovered through the appreciation and use of his intuitive and psychic abilities. He is now making that intellectual discovery.

Then the mind, the intellect, alters its focus, using its abilities automatically for intuitive ends, and its questioning abilities are freed from endless queries from the outside, so to speak, and it joins with the intuitions, seeking its answers freely in that greater realm.

The intellect then discovers that its own abilities were greatly limited before, because of the small scope within which its questions were asked. Ruburt is now coming to that kind of realization, and that kind of development—which is of course the only possible answer. Some intellects weary quicker than others, or quickly use up, say, a fairly limited scope, but Ruburt's has been restless and stubborn.

I am not making judgments now, but showing reactions—so the two of you hid the sessions from the beginning, for example. You tried to fit the sessions into the scientific context, as you thought was right, with the testing and so forth. None of that spoke of any great emotional exhibitionism, yet both of you feared it. Ruburt <u>has</u> pared down his abilities *(as I mentioned before the session)*. He has pared them down to those he could reasonably explain intellectually.

This means of course that his intellect is far more flexible than most—yet the intellect as you understand it has been conditioned to accept only a small portion of your intuitional reality. You concurred in a good bit of this, often through unspoken attitudes, and through invisible example, but you got your backs up against the world, with chips upon your shoulders.

This is rather an important session, and your dream contests represent your desires to pay more attention again to inner realities.

Ruburt felt he had to explain to the world, and he began to cut off experiences that he did not intellectually find decisive answers for. This does apply to the predictions and to his attitudes toward the mail—which are highly ambiguous.

(10:30.) Give us a moment.... In a way both of you wanted your worlds to meet. You have cut down on your own psychic experience until you finish *"Unknown,"* because you did not want to take the time to record dreams, and you did not want psychic events—either of you—to spill over into your daily lives and intrude upon your "work."

Again, a note: when Ruburt talks about his <u>work</u>, this is often a ruse, an excuse, to hold back from free, playful, intuitive or psychic experiences. You both like to use the word work to show others that you are not irresponsible, and that you <u>work</u> twice as hard as they do. This also means, however, that you inhibit natural, playful creativity and sometimes what I will call high art, because you are so obsessed with your images.

For a while you altered your schedules. This shook you up a bit psychically, and freed some energy, and Ruburt did very well typing *Seven*. You broke up some habitual negative patterns, and gave yourselves some different viewpoints. These viewpoints were barely noticed, and yet they also resulted in a loosening of some mental patterns, simply because you did not automatically do certain things because it was a certain time of day.

Sleeping five hours or so—for Ruburt, in any case—right now is good, because his body wants to move by then, and soreness and irritability begin toward morning as a rule for that reason and at this stage.

There are various reasons for the problems after a nap, but usually various feelings that he has not resolved during the day—often of guilt—come to the surface when he awakens.

He feels guilty, for one thing, that you prepare supper, but if he has not worked as much as he thinks he should have by then, that guilt is added. He feels it is the end of the normal working day for others, and therefore he should have put in so much time.

Creative work must transcend time, and when he is writing well, time is forgotten. His poem last night took a good full 20 minutes *(with amused irony)*. That cannot be compared in any way with the amount of work done by someone in a normal eight-hour day. Someone could work at a poem for eight hours, and have nothing. He wrote the poem because he felt like it—scandalous behavior—and also because he had expressed his feelings and written them down.

(Jane's poem is excellent, and concerns Jim Poett's interview for the Village Voice.*)*

Read this session carefully, and pay attention to it. Try to be somewhat daring in your ways together, and less cautious and inhibited. The session should give both of you important hints to release your own creativity, and when Ruburt is feeling blue about something, if he does not discuss it with you, he should write the feelings down at once.

End of session.

("A question?" I asked. As Seth, Jane nodded.

("What do you think of that reading Jane received in the mail today?" I referred to a reading by the medium, Elwood Babbitt, given for someone who had written Jane several months ago; the individual subsequently saw Babbitt, and sent Jane a copy of the long, rambling, very generalized material that could have applied to many people. We noted wryly that the correspondent made no mention of what EB had charged for the reading. Jane was scandalized and embarrassed by the reading. I was sorrowful and appalled. She repeated that there must be something wrong with her attitude toward affairs of that kind, but I said I didn't think so.

(The Babbitt reading is attached to this session.)

Give us a moment.... It is convention, in that the medium's insights are automatically translated into stylized versions that will be understood by those for whom he reads.

Both he and his customers follow the same psychic map. The readings give a certain comfort. They cannot be proven or disproven. The medium, for example, has not opened up into the higher intellect, for he will not question enough to truly discover the point where the intellect can go no further.

He is not besieged by doubts, either, and often his insights are good and helpful. On the other hand, many of his customers of course must look further, and despite themselves realize that this bit of truth is a pretty postcard, in James's words, and they yearn for some kind of a deeper originality—an authenticity, a spark of something that will be instantly recognized.

Ruburt can give them that—and "that" must of necessity appear out of context. It will not fit in with current theories, for the current theories by their nature must distort the truth they carry. <u>In those terms</u>, of course, some distortion is necessary, *(louder:)* yet there is a hint of the eternal—a snatch of timelessness. That can appear momentarily, and that is definite, if indefinable, as in my voice in this moment.

And now I bid you a fond good evening.
("Thank you, Seth. Good night."
(10:55 PM.)

DELETED SESSION
AUGUST 7, 1978   9:51 PM MONDAY

(Before the session I reminded Jane that we wanted something from Seth on her adverse reactions to the stronger-than-aspirin pills she's been experimenting with lately: Tylenol, etc. The only one that's seemingly compatible has turned out to be regular Anacin, beside the aspirin she's always used. I wondered whether her body didn't want to ingest the stronger stuff because it didn't feel it necessary, etc.

(We also discussed a letter Jane had received today from a young man who'd visited us unannounced a couple of months ago; he thinks he's being bugged by nasty voices from outer space; before that he'd insisted that Seth was speaking through him. He still refuses to consider that his problem is a psychological one, instead of disembodied, outside evil voices picking on him. I'd felt badly about his visit, since we certainly accorded him a hostile reception, and evidently had accomplished little.

(I ended up this evening wondering why nature would provide within its limitless possibilities that of such nasty ideas or creations—which, I told Jane, only meant that we had the power or ability to create such ungainly hassles. But to what end? There must still be much we don't know, I concluded —many things that Seth hasn't even touched upon yet, and that are undreamed of by us from our viewpoint. I mention this conversation here because you-know-who refers to it in passing in the session. I think that actually it's worth excerpting from the session and keeping in view for future reference and questioning.)

Now: *The Physical Universe As Idea Construction*: Ruburt's initial intuitive triumph.

All realities are the result of idea construction. Thinking is automatic. It is a process with which you are gifted. You can think of things that are distant, things that you have never seen. You can imagine events with which you have had no personal experience. You are used to dealing with concepts, so that your thinking is not restricted, for example, to the mental naming of an object—but you also inquire as to its origin, its meaning, its class. Your thinking itself is its own kind of invisible language, for you think before you learn language.

At that time you acquire the language of your people, and you learn to use mental concepts in a rather specialized way, and to further designate objects more specifically. Language therefore is bound to color your native thinking processes, so that it becomes almost impossible to wonder how you thought before you learned language.

Your mind is equipped with a certain mental understanding, as your body is equipped with an automatic physical understanding of its nature in relationship with the environment. Your physical senses correlate fairly quickly, so that consciously you are aware of your physical stance and relationship with the immediate physical world. Beneath this, there are other communications, not consciously recorded, so that the body reacts to temperature, air pressure, and so forth, and reacts accordingly.

In the same way, beneath your conscious use of language there lies a vast inner communication, a mental system upon whose basis language must rest. There you deal with ideas and concepts in a far different context, if you prefer, one that deals with similarities, complementary relationships, unities. This is the most complex of systems, in which each detail has meaning—not only because of its unique individual nature, but because of the greater meaning that any one detail has in the larger mental structure of the universe.

In that regard, each detail adds to the significance of the universe, and adds greater or different meaning to each other detail. These basic thought-processes, then, are too vast to be consciously apprehended, for they deal with meanings and relationships that reach before and after your life spans.

(10:05.) Those processes, however, contain the basic mental structures from which ideas and concepts as you understand them come, and they are also responsible for the inner mental and psychological processes, individually and worldwide, that form private and mass physical reality.

In that mental system, therefore, each detail is known with all of its probable variations, and in its relationship to all of the other multitudinous and indeed infinite living details that compose any given day. *(With dry amusement:)* There are a few rather interesting fields of endeavor that we have not mentioned thus far—a few million.

Now: this basic mental system provides the infant's natural mental environment, and nurtures it so that the infant is anything but strictly programmed mentally. It is provided with endless variations of probable reality systems, to which it will be able to mentally relate, and into whose framework it will be able to pour its curiosity.

I am hampered here by your <u>ideas</u> of ideas, to begin with. Again, you put the world and experience together in ways that you have learned so thoroughly that no other ways seem possible. Your beliefs about thoughts, for example, are a part of such learning, and they invisibly structure your understanding.

When I say "You create your own reality through your thoughts," you, meaning anyone, have a tendency to imagine each thought as a small brick, a psychological object, each one being formed into the structure of your experience. This can be an advantageous way of understanding certain principles—and I may have well hinted of such analogies myself. In your existence it is quite reasonable to visualize a desired event, for example, in the belief that the image and thought will help make the event physically real – and so it shall. It may also of course mean that other, perhaps more desirable events that you have not thought of may not happen—because you have been so specific, and perhaps determined your desire from your own level of understanding only—where the reservoirs of this deeper mental system might have been able to tell you that the event you want so badly is not, after all, to your best interest.

Your usual perception is of course blocked by time, and by your conscious understanding at any given point in your lives. The processes at this other level are so lightning fast, so inclusive, that they would not seem to carry any recognizable concepts, simply because the vast amount of information could not be followed or slowed for your attention.

At those basic levels direct knowing is involved, knowing itself in all of its infinite patterns, and that process alone involves unimaginable motion.

(10:25.) Nevertheless, that process is the foundation from which your mental life arises. Whenever you think anything—which is always—you are in touch with that foundation.

I have told you that your body knows how to grow, and surely that much should be obvious. The body knows which cells to activate and so forth, and how. In the same fashion your mind knows what thoughts are best for it to think, for it knows the great capacity of the individual human mental processes, and it "works" for mental and psychic fulfillment even as the body "works" for physical fulfillment.

Each person has a highly unique mental environment. For various reasons not to be gone into here, your people have learned not to trust their bodies or their minds. It seems to Ruburt that his thoughts are negative a good deal of the time—<u>naturally</u>—and that he must take effort to change them. Of course, instead it is the other way around: his thoughts are creative and exuberant—<u>naturally</u>—when he leaves himself alone, and the troublesome thoughts that <u>seem</u> so natural now are the results of acquired mental patterns as he began to distrust his own nature, as given many times.

It will help him to remind himself of this.

The mental processes at this deeper level, however, are different of course than your conscious ones, and in dreams, again, there are hints of a deeper kind of knowing, and a deeper kind of unity. When dreams appear bizarre it is only because, awake, you cannot follow the intricate creative unity that unites them. I am giving you this material for a reason, and I hope to carry it further, because I want both now to begin to have a feeling for the reality that exists behind your experience with concepts or ideas. And the information itself will help you intuitively apprehend some of the material just given.

(*10:35.*) Now give us a moment.... Any of the pills are all right, taken now and then—but the stronger ones provide overstimulations when taken often, and these caused Ruburt's difficulties. The less the better. He is also unused to taking medications. And that had something to do with the side effects. Otherwise, all I can do is to stress what I have said before. His desire to walk in the kitchen is excellent, and shows new determination.

<u>Physically speaking</u>, that walking is further activating all portions of the body—hence the new sensations in the right heel and ankle, and so forth. There is nothing standing in the way of Ruburt's normal walking—except the understanding that I am trying to give him, and that is dawning.

The material just given has also been given for that reason—for trusted, his mental life would blossom overnight. He became overly cautious <u>because he thought he should be that way</u>, though he was not by nature. He thought it was not mature or reasonable to trust people. He was afraid he was too vulnerable. He was afraid, too, of his own spontaneity, as I have so often said—when of course his spontaneity is the best insurance of protection, for the mind and body know when there is danger and when there is not. Forget then, both of you, imagined dangers of any kind, and all such projections.

End of session—

(*"Okay."*)

—and I bid you a fond good evening.

(*"Thank you. The same to you."*)

(*10:44 PM. Jane said she had "strong, definite feelings" about the material tonight, as if Seth was trying hard to reach her beneath usual levels of consciousness. She was very interested in reading the session when I had it typed. I told her I thought it was excellent. "I really felt it was great material, and that if you understood what it meant you'd understand a lot," she said. "You know what I mean?"*)

DELETED SESSION
AUGUST 9, 1978 9:21 PM WEDNESDAY

(*As we were eating lunch today Jane said she thought Seth would discuss the question of good and evil, re our conversation on those subjects the other day. Before the session I showed her a copy of my dream for last Monday morning—one that had been so unpleasant that I'd avoided writing it down until after supper tonight. It's on file in my notebook for August 7, 1978. In the dream I saw myself as a rather corpulent older individual wearing robes as they do in the Middle East; at an elaborate feast I watched mice being burned alive in a special gadget, before we skinned and ate their corpses. In the dream I swore off doing so ever again. The dream has stayed very vividly with me ever since I had it. Once I'd written it down, I saw that its subject matter fit in very well with the idea of good and evil, and told Jane I hoped Seth would use it in any discussion of his own.*

(*I had another question for Seth: What should Jane do about her walking on days when she doesn't feel like doing so—as today? I'd told her to forget it, to trust that her body would know when it wanted to walk. She's concerned, however, lest she find herself giving up on walking, at least to a greater degree than she now walks.*)

Now the universe <u>is</u> well-intended.

Its workings entail cooperative ventures literally beyond your comprehension—ventures in which each life, and each detail of each life, has a purpose, a well-intended purpose, so that when it <u>naturally</u> seeks its own good it also increases the good of all.

You have been considering the nature of good and evil, and in your dream you presented yourself with a capsule demonstration. It is good to eat, and each creature seeks food. In the world of nature you say there is a hunter and prey, and yet in that natural world "hunter and prey" are peculiarly suited to each other. The hunter is naturally equipped to kill in such and such a manner. The prey is most easily killed by such maneuvers.

Despite all of your knowledge about the animals, it has not really been suspected that the natural hunter-animal kills most mercifully. The animals follow the rule of good intentions, in which unconsciously, in your terms, the good of one does serve the good of all.

In that framework, necessary death is meted out in such a manner that each creature understands that its own death serves a greater purpose—and <u>further</u> understands that there is no malice involved (*whispering*).

To eat is good. To consume other creatures at your level of existence is natural. It is how the earth is replenished. To torture other creatures in the terms of this discussion is not at all "natural." The animals, however, are embarked upon a different avenue than you. The development of tools gave man options in the way and manner of killing his prey.

Your dream was an excellent rendition, for here you have men unaware of the mouse's dilemma to such an extent that it was beside the point—so taken for granted that it became invisible. The purpose to eat was good—well-intentioned. But the means were not those that would benefit all involved, for the mouse died no quick death.

A cat knows how to kill a mouse, and the consciousness of the mouse knows when to leave. Certain mechanisms are triggered that are inherent. They are not triggered as easily under conditions alien to the mouse's understanding of its and the hunter's biological natures.

In the dream you make a decision never to partake of such a feast again, and the decision simply represents the multitudinous like decisions that are made by individual people, when they finally recognize the fact that a given act, considered acceptable in the past, does not fit in with the overall intent of life at large. Such feasts were eaten often by the Arabs and the Turks.

(I was so surprised by this statement that I stared at Jane—whereupon, as Seth she thought I hadn't heard it properly and repeated it.)

The fire was supposed to burn away any disease, and mice were all too numerous. Acts which fit in with the good-intended universe, in which basically each life and detail, seeking its good, also works for the good of all others, bring forth what you call good acts—simple enough acts which are not well-intentioned in that light, toward the self or others "do not work right." They are flawed, unpleasant. They bring pain, sorrow, or illness to the self or to others, and they are often called evil acts.

In your system of reality, the other creatures cannot help but act with good intent—even if their intent is to kill their prey. Because of many reasons given throughout the material, mankind took himself out of that context. <u>Seemingly</u> he gave up a certain identification with nature, and as a result he will finally come to appreciate it from an entirely different viewpoint.

(9:44.) He will learn to be <u>consciously</u> well-intentioned. Again, simple enough. He will consciously seek his own good – not at the expense of others, for he will realize that he cannot achieve any good in that manner. You cannot kill a chicken, personally now, and eat it comfortably. You certainly cannot kill a cow by yourselves. Indirectly, however, you know that the slaughterhouses are cruel—that animals are not killed quickly or cleanly, <u>and to some extent</u> the psychic disquiet of those animals <u>is</u> consumed with their meat. Animals killed quickly and cleanly make better food.

On the other hand, because of your agricultural methods and so forth, many animals live, through breeding, who would not live otherwise—so those creatures are given life. When man learns to approach a well-intentioned psychological environment, he will then be following the inherent nature of all realities.

Acts not well-intentioned clash with the basic structures that form experience, and hence they do indeed appear in grotesque, fragmented or distorted form—often all the more reprehensible in contrast to their stated intent.

Now give us a moment.... As to Ruburt: first of all, he is at another stage, and one in which motion should be gently—persistently but gently—encouraged. His purpose and his psychological progress have led him to further activations, and as I have said several times, this means that sometimes he will feel like walking, and will do so with a relative amount of balance, and on other occasions, perhaps 20 minutes earlier or later, his walking might be uncomfortable and "worse" in performance.

Lately for example this is what is happening. The right side of the neck and shoulder area is further releasing. This is teasing the right arm and shoulder blade to greater freedom, and new positions, so minute, some of them, as not to be noticed. Those same changes, however, are repeated in the right hip, the entire right leg; that knee has loosened, and ligaments, tendons, as well as muscles in the heel and ankle area are being coaxed into new activity, and in areas that have been relatively unused before.

They are getting used to his weight, now, hence the feeling of soreness. He also experiences feelings of release in those same areas when sitting, however. He should not forget that.

He has been used to putting his full weight on that right leg, so he is more aware of the sensations. He has a tendency then to favor it for a while. The left knee has also loosened, and the entire back of the left leg, the altered position of the right leg however means that the left leg is also uncomfortable when he walks. It tries to release further, but the unaccustomed new positions of the right ankle make him feel insecure.

The arms have again further lengthened, and the shoulder blades are pulling apart more. It is not just lengthening, however, that is required, for the released muscles must learn to operate in new ways—and this has to do with the joints as well. His physical progress then is excellent.

He has been exercising because he wants to. Let him give himself the opportunity, as he has been, to walk twice a day, as far as he wants, or as briefly. Just so he allows the opportunity, for his own peace of mind, but do not force the body. You will not need to. Now he tries to walk when you are in the kitchen so as not to bother you, but there will be times when he will want to, and can simply call.

The gentle encouragement and the gentle stretching of the legs in his chair is excellent. They will gradually loosen and take his weight. And now after this weighty session I bid you a fond good evening—with the point that the eyes should show more improvement now as the neck ligaments are loosening.

End of session—unless you have a question.

("Are you saying that my dream had reincarnational connotations? I wondered about it when I wrote it down, but I didn't say so.")

I am saying if you ask me—and you have not—that your dream contained some important insights into your own questions, and that you might have interpreted it yourself.

("Well, I think I did to some extent.")

You could have "meditated" upon it. You do not appreciate your own dream, or your appreciation of it is too remote—and yes, it does contain some reincarnational data, for it shows you a moment in a life when a decision was made, even though the emotional disgust that you felt <u>at the time</u> was separated from you—for the mouse <u>at the time</u> stood not only for itself but also for the victims of war, burned bodies you had seen while soldiers went about the remains to see what loot might be left.

See what else you can get on your own.

("Thank you.")

End of session, and a fond good evening.

(10:12. I'd no sooner begun my closing notes than Seth returned.)

One small note that occurred to me: for whatever reasons—I will not discuss them now—Ruburt did not feel particularly that you needed or wanted his physical help in matters that you could perform more efficiently by yourself. To the contrary, he felt that he got in your way, got under foot, and that you preferred to do without such "help."

He did not feel encouraged in those directions in the kitchen. This was the result of his own situation, of course—and yet it is also a symptom of the joint situation as each of you set it up, for as he abdicated responsibilities, so you rationalized your fears, and did not encourage that kind of activity to the extent that you might have.

(Heartily:) End of session.

("Okay.")

(10:15 PM. Again, Jane was surprised at the early end of the session. Again, she thought the length of the session, or the time involved, had little to do with the quality of the material. She's had the same reactions following the last deleted session of Monday evening. She laughed. "I wonder if the sessions get better as I get better....")

DELETED SESSION
AUGUST 14, 1978 9:47 PM MONDAY

(I had several questions for Seth, which had grown out of the talk Jane and I had after breakfast. I could see through the day that they'd depressed her, however, so at session time when she mentioned them, I suggested we forget them. They're noted here, although I think that at least a good portion of tonight's material stemmed from remarks I made after supper, when I talked about not using my own abilities as much as I might have over the years.

(1. Why did Jane have to start using the typing table as an aid in walking, approximately a year ago from last June, when before that she could get around without it? 2. Why did Jane have to start using the chair on wheels to get around the house, starting last May? To us this was a regression from using the table, let alone from walking without any aid. 3. What part have all the delays involving Volume 2 of "Uknown" Reality played in all of this?)

Now, for openers: you are in your individual ways <u>perfectionists</u>. You judge yourselves too harshly. You think of yourselves as "you should be," and so you are not satisfied with the people that you are.

You judge the world harshly also. You do not thoroughly appreciate <u>emotionally</u> your part in the production of our material, or realize that its direction and so forth must be, and is, colored by your own unique characteristics as well as Ruburt's—and that <u>at certain levels</u>, the Seth material, as it exists, is a product of your lives together. Not as easily understood a product, perhaps, as a series of excellent paintings, not as easily categorized—and yet you are helping to paint a giant-sized picture of the psyche as it translates inner reality into the living fabric of the world.

Perhaps that does not seem to be what you had in mind as an artist. Perhaps it does not seem to be what you intended. You could have done conventionally well, with portraits, and with other kinds of paintings, with your technical knowledge, but as you learned more you kept trying to put more into your paintings, ever demanding more of yourself and of the art, and forcing upon yourself a kind of growth and development that <u>in a way</u> became larger than the art itself—so that the art, you felt, could never be adequate as an expression of the inner realities of which you became more and more certain.

Art was art, but it was also on your part a search for truth through the medium of painting. Whenever you feel that you have not used your abilities fully, you are doing two things: you are disapproving of yourself as you are, taking it for granted that you have gone astray in an important fashion, and you are also projecting that disapproval and "error" into the future.

Some of your paintings will be very well-known. Do not fall for the trashy concepts concerning age—particularly in relationship to art, for <u>there</u> there is far less correlation than there might seem to be, for example, in conventional terms in other areas of life.

Many of the most important art works have been done late in life, as you should know, and blossoming of the psyche cannot be given any age limit. You did not want buyers around, and you did not want the marketplace, and you wanted to progress at your own sweet rate—as you are. You did not want to settle for work of which others might approve, and get stuck at a certain level, even for money's sake; but you wanted to pursue your art in private, and you wanted it colored by its own vaster canvas of psychic endeavor.

Last week Ruburt did fairly well. He actually concentrated upon *Seven*, typed it creatively, walked several times a day, began to help with meals and with the house, and comparatively speaking you both had a fairly good week. Then, once again, you both began to concentrate upon the problem. Ruburt's legs activated themselves in rather strenuous fashion in bed. You both became frightened, and there is no need to <u>blame</u> yourselves.

Your whole civilization is immersed with the idea that the way to solve a problem—any problem, private or worldwide—is to exaggerate it, see its worst projection; and this, then, is supposed to make you take proper action. The approach unfortunately solves no problems, and only compounds them, whether the nation is trying to solve problems of energy, or social problems, or whether an individual is trying to overcome a dilemma.

You are so immersed in that method of problem solving, however, that it comes back to haunt you. At least you can be aware of it and alert. I will give you the answers to your questions, but they are not the way to solve your problem—and against all conventional knowledge, reviewing the mistakes of the past does not lead to wisdom.

(10:11.) When you become so worried, of course, you concentrate even further on the problem—how bad it is, and what will happen if it becomes worse in the future. The problem is, therefore, compounded to whatever degree—and when I give you both such reasons, then sometimes you use them, the two of you, to <u>add to</u> your private and joint self-disapproval.

The reasons for the table of course have to do with your ideas of the world, and with your perfectionism.

Now understand that I am using the term "perfectionism" in a comparative fashion—but you disapprove of defects of any kind, the both of you. *(Pause.)* Do you want this material?

(I nodded yes.)

I gave you portions of it in the past. At Ruburt's last visit to your dentist, both of you decided that his position was embarrassing, that it put you both in a bad light, that his condition spoke of invisible defects. Ruburt was frightened of going, had a very difficult time with the stairs, but made them. You said something like "It looks like you've had it, hon." He could have said, "Had it, shit," but he did not. You were embarrassed in the street. He was in people's way. You were impatient.

He was hurt and angry, but instead of thinking "I will walk all right, and be impatient with you sometime." he decided he would not be humiliated again, for he could no longer "pass" as normal.

You are compassionate toward others, and judge yourselves harshly. Ruburt felt he could not go out again until he could do so without embarrassing himself or you, and until he walked normally. If he walked all-right-enough in the house, however, then the time would come for another dentist visit or whatever. And he would have to go—so he would not walk that well in the house either—hence the table.

The fact is, neither of you wanted to appear on the street. You did not particularly want to be seen with Ruburt in his condition. You felt too sorry for him, and yet angry and embarrassed, and all of that was caused by concentrating upon the problem, projecting it in the future, in the definite belief, for all I have said, that that method of problem-solving works.

The belief is that if you frighten yourself badly enough through imagined projections and imagination, you will be frightened enough to change—but the nation or the individual following that method does not change for the better, but compounds the original condition, concentrates upon it until it looms larger than before. Such methods cause panic, national or individual.

You both thought Ruburt should hide in the house. You were too proud to show your defects, because in your eyes such defects are so horrendous, and Ruburt's condition becomes the symbol for all of man's physical distress, in your eyes.

The situation frightened him of course further, and you, so for the winter he largely sat in one chair in one room. <u>This</u> chair *(indicated)*, being used to get from room to room, was at that point creative, and it got him involved in the household again, and greatly added to the exercise given the legs over the entire day, for sometimes he walked to the bathroom three times in the winter, but for the rest of the day his motion was most limited.

He does need to put his full weight on his feet more, though last week was a good compromise for now—but overall the body has been more exercised. You must both be on guard against comparing his walking with normal walking.

Normal walking can gently be considered the goal. The legs are lengthening; the knees are loosening, and the feet. The discomforts, however, are the results of doubts, of fears, so that extra muscular tension for example is applied in any given case.

The leg and thigh discomforts in bed are definitely the result of concentrated periods of muscular exercise. The body wants to get up and move—either that, or a brief massage–but mainly the realization of the body's positive activity will help bring the discomfort to a halt.

(10:35.) Have Ruburt use last week as a basic model of operation, while adding to it. You can help when <u>you</u> are feeling confident enough, by reminding Ruburt when you see that he is bothered, that his body is healing itself. All of this, in which left alone it seems natural that the body will always take the worst rather than the better course, and that any problems are to be solved by stressing them.

The best way to protect yourselves from an enemy, for example, is to exaggerate your enemy's power and evil qualities, and this is somehow supposed to bring about peace. The way to solve a health problem, whether private or national, is to emphasize its existence, exaggerate its characteristics, and project into the future, and this is supposed to bring health.

Against all that conventional wisdom, what I have said sounds extremely simple, simplistic, Pollyannaish, until you try to do it. To solve a problem you begin to minimize its characteristics, diminish its importance, rob it of your attention, refuse it your energy. The method is the opposite, of course, of what you are taught. That is why it seems to be so impractical.

I have said this so many times —and I do realize it is difficult for you—but you cannot concentrate upon two things at once. So to the extent that you concentrate upon your pleasures, your accomplishments, and to the extent that you relate to the <u>psychic and biological moment</u>, you are refreshing yourselves. You are not projecting negatively, and you are allowing the problem to unwrinkle, unknot. You are denying it the energy of your attention that keeps it going. You do not spend time thinking that you have not used your abilities properly. You take it for granted that you <u>are</u> using them properly, and that allows them to fully develop.

You do not spend time worrying about what is going to happen to Ruburt's condition—meaning, how much worse he might get, either of you. Ruburt appreciates the motion that he has, and starts from there, and that motion will be increased. He concentrates upon what he can do, and enjoys it—and that will bring about beneficial projections.

I bid you a fond good evening.

("Okay.")

(10:47 PM.)

DELETED SESSION
AUGUST 16, 1978 9:22 PM WEDNESDAY

(The night was a very hot and humid one. I had the fan on, directed in Jane's general direction as she sat across the coffee table from me. I'd asked her earlier if she wanted to have a session, but she said she wanted to. As it was, the evening's work was rather brief—if extremely interesting.)

Now: I travel a long way in vital terms for our meetings, and those encounters have been going on for some time now.

The continuity should tell you something about our relationship, and also serve as a kind of reassurance. My presence, so to speak, has always been somewhat of a promise, as well as an actuality. For my presence and the sessions both do indeed imply a promise of knowledge beyond what is generally known, and, hopefully, of wisdom beyond that which is generally possessed. The sessions also imply the promise of a contact with a larger reality than your own—one large enough to contain the world that you normally recognize.

The sessions imply contact with an emotional and psychological existence that has its reality outside of your physical laws. The sessions imply the possibility of breakthroughs in the most important areas of human thought. The sessions themselves are like a vehicle that comes from beyond your time, yet you sit secure <u>in</u> your time—well strapped in, so to speak.

Before this life both of you decided upon the search for knowledge. Knowledge, of course, is not some thing that you find or discover. You must <u>become</u> knowledge. It is never apart from you. It is a process of self-discovery. You chose your environments, your interests, your families, friends, and associates forming bit by bit the details that would become the pictures of your lives.

You knew you would not be after conventional knowledge. To mix your purposes with the conventional family life would have been most difficult, so you chose situations that left you free until you met—that is, of property, children, or important ties.

You were gifted enough so that you would not starve in the marketplace *(humorously)*—and yet your gifts were also those that would fit in with your overall purposes of obtaining knowledge of the inner workings of nature, and the psyche. Both of you constantly question the world, and both of you in different ways protected yourselves, so that you would not be tempted by the world's usual ways.

You both believed in relating personally to the universe. You wanted some relative seclusion. The search for knowledge would mean often that you would be between beliefs, operating as you had been taught through training, and trying to operate according to the new knowledge. You know this, of course. The search for knowledge on your parts was personal. You would share what you learned with the world —but he who seeks knowledge must first of all be himself or herself, for most members of the world cannot follow such a course.

Ruburt found our last session extremely depressing, as he saw how the two of you conspired to bring about his physical condition. Though the primary "responsibility" is his, of course, yet each of you in the same fashion "conspired" to explore art, psychic realities, and the search for knowledge together. Each of you conspired to learn far more than might have seemed possible from your backgrounds, to sort through systems of beliefs. Each of you conspired to share your knowledge with the world, so that other lives were also enriched.

(9:43.) You simply overdid your ideas of security and protection. You tried to hang on to old beliefs "just to make sure" along the way. You kept the old ideas of problem solving, and were still hampered by old beliefs that told you not to trust yourselves.

It often seemed safer, even, to keep a certain distance from the material, lest you accept it too uncritically, and Ruburt's critical stance was usually simply an unneeded defense, so that he could keep footing in both worlds at once. You set yourselves these challenges, and in all of your lives you have been challenge-oriented. Sometimes you won out, and you did more often than not, and even when you seemingly failed you put the knowledge to use. Ruburt should ask for another reincarnational dream, and it will help both of you if you consider your situation from a larger context – for that context will throw illumination upon those areas where your comprehension is less than it might be *(with quiet amusement)*.

Ruburt has often felt that it was too late, and that you could not help him —for you would sabotage his efforts, as it seemed he himself did. Such feelings <u>should</u> be admitted. They are, however, the results of old hangovers, when he is reacting to conventional, quite limited knowledge filled with distortion, about the nature of the psyche, the nature of time—knowledge further polluted by methods of problem-solving that simply add to problems.

Your joint comprehension of this can bring about changes in Ruburt's condition that now, to you, would seem to be miracles. When you put the action of your mind in line with the knowledge I am giving you, you cannot help but solve your problems, because the solutions naturally arise.

My continuing "presence" serves to remind you of your ever-vital connections with other realities, and of your existence in those realities. New comprehensions <u>are</u> available at any time, new breakthroughs in any area, for those realities contain the sources of your world's action.

Do you have questions?

("No, I guess not.")

Then I bid you a fond good evening, with a note: I plan to finish our next book very shortly, and I hope this meets with your joint approval.

("Okay.")

A fond good evening.

DELETED SESSION
AUGUST 28, 1978 9:32 PM MONDAY

(No sessions were held last week. I've finished working on the last session for Volume 2 of "Unknown" Reality, and today began the last note for the book, on ESP class. Next I start going over what Jane has already done on the Intro and Epilogue. In the meantime, Sue W. has begun typing the appendixes.

(Friday evening Jane and I were visited by a psychologist [Ed Ostrander] from Cornell, after an exchange of letters over a period of several months. I'm afraid that the encounter was typical of others we've had with the members of academia, and once again we were rather taken by surprise. It wasn't until the next day that we realized the visit had upset us more than we knew, because of the various connotations aroused. Although we liked him personally, we came to understand that he used words as a barrier to any real communication, asked Jane few questions. At the same time he thought himself liberal-minded, he repeatedly couched Seth's ideas in the terms used by the respected, well-known members of his profession. He told us often that while he liked a good idea "no matter where it came from," he wouldn't use Seth's name in conversations with others, but would try to work in Seth's ideas under the guise of others' works. Jane and I were slow: we didn't realize that such thinking should have been challenged by us on the spot. Instead, we passively let it go by.

(In sum, we probably got exactly what we expected out of the deal, although it was certainly valuable as a reminder of how the psychic field and its members are regarded by the "straight" scientific community. Ed called himself a "closet" devotee of psychic matters. But Jane and I have seen the pattern demonstrated again and again: the visitor walks in the door, starts talking, usually about himself or herself, and seldom stops until leaving x-number of hours later. Although we now see that we should have said more—<u>interrupted</u> more—such behavior doesn't appear to be too easy for us, whether because of beliefs or what. But we don't really feel like confronting guests. At the same time, we end up wishing we'd done exactly that, so we feel caught in some ways that we don't think others have to bother with, or under-

stand in life.

(*By way of reactions, we thought of improving our behavior in any such future encounters, insistently if necessary, and of preparing for them by informing would-be visitors that they'd have to read a selected list of books beforehand. We would add that the books alone would indicate how different our thinking was from the usual, and that the visitor wouldn't find us agreeing with much of what they might want to say. Such an approach meant that we'd be hard to deal with, I suppose, but at least all would be forewarned.*

(Ideas of authority as represented by Ed were obviously involved. Jane actually reacted better to some of the things he said than I did, to her credit, but I'm sure we can do much better. Half the problem is that we don't see the people often enough to begin with. Even after all this time, then, we can still be caught unprepared.

(In connection with all of this, I came across the deleted session for December 18, 1974 while looking for something else yesterday. It fit in so well with the visit last Friday evening, concerning authority versus our interests, that I asked if Seth would comment on both the visit and that four-year-old session this evening.)

Now: you should reread Ruburt's library material in the *Cézanne* book, on authority and creativity, for it is excellent.

Authority, generally speaking, is necessary for society's survival—but it does not exist of itself. Authority is always vested in a person, organization, or whatever, by other people for a variety of reasons. But overall authority is meant to insure continuity, the status quo. It will always be "undermined" by creativity, and the search for another, newer version of reality.

You both grew up under certain authorities—the personal authority of the parents, and the greater authority—or Ruburt at least—of the church and state. For you, the church had little authority, but the state is vested with authority that must uphold the composite idea of reality generally held.

That particular authority of state, community, government, is a conglomeration of religious, scientific, and cultural opinions that are taken more or less as fact. Around them are grouped the universities and academies, the social organizations, down to the PTA or the Lion's Club.

In a manner of speaking, the stability of that authority, however misguided, provided a <u>relatively</u> safe framework in which you could both grow into maturity. Many new versions of reality appear first in art or fiction, and in such a way new ideas are spread through a society, while no threatening advances are made upon the world of fact. In any society, as young people come to maturity, they begin to weigh their individualistic version of reality against the adult authoritative one, and in one way or another, as they attain adulthood, they change the system to whatever degree.

The authoritative world offers security and a certain amount of safety even in the spreading of new ideas, provided they remain in the artistic realm. Most people settle for following authority—particularly in the professional aspects of their lives, the community affiliations, and so forth, while here and there insisting upon a kind of private creativity that does not threaten the larger beliefs of the structure.

Fellowship is important even to the animals, and your species is highly social. To be ostracized, for example, is no small matter. That is why individuals with ideas counter to the system band together in groups of all kinds, whether or not their particular ideas happen to agree with the group with whom they become affiliated. At least they are not alone. Often they form their own small authoritative structure. Within it certain ideas predominate that are taboo outside.

Academic people do like structures, and to some extent mass learning experiences of course require them. At certain times universities are avant-garde, and in other periods of history they are instead highly conservative. Contacts with so-called authorities are good for both of you, so that you can see that such authorities are simply people. You expect more of them than you do others, because you are still blinded by the ideas of authority.

Your friend—Professor "Crazies"—thought himself on the one hand very avant-garde to come here, and on the other he felt the need to protect himself, to maintain the stance of a professor. You should indeed have spoken more freely, but you also should have seen him simply as an individual, and not as a symbol of a school, or a structure, or as a scientist.

(9:52.) Now when you freely communicate ideas that are threatening or frightening, or even strange, <u>to some extent</u> you are attacking the heart of the authoritative structure. You are telling it to change, when all of its instincts, you see, are to maintain stability, and in your country, at least, that stability has been large enough and flexible enough so that you are being financially rewarded, to whatever degree, for promoting ideas that run counter to the deepest beliefs of that system.

When this happens, you become part of a creative surge. Enough people <u>are</u> interested, or the books would not be read, so emotion grows. Many of those people, however, in say businesses or professions, would automatically try to grasp the new ideas with one hand, while protecting themselves from any consequences with the other: "I know these ideas seem crazy, but -" or, in the case of your professor, "I collect my crazies, but those people are authentic."

You can best help in such situations by treating each person as an individual. Do not expect too much. To expect too much is to grant authority a basic authority that it does not possess.

Again, that library material fits in excellently here. The ideas that we are promoting would indeed change your society—and to some extent they are—for they are altering your readers' ideas about reality, and challenging the concepts of science, religion, and to a lesser degree, of government itself.

Again, you both intended this. You knew it would be difficult. You began before our sessions even, in your private lives before you met. Many individuals come into a world for the purpose of changing it for the better, and there is no more efficient way of doing that than by the promotion of ideas—for no exterior altered circumstances can ever be applied from without unless the inner foundations have been laid.

You are in your ways conscientious persons. You would have ordinarily returned your stock to the earth in terms of children, and yet instead decided upon bringing forth a new birth of ideas, so that your extended family is the family of your readership. Those readers teach their children, and so you help create a new mental and psychic atmosphere that in physical terms will long outlast this life.

Ruburt dislikes authority. He lived under the authority of Welfare, as well as the church. That dislike was to serve as an impetus, as it did, but the adult should see—the adult Ruburt—that there is no authority in those terms. There is nothing to fight in those terms. The authorities are simply people doing their best to preserve a status quo—with which many are already dissatisfied. Their authority becomes a trap for them, for to preserve it they must keep themselves in ignorance.

(10:10.) The dissenting factions in your own country are quite healthy, for they are held together by a string of authority that loops and unloops, yet is flexible enough so that many completely contrary ideas can dangle side by side.

Religious authority, when completely exercised, can be disastrous, for it sets up an unyielding set of principles as absolute truth, and any dissension is considered dangerous. *(Amused:)* With my nearly forgotten experience as a minor pope, I can say I would trust a crooked politician far better than a holy but fanatic religious leader.

In the deepest of terms, each person must be his or her own authority, and equally respect but not bow down to, the same innate psychic authority within each other living individual. That should be the basis for your democracy.

Now in our sessions I must unfortunately try to explain the greater aspects of reality in terms of a Framework 1 culture, with its psychic conventions. I must go against the authority, not only of the so-called straight system, but against the authority of the conventionalized occult in its multitudinous variations.

<u>There</u>, I lived in the land people called Atlantis in your past. The Atlantis, however, as it is known in myth and pseudo-fact, is a psychic structure from the future that sheds its light backward into the past, and illuminates not one but several past cultures, which taken together, become in your terms a conglomerate Atlantis.

The Atlanteans, so-called for example, are supposed to be coming back now. All concepts and ideas in the first place, referring to a continuous forward progression of time distort all reincarnational experiences as a rule. It is almost impossible to describe some of what I know. Simple facts to me sometimes appear quite clearly in the material I give you—but then I perceive that the particular information escapes you completely. I can say that I traveled in Rome at about the time of Christ. To me there is no contradiction between that statement and the statement that the reality of that Rome is even now being affected by present, current concepts and beliefs. The past changes, even as in your terms, say, a river does—only the changes go out in all directions. Atlantis is as real as tomorrow is—and <u>that</u> is a loaded statement.

(10:23.) Give us a moment... When you speak of reincarnation, the past is usually considered, as you have yourself often noted. I told you that <u>in certain terms</u> this was the last life for each of you, your breaking-off points. But that does not mean there are not future lives in earthly terms for you. If all of your lives are looked at like a Ferris wheel, then this is the seat you are in when you get off, though some of the other boxes or seats may be labeled future or past.

<u>In certain terms</u> then, and following a given line of probabilities, in future lives you know the outcome of your work now, and you can also ask for advice from your future selves, who are very actively interested, since their reality is so involved with your own. If it were not for such facts, then again in certain terms these present sessions would not be held. Whenever you come into difficulties, it is because you are still relying upon Framework 1's authority, in which normal cause and effect operates, in which problems are solved by exaggerating them, and in which magical changes or alterations are considered out of context to normal living. "Magical" changes happen all the time. Your very existence is proof of that, for it is a mystery to Framework 1's understanding. Framework 1 looks to time, and particularly the past, as authority.

Ruburt's condition <u>can</u> change overnight, in literally dazzling improvements, if only the "authority" of Framework 1 is forgotten—as it is so often in your creative lives.

I have said what I wanted to say. I will end the session unless you have a question.

("I guess not.")
(Loudly:) Then I bid you an authoritatively fond good evening.
("Thank you very much.")
(10:37 PM.)

THE SETH AUDIO COLLECTION

RARE RECORDINGS OF SETH SPEAKING through Jane Roberts are now available on audiocassette and CD. These Seth sessions were recorded by Jane's student, Rick Stack, during Jane's classes in Elmira, New York, in the 1970's. The majority of these selections have never been published in any form. Volume I, described below, is a collection of some of the best of Seth's comments gleaned from over 120 Seth Sessions. Additional selections from The Seth Audio Collection are also available. For information ask for our free catalogue.

Volume I of The Seth Audio Collection consists of six (1-hour) cassettes plus a 34-page booklet of Seth transcripts. Topics covered in Volume I include:

- Creating your own reality – How to free yourself from limiting beliefs and create the life you want.
- Dreams and out-of-body experiences.
- Reincarnation and Simultaneous Time.
- Connecting with your inner self.
- Spontaneity–Letting yourself go with the flow of your being.
- Creating abundance in every area of your life.
- Parallel (probable) universes and exploring other dimensions of reality.
- Spiritual healing, how to handle emotions, overcoming depression and much more.

FOR A FREE CATALOGUE of Seth related products including a detailed description of The Seth Audio Collection, please send your request to the address below.

ORDER INFORMATION:
If you would like to order a copy of The Seth Audio Collection Volume I, please send your name and address, with a check or money order payable to New Awareness Network, Inc. for $60 (Tapes), or $70 (CD's) plus shipping charges. United States residents in NY must add sales tax.

Shipping charges: U.S.—$6.00, Canada—$7, Europe—$17, Australia & Asia—$19

Rates are UPS for U.S. & Airmail for International—Allow 2 weeks for delivery
Alternate Shipping—Surface—$9.00 to anywhere in the world—Allow 5-8 weeks

Mail to:	NEW AWARENESS NETWORK INC.
P.O. BOX 192,
Manhasset, New York 11030
(516) 869-9108 between 9:00-5:00 p.m. Monday-Friday EST
Visit us on the Internet—www.sethcenter.com

Books by Jane Roberts from Amber-Allen Publishing

Seth Speaks: The Eternal Validity of the Soul. This essential guide to conscious living clearly and powerfully articulates the furthest reaches of human potential, and the concept that each of us creates our own reality.

The Nature of Personal Reality: Specific, Practical Techniques for Solving Everyday Problems and Enriching the Life You Know.. In this perennial bestseller, Seth challenges our assumptions about the nature of reality and stresses the individual's capacity for conscious action.

The Individual and the Nature of Mass Events. Seth explores the connection between personal beliefs and world events, how our realities merge and combine "to form mass reactions such as the overthrow of governments, the birth of a new religion, wars, epidemics, earthquakes, and new periods of art, architecture, and technology."

The Magical Approach: Seth Speaks About the Art of Creative Living. Seth reveals the true, magical nature of our deepest levels of being, and explains how to live our lives spontaneously, creatively, and according to our own natural rhythms.

The Oversoul Seven Trilogy (The Education of Oversoul Seven, The Further Education of Oversoul Seven, Oversoul Seven and the Museum of Time). Inspired by Jane's own experiences with the Seth Material, the adventures of Oversoul Seven are an intriguing fantasy, a mind-altering exploration of our inner being, and a vibrant celebration of life.

The Nature of the Psyche. Seth reveals a startling new concept of self, answering questions about the inner reality that exists apart from time, the origins and powers of dreams, human sexuality, and how we choose our physical death.

The "Unknown" Reality, Volumes One and Two. Seth reveals the multidimensional nature of the human soul, the dazzling labyrinths of unseen probabilities involved in any decision, and how probable realities combine to create the waking life we know.

Dreams, "Evolution," and Value Fulfillment, Volumes One and Two. Seth discusses the material world as an ongoing self-creation—the product of a conscious, self-aware and thoroughly animate universe, where virtually every possibility not only exists, but is constantly encouraged to achieve its highest potential.

The Way Toward Health. Woven through the poignant story of Jane Roberts' final days are Seth's teachings about self-healing and the mind's effect upon physical health.

Available in bookstores everywhere.